T0298956

PREVENTION AND EARLY INTERVENTION

Individual Differences as
Risk Factors for the
Mental Health of Children
A Festschrift for
Stella Chess and Alexander Thomas

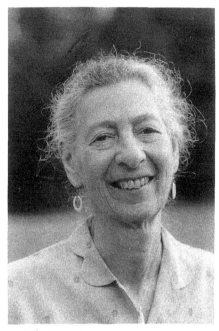

Stella Chess

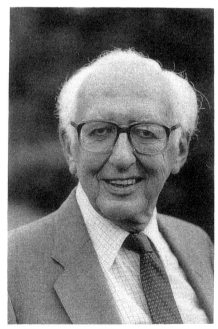

Alexander Thomas

PREVENTION AND EARLY INTERVENTION

Individual Differences as Risk Factors for the Mental Health of Children

A Festschrift for
Stella Chess and Alexander Thomas

Edited by

WILLIAM B. CAREY, M.D.

and

SEAN C. McDEVITT, Ph.D.

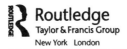

Routledge
Taylor & Francis Group
New York   London

Routledge is an imprint of the
Taylor & Francis Group, an informa business

Library of Congress Cataloging-in-Publication Data
Prevention and early intervention: individual differences as risk factors for the mental health of children: a festschrift for Stella Chess
and Alexander Thomas / edited by William B. Carey and Sean C.
McDevitt.
    p. cm.
    Includes bibliographical references and indexes.
    ISBN 0-87630-723-3
    1. Child mental health.   2. Individual differences in children.
3. Mental illness—Risk factors.   4. Temperament in children.
5. Child psychopathology—Prevention.   I. Chess, Stella.
II. Thomas, Alexander   III. Carey, William B.
IV. McDevitt, S.C. (Sean Conway)
RJ499.P7126 1993
618.92'89—dc20   93-25940
                                          CIP

Published by
BRUNNER/MAZEL, INC.
19 Union Square West
New York, New York 10003

Manufactured in the United States of America

10 9 8 7 6 5 4 3 2 1

CONTENTS

FOREWORD

We are honored and delighted to have the opportunity to write the foreword for this Festschrift honoring Stella Chess and Alexander Thomas for both personal and professional reasons. Alex and Stella provided us with our earliest research experiences, one of us (P.C.) as research assistant and the other (J.C.) as statistical consultant on the New York Longitudinal Study. And this proud association has continued over the many intervening years to the present day.

It is hardly an exaggeration to say that empirically based modern American child psychiatry began with Stella Chess and Alexander Thomas. They instituted and carefully nurtured a dialogue between the fields of child development and child psychiatry that has immeasurably enriched and made more useful the work of each.

Their work on temperament and their promotion of the idea that important life outcomes are the product of ongoing interactions between the child's behavioral style and the complimentarity or lack of fit of the parenting environment reflect an American emphasis on individuality. This conception of the individual provides such an appropriately complex ontology as to allow for the full variety of phenotypes. The idea of "goodness of fit" of the environment is sufficiently straightforward as to be compelling even to the unsophisticated and sufficiently difficult to describe in detail that we can expect this task to occupy researchers a number of years into the future.

With the New York Longitudinal Study they recognized early the essential need for longitudinal data beginning with early childhood and lasting into middle adulthood. Such comprehensiveness was necessary in order to answer questions involving the complex interactions of systems. Perhaps uniquely in this study, a clinical level of appreciation of the life course of each subject was made possible by the close connection between researchers and subjects. Their knowledge and personal investment in every phase of their subjects' lives have been generative of new lines of inquiry. That landmark study, despite its limitations as to sample (of which they are most aware), has nevertheless been so informative and challenging as to inspire a whole series of longitudinal studies designed to answer the questions they raised.

Perhaps nothing characterizes the tenor of their thinking and interactions more than the respect in which they hold children, parents, and colleagues. This respect led them to appreciate the contribution of children to their own development, at a time when children were predominantely viewed as objects to be acted upon. Respect for the efforts and intentions of parents led them to question the prevailing theories that blamed parents, particularly mothers, for negative outcomes of their children, and to look for a way of helping parents to understand how they could better adapt to the individualities of their children. Respect for their colleagues led them to entertain and be receptive to the perspectives of those who had been trained into very different ways of thinking about the content and methods of research on children.

That respect and affection is returned in full measure by both families and colleagues, including those represented in this volume and many others. Above all, we learned from them the importance of the highest quality of empathic, insightful clinical thinking to the research enterprise.

PATRICIA COHEN, PH.D.
Professor of Epidemiology
School of Public Health
Columbia University

JACOB COHEN, PH.D.
Professor of Psychology
New York University

ABOUT THE CONTRIBUTORS

Catherine J. Andersen, M.Ed. Executive Director, Difficult Child Support Association of B.C., Delta, British Columbia, Canada

Naleen N. Andrade, M.D. Department of Psychiatry, University of Hawaii, Honolulu, Hawaii

James R. Cameron, Ph.D. Preventive Ounce, Oakland, California

William B. Carey, M.D. Director of Behavioral Pediatrics, Division of General Pediatrics, Children's Hospital of Philadelphia; Clinical Professor of Pediatrics, University of Pennsylvania School of Medicine.

A.D.B. Clarke, Ph.D. Emeritus Professor, School of Education, University of Hull, U.K.

Ann M. Clarke, Ph.D. Emeritus Professor, Department of Psychology, University of Hull, U.K.

Marten deVries, M.D. Department of Social Psychiatry, University of Limburg, Maastricht, The Netherlands

Judith Dunn, Ph.D. Distinguished Professor of Human Development, Department of Human Development and Family Studies, College of Health and Human Development, Pennsylvania State University, University Park, Pennsylvania

Leon Eisenberg, M.D. Presley Professor of Social Medicine and Professor of Psychiatry, Emeritus, Department of Social Medicine, Harvard Medical School, Boston, Massachusetts

Andrzej Eliasz, Ph.D. Institute of Psychology, Polish Academy of Sciences, Warsaw, Poland

Lena Gaddis, Ph.D. University of Northern Arizona, Flagstaff, Arizona

Anita L. Gerhard, M.D. Department of Psychiatry, University of Hawaii, Honolulu, Hawaii

Edmund W. Gordon, Ed.D. John M. Musser Professor of Psychology, Emeritus, Yale University, New Haven, Connecticut; Professor of Psychology, City University of New York

Nancy W. Hall, M.S., M.Phil. Department of Psychology, Yale University, New Haven, Connecticut

Robin Hansen, M.D. Department of Pediatrics, University of California, Davis

Sara Harkness, Ph.D., MPH. Professor of Human Development and Anthropology, College of Health and Human Development, Pennsylvania State University, University Park, Pennsylvania

Mahin Hassibi, M.D. Clinical Professor of Psychiatry, New York Medical College, New York City

Margaret E. Hertzig, M.D. Associate Professor of Psychiatry, Cornell University Medical College, New York City; Director, Child and Adolescent Outpatient Department, Payne Whitney Clinic, New York City

Jerome Kagan, Ph.D. Professor of Psychology, Department of Psychology, Harvard University, Cambridge, Massachusetts

Barbara K. Keogh, Ph.D. Professor of Educational Psychology, Graduate School of Education, University of California, Los Angeles

Jacqueline V. Lerner, Ph.D. Professor of Psychology, Department of Psychology, Michigan State University, East Lansing, Michigan

Richard M. Lerner, Ph.D. Director, Institute for Children, Youth and Families, Michigan State University, East Lansing, Michigan

Melvin Lewis, MB, BS, FRCPsych, DCH, Yale Child Study Center, New Haven, Connecticut

Roy P. Martin, Ph.D. Department of Educational Psychology, University of Georgia, Athens, Georgia

Michel Maziade, M.D. Le Centre de Recherche, Université Laval Robert-Giffard, Beauport, Québec, Canada

John F. McDermott, Jr., M.D. Professor and Chair, Department of Psychiatry, John A. Burns School of Medicine, University of Hawaii, Honolulu, Hawaii

Sean C. McDevitt, Ph.D. Private practice in Scottsdale, Arizona.

Barbara Medoff-Cooper, Ph.D., C.R.N.P. University of Pennsylvania School of Nursing, Philadelphia, Pennsylvania

Stephen Olejnik, Ph.D. Department of Educational Psychology, University of Georgia, Athens, Georgia

Robert Plomin, Ph.D. Director, Center for Developmental and Health Genetics, Pennsylvania State University, University Park, Pennsylvania

David Rice, Ph.D. Preventive Ounce, Oakland, California

David Rosen, M.D. Department of Psychiatry, Kaiser Permanente, San Rafael, California

Michael Rutter, M.D., FRS. Professor of Child Psychiatry, Department of Child and Adolescent Psychiatry, Institute of Psychiatry, De Crespigny Park, London

Sandra Scarr, Ph.D. Commonwealth Professor of Psychology, University of Virginia, Charlottesville, Virginia

Bill Smith, M.S. Center for Human Development, La Grande, Oregon

Jan Strelau, Ph.D. Department of Psychology, University of Warsaw, Poland

Charles M. Super, Ph.D. Department of Human Development and Family

Studies, College of Health and Human Development, Pennsylvania State University, University Park, Pennsylvania
Edward Zigler, Ph.D. Department of Psychology, Yale University, New Haven, Connecticut

PART I

INTRODUCTION

1

INTRODUCTION

Sean C. McDevitt

A moment of inspiration is an ethereal event: unplanned, enriching, energizing. The life work of Stella Chess and Alex Thomas has provided that cherished moment of inspiration to countless students of child health and development. Their research, review, and theorizing have led the field toward a new era of understanding of the evolution of behavior from infancy into later life. (See the NYLS bibliography in the Appendix for a complete listing.) More importantly, they have recast our view of how to identify and help those whose healthy development has been jeopardized by conflict and discordance. The purpose of this festschrift is to honor the individuals who have inspired us and their ideas.

Behavioral development in the 1950s was understood either as a function of environmental contingencies à la B. F. Skinner or from the psychodynamic perspective of Freud and his disciples. Although diametrically opposed in philosophy, both theories viewed the infant as primarily motivated to obtain pleasure and avoid pain. Behavior was seen as motivated by this principle. The idea of primary reaction patterns, later called temperament, which were stylistic and unmotivated, provided a new path for the study of aspects of behavior that were mediators of the influence of environmental factors. Furthermore, these fundamental elements of personality seemed to insulate the child or, alternatively, make him or her more vulnerable to stress. Ideas that 35 years later seem self-evident were unorthodox and even suspect in those years.

The implications of these ideas for clinical practice were as enormous as they were for research in development. Those of us trained in child guidance prior to 1980 recall that the focus of treatment at that time was based on the notion that children developed psychopathology because of how they were mishandled by their parents, teachers, families, and so on. The goal of many a treatment plan was to identify and help the mother work through her unconscious conflicts about the child. *Mal de mère* was so prevalent that even infantile autism was thought to have been caused by "refrigerator mothers"! The notion that child–environment relationships were interactional and that there were important elements on both sides of the equation literally unfettered helping professionals from a focus on resistances, interpretation, and unconscious hostility. In its place, Stella, Alex, and their like-minded colleagues began to develop a clinical approach based on information, instruction, and consideration of interactional elements. This realignment put parents in partnership with the professional to influence change and took clinicians out of competition with parents.

As research findings regarding temperament–environment interaction began to be aggregated from studies throughout the United States and elsewhere, it became apparent that the empirical results would not be accounted for on the basis of a simple unidimensional model, no matter how timely. What was needed was a process approach that unified the findings by linking the observations to their functional outcome. Thus the "goodness-of-fit" notion was explicated to conceptualize the interplay of situational factors and their relative match or mismatch with the characteristics of the individual. As measures of individuals and environmental factors have evolved, tests of the goodness-of-fit model are playing an increasingly important role in developmental research. In clinical research, the concept of temperament risk factors (mismatches between temperament and environmental conditions) has been proposed to investigate the importance of these conflicts and resulting stressful reactions on development and behavior.

To understand the influence of Alex and Stella on their field, one has to know who they are and the beliefs they have brought to it. In their work as parents, physicians, scholars, and partners with one another, they have reflected their own individuality as well as common values. Stella has a gift for taking an observation or vignette and using it to instruct or to make a point that holds truths far beyond the example that illustrates it. Alex, the great synthesizer, finds elements of commonality in viewpoint between disparate results and upholds both findings by showing the value of each to its own application. Their common focus is a practical, useful, objective, humanistic view of children and their families. They study ideas to understand people, not as ends in themselves.

The topic of this book is the role of individual differences in prevention and early intervention. It is a suitable area for honoring Stella and Alex's work, though it isn't the only topic that could have been chosen. The contributors to this volume were selected, through the editors' consultation with several individuals, according to the pertinence of their work for developing this particular theme. There are many, many important scholars and clinicians who could not be included because of space and topical considerations. The editors apologize in advance to those worthy individuals, whose work can be found in any general review of this area of investigation and in the reference lists of the chapters of this volume. We know that you feel no less grateful to Stella and Alex than those who were included, and we wish we could have had a longer book. The editors also wish two of our esteemed colleagues could have lived to read this tribute: Herbert Birch and Ronald Wilson. Their premature deaths undoubtedly have diminished our collective accomplishments in this area. We believe that they would have wanted to contribute to this book, too.

A brief overview of the contributions that make up this collection of essays shows how widespread the impact of Alex and Stella's ideas has been. The contributors include clinical, research, and social psychiatrists; pediatricians; clinical nurse practitioners; clinical, developmental, and educational psychologists; an anthropologist; and assorted others. Along with the professor from Harvard is a parent from British Columbia. The psychologist from Poland is in the same company as the parent counselor from Oregon. The Pavlovian and the factor analyst discuss issues with the behavioral geneticist and the day-care researcher. All have been influenced by the same concepts of individual differences in temperament. It is a tribute to the fundamental appeal of Stella and Alex's work that it has captured the attention of such a diverse, international group of individuals.

This volume is organized around the foundations, research findings, and practical applications of individual differences on the mental health of children, both for prevention and intervention. William Carey's summary and conclusion highlight the important issues and findings on this topic of importance to behavioral scientists and practitioners. As emphasized in the New York Longitudinal Study (NYLS), not only the well-established fact but also statements of the possibilities for further investigation have been encouraged. Also as in the NYLS, both what is known and how that can be used to help children and their families are emphasized.

In large part the tribute to Thomas and Chess in this volume is based not on what they have done themselves but on the manner in which their work has inspired others to think differently about important issues in the areas of personality development, clinical practice, and the genetic and biological origins of behavior. The range of influence of the NYLS and the other work of that group is demonstrated by the breadth of contributions to this volume. The chapter by Mahin Hassibi, although biographical in nature, identifies a number of threads that have been woven into the fabric of their work. Many will be surprised to learn how Stella and Alex's personal experience as parents planted the seeds of innovations in research and practice that blossom in their work. That notwithstanding, we should all be pleased that Stella heeded Lauretta Bender's advice to stand up and "say who you are and then what you think and why."

TEMPERAMENT CONCEPT AND THEORY

Theoretical and conceptual issues that were only implicit in the NYLS are now clarified by decades of research. Michael Rutter reviews the theoretical underpinnings and empirical findings to date regarding the role of temperament in development and as a risk factor for behavioral disorder, and indicates how much more needs to be understood regarding the mechanisms that underly temperamental differences, including some of the methodological issues that plague investigators. Jerome Kagan's chapter examines some of the work that is directed at the neural substrates that may result in observed differences in behavior, primarily in inhibition but possibly in other individual areas of personality as well. Kagan's argument that the centers of temperament can be localized in brain structures or analyzed in the biochemistry of neural transmission represents a major step beyond the early NYLS focus on reliably observed external behavior. It shows the progress of theoreticians in the field that these new levels of understanding can be explored empirically. Jan Strelau's chapter, taken from his Pavlovian tradition, highlights the influence of the New York group on Eastern European scientists who have been studying differences in temperamental reactivity for many decades. This chapter is remarkable in its focus on the practical implications of temperament for health and educational success and for the adoption of a "temperament risk factors" model of assessing outcome. Judith Dunn's report on sibling relationships indicates how studies support the notion that individual differences in temperament can affect the quality of relationships developed by family members with one another—rejecting the simplistic view that parents account for how these roles evolve. The focus on the processes of development and adaptation shows how new models lead to fresh areas of inquiry. The NYLS clinical vignettes regarding family relationships and the impact of temperament on their functioning are now being studied empirically by developmental researchers. Roy Martin's chapter with Stephen Olejnik and Lena Gaddis on the importance of temperamental individuality in scholastic ability and academic achievement is notable for its theoretical analysis as well as the sophistication of its statistical model. Whereas early studies simply correlated IQ and temperament, the current state of the art has become quite complex. Martin's previous work has included an educational emphasis on application of temperamental characteristics; his theoretical model builds on this foundation.

Michel Maziade's work on the role of extremes in temperament for later adjustment is a classic example of building on a fresh concept suggested by the early NYLS work. Maziade's investigations show how, with the use of a carefully sampled group of children representative of different levels of a population, high-risk temperament groups can be shown to develop internalizing or externalizing disorders, but only when the environmental factors indicated a lack of attenuation of the extreme. The robustness of the clinical observations of the NYLS can be savored by those who recall the critics who stated that their findings wouldn't stand up to replication in representative samples of subjects.

DEVELOPMENT AND DEVELOPMENTAL RISK

In the NYLS a major focus was the role of temperament as one of many aspects of development and how behavioral individuality fit into the overall pattern of growth and adjustment. The chapter by Ann and Alan Clarke explicates the major lines of development, including biological and psychosocial trajectories, transactions, and encounters. Within this system cognitive, scholastic, and familial factors shape how they affect overall adjustment. The Clarkes' systemic view of temperamental differences and behavioral adjustment put these facets into perspective with the other major lines of development.

Nontemperamental individual differences can also have profound implications for developmental outcome. The chapter by Margaret Hertzig, one of the original NYLS group, shows the influence of biological and social risk factors at work in low-birth-weight infants. Particularly important in the findings is the interaction between the risk factors for individuals and the development of care plans that must take into account the relative salience of these specific factors.

The contribution by Melvin Lewis on chronic illness as a psychological risk factor shows the interaction between illness, a nontemperamental factor, and increased incidence of behavioral and emotional disorders. In addition, the presence of certain elements such as pain may increase the need for support and intervention by parents and hospital staff. Lewis indicates some of the similarities between management of chronic illness and the goodness-of-fit model of Thomas and Chess.

TEMPERAMENT AND CULTURAL CONTEXT

Three chapters deal with how differences in cultural environment and individual differences can interact to produce concordant or discordant relationships. Charles Super and Sara Harkness have taken the temperament–environment interaction idea to its inevitable abstraction, the cultural/developmental niche. Citing African studies as well as clinical experience, they examine the importance of parental belief systems for altering discordant interactions. To clinicians it may be exciting to see the similarity in the process of family change between Super and Harkness's examples and those in the accounts of the NYLS. Marten deVries uses cross-cultural comparisons to demonstrate the real-world complexity inherent in evaluating the inter-actions of individuals with family, culture, development, and other influences needed to complete the predictive equations. One senses humility similar to that of the NYLS researchers, who were faced with similar complexities in just one culture. Edmund Gordon considers the likely pathways to understanding the bio-logical substrates of temperament's influence by culture. The epigenetic, interac-tionist perspective may reveal differing levels of biological influence and expression over time, as well as variable influence by cultural factors. The consideration of these issues alone indicates the forward movement in the understanding of the role of biologically based styles of behavior on development. The chapter by Anita Gerhard, John McDermott, and Naleen Andrade examines the content of culture and how it may balance or imbalance the relationship between individual differences and interaction within families and social groups. The point, that the predominant cultural view may intersect with the adjustment of individuals whose behavior is discordant with it, is a convincing one. Although admittedly speculative regarding temperamental differences, some comparative cultural research has been done to reveal the role of individual differences in separate cultures.

INDIVIDUAL DIFFERENCES AND THE ENVIRONMENT: GOODNESS OF FIT

While the original nine dimensions proposed by the NYLS have been known for three decades, the concept of goodness of fit as a process of interaction was introduced much later. Relatively fewer studies have been completed examining the model directly. A notable exception is the work of Jacqueline and Richard Lerner, whose chapter reviewing several of these investigations indicates the fruitfulness of this direction for research. The recognition of multiple levels of interrelationships between persons and contexts, and the need to overcome methodological problems inherent in looking at the dynamic interplay between them, is an important step in providing concrete examples of how to study goodness of fit.

The interaction of genes and environment has been a focus of research since the organism–environment debates of the 1960s. The outcome of that debate, a more general acceptance of interactionism, has facilitated the scrutiny of behavioral genetic influences through studies of individual differences such as IQ and tem-perament. The chapters by Sandra Scarr and Robert Plomin indicate the impact of the NYLS on two of the most active researchers in this field. Scarr's view of environmental influence, as a measure of specific subtypes of environmental var-iation toward which the genotype gravitates, indicates that individual differences may *define* what constitutes environment. Plomin's theses on genetic contribu-tions are in accord with Scarr's but include the fascinating additional hypothesis that environmental influences within a family are not shared by sibs, or at least do not have the same effect on children in the same family. As empirical results tend to do, this finding raises many new, interesting issues in the area of family development that reach well beyond the clinician's observations in practice. Both authors document the impact of the NYLS on their thinking.

ASSESSMENT OF INDIVIDUAL DIFFERENCES

A major longitudinal research project is a risky place to become an innovator in technique or methodological design. As new questions and needs become apparent, only the most ardent will improvise to answer an important question rather than jeopardize the validity of later predictions based on an unsharpened tool. Yet, the NYLS researchers repeatedly emphasized the value of finding data analyses that would answer meaningful questions.

Almost as risky as inventing new methods is resurrecting discredited ones. Although the NYLS originally used structured interviews to collect temperament data, the method was felt to be laborious and inefficient. The use of a questionnaire to collect observational ratings by care givers (in historical sequence: mothers, parents, caretakers) was felt, in both the clinical and the research communities, to be of questionable reliability and hopelessly invalid. Still controversial to some, the assessment of temperament by care giver rating has developed by virtue of an increasingly sophisticated technology of design and review based on evidence comparing behavioral ratings, observations, and questionnaire use. My own (Sean McDevitt's) review of temperament questionnaires shows the progress in assessment techniques as well as areas that still need further refinement in the quest for reliable, valid temperament data that can be obtained in both applied and research settings.

PREVENTION AND INTERVENTION STRATEGIES
IN APPLIED SETTINGS

Few clinicians can read the work of Thomas and Chess and fail to see the immediate implications for their own work with children and their families. Although the relationship between research and practice is a dialectical one, few have synthesized them as well as the NYLS group. The value of this example for later practice is seen in the chapters under intervention and prevention. Barbara Medoff-Cooper's chapter reviews the current findings on "at-risk" infants and relates the nature of the evolving role of the professional in the newborn nursery. Interestingly, both the infants and the care givers are the focus of clinical intervention throughout observation, assessment, and teaching aspects. Carey's contribution on the role of the professional in the primary medical care setting offers a template for practice by pediatricians, with clinical examples demonstrating the utilization of intervention strategies in actual cases. It is probably the most impressive statement to date on the role of the physician in dealing with stressful child–environment interaction, including limitations on behavioral practice in primary care. James Cameron, David Rice, Robin Hansen, and David Rosen have developed a novel application of temperament assessment and intervention. Working with teams of physicians, nurses, and counselors in an HMO (health maintenance organization) setting, they demonstrate in their research the interconnection between patient acceptance, validity, and clinical intervention through anticipatory guidance. This research, practice, evaluation loop offers constant feedback and improvement of prevention efforts for young children and parents.

Beyond the clinical domain of primary care, temperamental issues continue to be seen as influential in educational settings. Edward Zigler's chapter with Nancy Hall explores the day-care setting and emphasizes the role of temperamental differences in out-of-home environments. Individual adjustment to new circumstances depends on these factors, and how the care givers relate to child characteristics. The social policy implications for the availability and quality of day care in the United States are far-reaching.

Barbara Keogh's work on the teachability concept in schools has integrated temperament with several other sources of teacher perception to apply the goodness-of-fit notion to the classroom. A common thread seen throughout this section is also noted here: that increasing sensitivity to a child's temperament can improve the quality of interaction between the child and the teacher (care giver, parent, etc.).

In the NYLS the parent counseling given to participants was usually based on problems that did not involve a major behavioral disorder. Thus the guidance required was based on brief counseling and didn't require intensive psychiatric training. Two chapters in this section highlight the extension of parent counseling utilizing other parents and paraprofessionals in helping roles. On the community level, Bill Smith's program for parent-to-parent assistance in handling difficult temperament illustrates the power of the temperament concept in training counselors to provide support and guidance for those who must care for a difficult youngster day after day without respite. Catherine Andersen's description of the parent support groups in western Canada indicates the value of programs run by parents for themselves and others to receive support and assistance in handling behaviorally difficult children. The sharing of ideas and experiences, and educating parents about temperament, have proved useful to many beleaguered parents.

ADVOCACY

Finally, the chapter on social advocacy by Leon Eisenberg calls for a spirit of alliance, with the goal of promoting the health of the public through social justice, a hallmark of the careers of Alex and Stella. Both have been advocates of human rights and social responsibility in this country, a facet of their humanism that many may not have appreciated. Eisenberg, their longtime colleague, pays tribute to their efforts and apprises us of their ongoing commitment to this cause.

The seed of Alex and Stella's work has grown a trunk with many branches, each growing and dividing into new offshoots. While it is pleasing to see how the tree has grown and put down deep roots, it is just as important to note that it continues to grow in many directions, that it has cast its own seeds, and that those others now are growing also.

2

Biographical Sketch of Alexander Thomas and Stella Chess

Mahin Hassibi

Stella Chess and Alexander Thomas are both native New Yorkers. Born 2 months apart in 1914, they share roots in immigrant families—their parents having come to this country with their own families from Eastern Europe—but of more significance is their shared value system, with its emphasis on education, self-reliance, and independence. Alex's father had a small business, while Stella's father was a lawyer. Although Alex and Stella traveled in different circles and moved at different tempos, eventually their terms in New York University Medical School overlapped long enough for them to meet and marry.

A precocious boy, Alex finished high school at age 14, and entered City College in New York shortly thereafter. By 18, he had managed to receive his B.S. degree magna cum laude while also being the family's breadwinner during the Depression, when his father was in financial trouble. Studying during the day and working as switchboard operator at a hospital at night, Alex discovered a love for medicine, and a talent for organization as he was given the responsibility for arranging the on-call and the vacation schedules for the doctors.

Stella's mother was a schoolteacher, which may account for her love of teaching and her ease in dealing with all teachers. Stella began her teaching career at age 4 when, having memorized her older sister's primer, she taught her grandmother, who spoke but did not read English, how to read. The fact that she herself was a nonreader and dyslexic was a later discovery, and of no import, either to her or her grandmother. Her mother had to wait for Stella's shock at her own inability to read by the third grade before she agreed to tutoring. Awarded a scholarship to a private school, Stella often chose to follow her own interests rather than the expected, gender-typed activities. She took woodworking rather than cooking classes, having to find many unanswerable arguments for whomever felt that she should do otherwise. During summers she worked as a camp counselor as soon as it was possible for her to do so, and came to the happy and significant conclusion that she liked children and they liked her. Once, when a group of older teenagers complained that she had overscheduled their evenings, she suggested that they go on strike. She then spent hours teaching them how to choose slogans, prepare placards, and march up and down chanting their grievances against her.

Stella attended Smith College in Massachusetts and managed to take her preferred courses without bothering with the prerequisite classes. She believed that teachers like to teach students who are enthusiastic about learning. Therefore, she would ask them to sign her petitions to enter advanced courses for which she had not wished to take the elementary requirements, and they invariably did. She remembers college as an intellectually exciting time and a good preparation for New York University Medical School, which she entered in 1935. She was happy to be accepted on her merits rather than as part of the sex and religious quotas of the other medical schools in the city.

For Alex medical school was a liberating experience both personally and intellectually. He felt at home with his peers, and was involved in the intense political and intellectual debates of the time. He also met Stella, which he ranks as one of the few truly important events of his personal life. Graduating with Alpha Omega Alpha honors in 1936, Alex began a 3-year postgraduate training in laboratory and internal medicine at Mount Sinai Hospital in New York City. He did clinical research and published papers on purulent meningitis and on suppurative and necrosuppurative bronchopneumonia in children in the journal of Mount Sinai Hospital (Thomas, 1939, 1941).

During medical school. Alex had felt no particular interest in psychiatry. However, once he began to practice medicine in New York City, he noted that some patients masked their emotional problems by complaining about physical symptoms. With a budding curiosity in psychiatry, Alex volunteered for the army in 1942, and once enlisted he seized the opportunity to care for patients with psychiatric as well as other medical problems. He had to teach himself psychiatry in order to treat his patients. By the time of his discharge in 1946, his interest in and fascination with psychiatry resulted in the decision to undertake formal training in the field, which he did as a resident in psychiatry at Bellevue Hospital. Because at the time psychoanalytic experience was viewed as a desirable addition to training in psychiatry, he arranged for the necessary training and personal analysis.

For Stella the choice of psychiatry in general, and child psychiatry in particular, was made during medical school when once she attended a lecture by Lauretta

Bender. Dr. Bender was the director of the children's unit at Bellevue Psychiatric Hospital and one of the pioneers in child psychiatry. Stella was impressed by the way that Dr. Bender viewed children and their problems. Having worked with youngsters in summer camp, Stella had come to conclude that children responded best to those who treated them with respect. She noted that Dr. Bender described psychiatrically ill children as worthy individuals attempting to cope with specific issues of their lives with different degrees of success. Characteristically, she set to work arranging to spend time on Dr. Bender's unit in Bellevue during her third and fourth year of medical school, whenever she could spare the time. Her project involved studying children with language disorders. Upon completion of her research, she informed Dr. Bender that the results did not support the then authoritative views in the field and asked her advice as to how to report them. Dr. Bender advised her: "First, say who you are and then what you think and why." Dr. Chess never again hesitated to contradict authoritative views with ease and self-confidence. At times one is left with the distinct impression that she has no doubts that all current opinions deserve to be challenged and probably will be found wanting.

Following her training in psychiatry, Stella began work as a child psychiatrist at Northside Center for Child Development, while Alex was busy as a part-time instructor in psychiatry at NYU Medical School and Bellevue, and with a flourishing practice in psychiatry and psychoanalysis, seeing patients four or five times a week as the model dictated. However, he soon discovered that sitting face to face with some patients was more helpful than using the couch, and that for some people once or twice a week sufficed for psychotherapy, while others needed to resolve their problems jointly with their spouses present. With his background in internal medicine it came naturally to him that his own understanding of patients' needs was a better guide in the practice of psychiatry than were the customary notions based on theoretical considerations. He therefore began modifying his techniques and shared his innovative ideas with others, hoping to liberate the practitioner from the rigidity imposed by the orthodox theoreticians of psychoanalysis (Thomas, 1956).

By the early 1950s, Alex and Stella had a good-sized family: two adopted children and two homegrown. The three boys and one girl kept their parents supplied with examples of their differences in every facet of life. They attended few out-of-town conferences and passed over some professional opportunities because for both being with their children was their highest priority. Meanwhile, Dr. Chess was hard at work attempting to find direct links between parents' child-rearing practices and attitudes and their children's problems and psychopathology. She had already published the two papers "Developmental Language Disability as a Factor in Personality Distortion in Childhood" (Chess, 1944) and "Factors Influencing the Adaptation of Organically Handicapped Children (Chess, 1951).

By now discussions and exchange of opinion and observations between her and Alex had convinced both of them that the current views of pathogenesis of behavioral abnormalities did not adequately account for their own observations of patients and their families. Finally, one evening in 1956, as they were coming from a meeting where Stella had presented a case and continuing to discuss the child and his problems, it became clear to them that the child's behavioral and emotional problems were largely caused by his physical characteristics and their effects on his interaction with peers and teachers rather than solely by his parents' activities and attitudes. The clarity of presentation finally brought the point home with intensity and conviction, and they began to formulate their own hypothesis.

Well acquainted with the psychiatric thinking and literature and imbued with justified confidence in their own observations, Stella and Alex came to conclude that major areas in child development, both normal and pathological, remained unexplored and uncharted. Furthermore, it became clear to them that the strong adherence to current theories had resulted in premature closure of many issues to the detriment of scientific inquiries and progress. An important example of such subjects was the role of individuality of responsiveness to forces in the environment, even those viewed as universal factors according to psychoanalytic theory.

The story of the birth of the New York Longitudinal Study, as told by Chess and Thomas, is an example of the process by which a creative enterprise is conceived, the increasing enthusiasm and the apprehension that accompanies each step, and the resolve with which the idea is pursued. Stella and Alex knew very well that children reacted differently even as very young infants. Friends with newborn babies agreed wholeheartedly when this question was raised. However, these anecdotal observations required a systemic design in order to be of any value in providing a basis for scientific study and empirical conclusion. As clinicians, they felt inadequately equipped to design a scientifically appropriate research project. Their consultations with professionals left them with a sense of the difficulty of the task as well as the significance and the value of such an undertaking. Fortunately, friends and colleagues with small children volunteered to participate, and the naturalistic method of recording the observed behavior, selected by trial and error, proved to be the ideal method for the purpose. Multiple descriptive interviews of the first year of 20 babies were obtained before Dr. Herbert Birch, a researcher and scholar with background in research in animal and human behavior, joined them to design a method for quantifying the data.

By the late 1950s, when their first paper on individual differences in responsiveness to the environment appeared in the literature (Thomas & Chess, 1959), a remarkable amount of behavioral data on early childhood had been collected in a systematic manner, and the foundation for the introduction of a new conceptual framework into child development, developmental psychology, and psychiatry had been laid. In the matter-of-fact way so characteristic of them, Alex and Stella credit Michael Rutter, the British child psychiatrist, with suggesting the more elegant word "temperament" instead of "primary reaction patterns."

Like other pioneers, Chess and Thomas met with indifference within psychiatry when their early papers were published. When their work could no longer be ignored, they were criticized for attempting to discredit psychodynamic theory by reducing the complexity of development to observable fragments of behavior. However, the fact that their findings were replicable and their conclusions had the potential of opening new and fruitful avenues of research and study was welcomed in many quarters and finally overcame the resistance within the field. As the eminent Harvard pediatrician Berry Brazelton wrote, Chess and Thomas's work "made it 'de rigueur' to think of different styles of development in children" (Brazelton,1969, p. 125). The scientific community's acceptance of the importance of their endeavor came when the National Institute of Mental Health decided to give financial support to the New York Longitudinal Study, and the team of Chess, Thomas, and Birch received the first of a number of grants starting in 1960.

Coming from a politically liberal background, both Stella and Alex have felt a deep commitment to working against bias and discrimination in all forms and appearances. Stella began her public career as a consultant to what was then called the Colored Orphan Asylum because she had been certain that working with privileged children in private practice would not fulfill her strong desire to serve all needy children. Later on she moved to the North Side Center for Child Development, a private clinic serving poor and minority children. The designers of the study of temperament had envisioned using only middle-class children because the were well acquainted with damage and distortions of normal development caused by unfavorable social circumstances and poverty. However, once the temperamental issues were delineated, Alex and Stella found it natural to use the same concepts and strategies in studying and understanding the Puerto Rican children and their families in New York City. These were the first cross-cultural studies of temperamental styles and their roles in normal and abnormal development.

Alex's interest in institutions and their practices and his insight into their policies and subsequent impact on society were the basis of his book coauthored with Samuel Sillen, called *Racism and Psychiatry*. In this book they advocate eloquently and strongly for an all-out effort by organized psychiatry for recruitment and training of minority students as researchers and practitioners in psychiatry in order to ensure the cultural validity and the relevance of psychiatric knowledge and practice for minority groups (Thomas & Sillen, 1972).

Those who know Stella have heard her say that ideally everything must serve more than one purpose. Her own tragic firsthand experiences with her daughter, who became neurologically impaired by meningitis in early childhood, gave her considerable knowledge and perspective on raising a handicapped child. The insight and the understanding proved immensely helpful and relevant when in 1965 she was invited as a coinvestigator with Drs. Saul Krugman and Louis Cooper to study the consequences of congenital rubella. The research project of the New York University—Bellevue Hospital department of pediatrics was designed to study the various known sequelas of congenital rubella, including the lesser known and rarely studied psychiatric consequences. This project followed the 1964–1965 rubella epidemic. Dr. Chess's findings not only revealed the alarmingly high rate of cognitive, behavioral, and psychological deficits and abnormalities caused by congenital rubella but, of equal importance for the field, confirmed that the syndrome of autism in childhood can result from an identifiable brain pathology. Dr. Chess could now point out that the brain disease, and not the "refrigerator mother," had caused the behavioral picture of autism. It now seems reasonable to assume that in a not-too-distant future, schizophrenia will also be shown that to have an organic etiology, as Dr. Chess predicted it would be some time ago (Chess, 1963).

Alex depicts Stella's thinking style as vivid, detailed, and descriptive, while he is personally more at ease with abstraction and generalization. In the design of the Longitudinal Studies, the requirement for the voluminous description of activities of the child and the caretaker is the result of Stella's insistence on having adequate observable facts as the basis for abstract generalization. Furthermore, with her remarkable memory for details, she is able to provide numerous examples of observed data to dismiss or entertain new interpretations or explanation of their findings. Indeed, once Stella has agreed that a conceptual formulation is plausible, Alex can safely assume that their data include many examples in support of the concept under discussion.

Dr. Chess has practiced what she has preached in her books for parents, namely, to have fun with and enjoy children. With them she is the observer who is fascinated by every move and statement and is amazed at her own good fortune at being able to participate. As a grandmother with grandchildren of various ages, she can look forward to many opportunities to be with children in the future. It is an article of faith with her that children like her, and she knows that she takes great pleasure in their company.

For Alex, a proud father of three successful sons in various professions, charming the women of the family is a delightful hobby. After he lost his mother at an early age, Alex, it is said by his brothers and sister, managed to charm their stepmother to marry their father. Alex talks about the early illness of his and Stella's daughter, her subsequent handicap, and her premature death with a sense of loss and profound sadness.

Dr. Chess has been a professor of child psychiatry at New York University School of Medicine since 1970. However, her contribution to the training of child psychiatrists and the teaching of child psychiatry goes back much farther. She wrote the second textbook of child psychiatry in the United States (*An Introduction to Child Psychiatry*, 1959) and trained several generations of child psychiatrists in her capacity as professor and the director of the division of child psychiatry at the New York Medical College, before moving to the New York University Medical School in 1965. During her productive years with New York University, Dr. Chess established a child psychiatry clinic within the pediatrics department at Bellevue Hospital in order to meet the needs of physicians and their patients efficiently and adequately and to see children where it can be done most easily.

Dr. Thomas has been associated with the department of psychiatry of the New York University School of Medicine since he finished his training in 1949. He taught medical students, supervised residents, and was involved in various aspects of the academic and administration plans of the medical school, achieving full professorship in 1966. Because of his managerial and organizational skills and his considerable ability in interpersonal diplomacy, he was appointed director of the Bellevue Psychiatric Hospital in 1968, a difficult job that he performed with distinction for a decade. Another of Dr. Thomas's contributions to organized psychiatry has been his involvement with the New York District Branch of the American Psychiatric Association, he was president in 1973–1974.

During their very fruitful professional lives, Drs. Chess and Thomas have encouraged many young investigators in formulating research concepts, and generously given of their time to help researchers and practitioners understand and apply their findings. Their efforts toward educating the public and helping parents and children have taken the form of writing several books and many articles for the nonprofessional audience.

In addition to having received many awards and honors for outstanding contribution to the knowledge of child development and the practice of child psychiatry, Dr. Chess and Dr. Thomas have both held offices on the editorial boards of professional journals and on the boards of directors of many associations. They have served as consultants on various scientific advisory boards, and have managed to influence the field and its direction.

Another significant contribution by which Chess and Thomas have enriched the profession is the editing since 1968 of *Annual Progress in Child Psychiatry and Child Development*, which has required close and conscientious reading of all the important journals in child development, child psychology, pediatrics, and psychopathology published in English and has earned them the gratitude of all the workers in the field.

The seminal importance of Chess and Thomas's work is not limited to description and scientific documentation of temperament. In an impressive number of books, chapters for books, and articles for professional journals, they have raised fundamental issues about the dynamics of psychological and behavioral development and provided a theoretical basis for new thinking about the etiology and evolution of behavioral pathology. Their influence on the field and its direction is attested to by the number of researchers studying temperament, not only in the United States but also in Europe, the Far East, and India. Cognizant of many interacting forces that impinge on the individual from the moment of conception, they have limited their discussion to the role of temperamental styles in shaping and modifying the experiential dimension of interaction between the individual and the environment. Their findings and ideas have by now influenced and informed not only the theoretical debates about personality development but also all discussions about child-rearing practices. They have seen the early skepticism of the profession give way to slow acceptance and final incorporation to the degree that their ideas are now treated as an integral part of the collective knowledge of developmental psychology.

Stella and Alex are now in their late seventies, and retirement has meant a much lighter schedule outside their home. Their long relationship remains an example of "goodness of fit." Although inevitable physical frailties and ailments have placed limits on the their activities, they maintain an active interest in their work. It is a good bet that Alex and Stella have read the latest paper on developmental issues, plan to attend the next conference on temperament, are aware of the goings on in the lives of many of their research subjects, and provide necessary consultation to them about their own children. Their voluminous body of data is a source of continous intellectual challenge and productive thinking. Currently, Stella is busy at work looking into the possibility that socialization will modify the degree of expression of temperamental qualities, while Alex is puzzling out the role that self-awareness and cognitive mechanisms play in individuals' coping with their own temperamental styles.

REFERENCES

Brazelton, T. B. (1969). *Infants and mothers: Differences in development.* New York: Delacorte Press.

Chess, S. (1944). Developmental language disability as a factor in personality distortion in childhood. *American Journal of Orthopsychiatry, 14* (3), 483–490.

Chess, S. (1951). Factors influencing the adaptation of organically handicapped children. *American Journal of Orthopsychiatry, 21,* 827–837.

Chess, S. (1963). Mal de mere [Editorial]. *American Journal of Orthopsychiatry, 34,* 613–614.

Thomas, A. (1939). Purulent meningitis produced by the minute hemolytic streptococcus and b. coli. *Journal of Mt. Sinai Hospital, 5,* 702–704.

Thomas, A. (1941). Suppurative and necrosuppurative bronchopneumonia in children. *Journal of Mt. Sinai Hospital, 18,* 26–28.

Thomas, A. (1956). Simultaneous psychotherapy with marital partners. *American Journal of Psychiatry, 10,* 716–724.

Thomas, A., & Chess, S. (1959). Longitudinal study of primary reaction patterns in children. *Comprehensive Psychiatry, 1,* 103–107.

Thomas, A., & Sillen, S. (1972). *Racism and psychiatry.* New York: Brunner/Mazel.

PART II

INDIVIDUAL DIFFERENCES AS RISK FACTORS: TEMPERAMENT

3

Temperament: Changing Concepts and Implications

Michael Rutter

Concepts of temperament and of constitutional differences in personality characteristics go back 2,000 years to the time of Hippocrates (Garrison & Earls, 1987). Modern views on the linking of physiological and behavioral features derive from Pavlov's typology of nervous systems and from its extension and modification in terms of theories proposed by Hans Eysenck, Jeffrey Gray, Auke Tellegen, Robert Cloninger, and others (see Rutter, 1989). Yet, despite the importance of all of these, the notion of temperamental differences largely caught the public and professional imagination through the writings of Stella Chess and Alexander Thomas (Thomas, Chess, Birch, Hertzig, & Korn, 1963; Thomas & Chess, 1977; Chess & Thomas, 1984), together with Herbert Birch and other colleagues. Their papers stood out in terms of both the extent to which their ideas were closely tied to children's observable behavior in everyday situations and the obvious clinical relevance of the individual differences that they highlighted. At a time when American psychiatry was dominated by psychoanalytic concepts of intrapsychic conflict, they emphasized that children's behavior was shaped by crucial stylistic components (the "how" of behavior), as well as by motivational concerns (the "why" component), content (the "what" element), and maturational level. Their propositions were out of keeping with the zeitgeist of the 1950s and 1960s and, therefore, seemed revolutionary at the time. It is a measure of their achievement that their main message now seems obvious, self-evident, and no longer controversial. Moreover, their concepts have led to the establishment of a body of research on temperament and on other individual differences far too large to summarize succinctly here (see Kohnstamm, Bates, & Rothbart, 1989).

I am delighted to have this opportunity to express my personal gratitude to Stella and Alex for their generous sharing of ideas and positive encouragement of my development as a young investigator during a most formative year working with them during 1961–1962. My own thinking was greatly influenced by numerous stimulating discussions (and indeed arguments, too, because friendly dispute plays a major role in clarifying one's own concepts), and it has been deeply rewarding to remain involved in the continuing process of evolving concepts concerning the role of temperament in development. In that connection, it should be noted that the mark of greatness in any new idea is to be found *not* in the extent to which it proves correct in all its details but rather in the extent to which it fosters new research that carries the whole field forward. It is obvious that the Chess/Thomas writings on temperament rate very high by that criterion, and deservedly so.

EVOLVING CONCEPTS OF TEMPERAMENT

Their initial concept of temperament was concerned with behavioral propensities that were already evident in infancy and that were a reflection of the constitutional makeup of the individual child. It came to be generally accepted that temperamental characteristics are manifest very early in life, are strongly heritable, and are stable over time. Yet there are good reasons for questioning each of these criteria. To begin with, the assumption that constitutional features are necessarily evident in infancy is clearly mistaken. The propensity for language is a biologically determined species-typical skill, but it takes time to develop and it is not apparent in early infancy. Similarly, the menarche is a constitutional feature, variations in the timing of which involve a strong genetic component (Meyer, Eaves, Heath, & Martin, 1991), but it does not occur until adolescence. The general expectation that genetic influences are maximal at birth and diminish in importance thereafter, as the environment has an ever-increasing opportunity to shape development, is also wrong (Plomin, 1986; Rutter & Rutter, 1993). To the contrary, heritability for most characteristices *increases* as children grow older, at least up to middle childhood. On the whole, monozygotic twins remain alike to a roughly similar degree as they grow older, whereas dizygotic twins tend to grow apart. Probably this tendency comes about for several rather different reasons. Intrauterine and perinatal environmental influences tend to be maximal in infancy, with their impact fading thereafter. Genetic factors influence developmental course and pattern, and not just individual differences at birth. Also, genetic factors operate in part through their impact on the selecting and shaping of environments, and on susceptibility to particular environmental influences. Nature and nurture are not as separate as used to be thought (Rutter, 1991); because nature plays a role in determining exposure, and response, to nurture, it tends to make a cumulative impact over time.

It is, in any case, unnecessarily restrictive to confine "constitutional" features to those that are genetically determined. Neural development is "driven" by experiential input (Blakemore, 1991); prenatal androgens influence both neural organization and behavioral qualities (Arnold & Gorski, 1984; Mayer-Bahlberg, Ehrhardt, & Feldman, 1986); early stress experiences bring about lasting changes in the neuroendocrine system and in emotional responses (Hennessy & Levine, 1979; Hunt, 1979); and early nutrition influences later metabolic functioning (Mott, Lewis, & McGill, 1991). In all these examples, environmental factors influence the biological constitution, but the endproduct is no less "constitutional" for that reason.

The expectation that temperament should be stable over time reflects the view that constitutional features should not alter over the course of development. Although, on the face of it, that sounds reasonable, it ignores the fact that development is necessarily concerned with change in the constitution, as well as in behavioral functioning (Rutter & Rutter, 1993). Development, of course, involves continuities as well as discontinuities, so that some sort of consistency is to be expected. However, such consistency takes several different forms, and it cannot simply be equated with high correlations over time (Rutter, 1992).

If the concept of temperament cannot be reduced to stylistic behavioral qualities that are strongly genetic, established early in life, and stable over the period of development, what should the concept comprise? Whereas there is no universal agreement on a concise formula or criterion, certain elements would be agreed on by most people in the field. First, temperament concerns those individual behavioral qualities that a person brings to a range of situations and that characterize that person's interactional style; in other words, cross-situational pervasiveness is a necessary feature. However, that does not mean that it will be shown identically in all situations. It was a mark of Chess and Thomas's foresight that they appreciated that some characteristics might be demonstrated most clearly in new, stressful, or challenging situations. That was inherent in their dimensions of approach-withdrawal to new situations and of adaptability to them. It is also apparent in Kagan, Reznick, and Snidman's (1989) focus on behavioral inhibition and Higley and Suomi's (1989) studies of similar features in monkeys. In both cases, individuals who stand out from the crowd in their inhibited response to challenge situations appear unremarkable in more ordinary day-to-day circumstances.

That recognition is important in its implication that temperamental features may need to be tapped through assessments of how people respond to unfamiliar situations, and ordinarily will need to involve assessments across a range of situations. However, two other considerations must also be taken into account. On the one hand, there is a need to decide whether a particular characteristic concerns responses only to a particular class or classes of situation. For example, the characteristic of "sociability," which constitutes one of the features in most people's lists of fundamental temperamental characteristics, is confined to responses to social situations. On the other hand, even with the best of concepts and the best of operationalizations of a particular behavioral measure, it has to be accepted that temperamental qualities are abstractions and not directly observable discrete behaviors (Rutter, Birch, Thomas, & Chess, 1964; Rutter, 1987a, 1989). The *latent* variable of temperament comprises that aspect of behavioral style that reflects the "person" contribution (rather than relationship or situational aspects) and that is indeed stylistic (i.e., does not concern the content or motivation of the behavior). Thus, inhibition in social situations is a temperamental feature, but refusal to enter the school building because of panic or fear of encountering a particular person who is disliked is not. The problem is that the very best of measures will include unwanted, as well as wanted, components. Thus, even very well thought-out measures will include some degree of error, perceptual bias, relationship qualities, situation specificities, and cognitive-motivational components. The nature of a person's response to a social situation will necessarily be influenced by the cognitive processing of the situation, and by the person's self-concept, as well as by temperamental qualities. There is no ready solution to the problem of how to get closest to the latent construct as conceptualized. Clearly, multiple measuring devices and multiple situations help to overcome biases, errors, and situation specificities. However, there is much to be said for the use of statistical procedures, such as structural equation modeling, that can partition and measure the different components and not just reduce the influence of the unwanted ones (Rutter & Pickles, 1990). In addition, there may also be advantages in including physiological, or other nonbehavioral, features in the triangulation of measurement, as done by Kagan and associates (1989) in their assessment of behavioral inhibition. The point of this addition is not to provide a more "basic" constitutional component on the grounds that laboratory measures are always more "basic" than behavioral ones. As numerous examples illustrate, there is a two-way traffic between biological functioning and psychosocial features (Rutter, 1986). Thus, sex hormones are influenced by whether a person becomes socially dominant or submissive, as well as hormones influencing assertive behavior.

The second issue concerns the supposed strong heritability of temperamental features. Of course, it would be reasonable to expect that there should be a substantial genetic component and that is indeed what has been found empirically. However, most human behavior involves a heritability within the 30% to 60% range, and temperamental characteristics do *not* stand out as being more heritable than other features (Plomin, 1986). In any case, putting things around the other way, it is not reasonable to expect that constitutional features would be immune from environmental influences, and they are not. The key issue is a different one; namely, whether the genetic component involved in temperament is *different* from that involved in the psychiatric disorders to which it predisposes. Curiously, we know next to nothing on that very important matter—partly, because in most studies the measures of temperament and of disorder have been too confounded for the question to be tackled adequately.

A third consideration involves the choice of traits to be included under the umbrella of temperament. Some theorists have sought to make the choice in terms of those characteristics that have a clear neurobiological origin. The approach is reasonable in view of the wish to focus on features that are strongly constitutional. However, the empirical evidence so far on neurobiological origins is not such as to lead to a clear choice of dimensions (although such evidence as there is leads in much the same direction as other approaches—see below). Clearly, it is desirable to reduce the almost infinite list of human traits to a more manageable, small number. Basically, three main approaches have been adopted. First, factor analysis may be used to derive dimensions on the basis of intercorrelations between behavioral features. Although the method is much favored by psychometricians, and although it does have the distinct advantage of drawing out key common elements, it does not seem a satisfactory criterion on its own because it involves no test of external validity (Rutter, 1982). Chess and Thomas used a more clinically oriented inductive approach in order to select features that seemed to differentiate children most clearly in meaningful aspects of their response to everyday situations. Although their system proved popular with clinically oriented investigators, several of the original nine traits have not stood the test of time and there has been an increasing tendency to turn to behavioral composites of one kind or another. Of these, the Chess/Thomas concept of the "difficult child" has proved most popular because it has been shown to predict psychiatric disorder (Maziade et al., 1990). Obviously, this provides the much-needed external validity. However, there has been an understandable reluctance to define a *personal* constitutional trait in terms of its propensity to engender negative responses from other people (if only because different features may aggravate different people and because there has not emerged a satisfactory unifying feature of just what characterizes the personal style that gives rise to the interpersonal difficulties). Bates (1989) has argued that it may involve two separate components: sensation seeking and high sensitivity to aversive stimuli; the suggestion is plausible, but it does imply rather different consequences for the two components. It would be premature to draw firm conclusions on the key temperamental features, but the eventual list will probably include features such as emotionality, activity, sociability, impulsivity or sensation seeking, and high sensitivity to aversive stimuli—possibly plus aggressivity.

CLINICAL AND DEVELOPMENTAL IMPLICATIONS

Temperamental qualities have been of interest mainly because of expectations that they may play a role in the development of personality and of personality disorder (Rutter, 1987a) and that, at least at extremes, certain of them may constitute risk factors for psychiatric disorder (Rutter, 1989; Garrison & Earls, 1987; Bates, 1989). Because the term "temperament" has usually been applied to children and "personality" to adults, it might be supposed that the former simply evolves into the latter. However, that supposition overlooks the many facets of personality. There is every reason to suppose that in adulthood, as in childhood, everyday functioning is influenced by basic stylistic components. Thus, some people are generally more (or less) sociable or emotional than others. There is no reason to avoid calling these temperamental characteristics just because a person is adult. However, everyday functioning is also influenced by self-concepts, by social cognitions, and by values and attitudes (Rutter, 1987b). Humans are thinking beings, and as such their personality will be shaped by the ways in which they deal with the temperamental qualities with which they have been endowed, and by the views of themselves and their social worlds that they acquire. Thus, we characterize ourselves and other people in terms of self-esteem, self-confidence, and self-efficacy, as well as by attributes such as suspiciousness, conscientiousness, empathy, and trustworthiness. It seems reasonable to suppose these qualities will be shaped, in part, by temperamental qualities such as sociability and emotionality, but there is a remarkable paucity of research on the developmental processes involved or, indeed, on the relative strength of different influences on the evolution of self-concepts. That remains a priority need on the research agenda for the future. Chess and Thomas have usefully laid out some of the issues to be taken into consideration in the application of temperamental concepts to adults and in thinking about personality development more generally (Thomas & Chess, 1980; Chess & Thomas, 1990), but systematic investigation of the issues has scarcely begun as yet.

There is a comparable lack of understanding of the connections between temperament and personality disorder (Rutter, 1987a). Indeed, there is a lack of agreement on the basic question of just how personality disorder should be conceptualized. Frequently, personality disorder has been viewed as a pervasive and persistent pattern of social malfunction that has arisen on the basis of the individual's being extreme on some particular trait (see Tyrer, 1988). Thus, many personality disorder categories are named on that basis, with adjectives such as paranoid, anxious, depressive, or obsessional. However, it is apparent that, in many ways, these represent subclinical varieties of some form of psychiatric disorder at least as much as trait extremes. It is also apparent that by no means all individuals with pervasive, persistent social malfunction have any extreme trait; equally, not all people who exhibit unusually marked personality characteristics are impaired in their social functioning. Although there is a clear need to retain personality disorder categories, it is also apparent that something of a rethink on their conceptualization is required. It is by no means self-evident that temperamental features will be found to play a major role in the development of such disorders.

By contrast, their importance as risk factors for child psychiatric disorders seems somewhat more secure (Garrison & Earls, 1987), although knowledge is still lacking on numerous key issues. Thus, the early findings from the Chess/Thomas longitudinal study (Rutter et al., 1964), as well as those from other later investigations (e.g., Graham, Rutter, & George, 1973; Porter & Collins, 1982; Maziade, 1989), have tended to show associations between behavioral constellations of one type or another (usually some variant on the so-called difficult child complex) and disruptive behavior disorder. On the whole, *individual* temperamental characteristics have not been found to constitute major risk factors for child psychiatric disorder; equally, fewer links with temperament have been found for nondisruptive types of disorder. The connection between behavioral inhibition and anxiety disorders may constitute an exception (Kagan et al., 1989), but so far the evidence on this association is distinctly limited.

These results raise important questions on mechanisms, and also give rise to methodological queries. Many of the studies have relied on a single questionnaire measure of temperament; for the reasons discussed already, it seems extremely doubtful that these are adequate for the purpose. If the construct concerns a pervasive behavioral style, multiple measures covering several settings would seem to be desirable, if not essential. There are also continuing uncertainties on the best way to subdivide temperamental characteristics. In particular, outside of the realm of behavioral inhibition, rather little use has been made of combinations of physiological and behavioral features—a combination that seems highly desirable on conceptual grounds as well as on the empirical evidence that it may be a better risk indicator. Finally, much of the research has been concerned with variations within the normal range rather than with the effects of extremes. It may well be that it is only the latter that constitute significant psychiatric risk factors. It is obvious that improvements in the quality, as well as the quantity, of research on this topic are needed.

Nevertheless, even with those caveats, the findings to date require a critical appraisal of the possible risk mechanisms that may be involved. The first possibility is that the supposed temperamental trait is actually no more than a subclinical manifestation of the disorder for which it is supposed to constitute a risk (Stevenson & Graham, 1982). That could be the case with respect to disorders for which the symptom pattern seems to overlap with the extreme of the trait; for example, behavioral inhibition and generalized anxiety disorders or the "difficult child" constellation and oppositional defiant disorder. Nevertheless, it seems unlikely that that constitutes a general explanation, if only because the symptoms of most disorders do not constitute extremes on any temperamental characteristic (Rutter, 1987a). However, what are needed to resolve the issue are genetic designs with adequate multimethod assessment of both temperament and disorder in order to determine whether the *same* genetic and environmental influences apply to both (Rutter, Simonoff, & Silberg, 1993).

A second possibility is that the temperamental feature involves an increased susceptibility to psychosocial adversities. There are many examples in biology and medicine of person–environment interactions (Rutter & Pickles, 1991), and certainly it is quite plausible that temperamental attributes *could* create a psychiatric risk through this mechanism. Behavioral inhibition is characterized by an unusually marked response to stress and challenge, and this might make it more likely that children with this feature would develop focused fears or generalized depression. However, whether or not it in fact functions in this way is quite unknown. Conversely, it has been found that an unusually *low* physiological reactivity is associated with an increased risk for recidivist criminality (Magnusson, 1988); perhaps this arises because the features render children less responsive to normal social controls. There is also some evidence that "difficultness" mainly leads to disorder when there are associated psychosocial adversities (Maziade, 1989; Maziade et al., 1990). However, few studies have tested for interaction vulnerability mechanisms of this type, and their importance is not known.

Another alternative is that temperament makes its impact through its influence on interpersonal interactions. This mechanism is suggested by the general body of evidence, both naturalistic and experimental, that how people behave toward others influences how others behave toward them. Thus, Dodge (1980) showed that aggressive boys tended to elicit hostile behavior from their peers, and Brunk and Henggeler (1984) showed that adults behaved differently, even in neutral or ambiguous circumstances, toward children who behaved in a compliant rather than oppositional manner. Similarly, we found that when parents are depressed and irritable, they are more likely to behave particularly negatively toward those of their children who exhibit difficult temperamental characteristics (Rutter, 1978). It is clear that even apparently familywide influences (such as discord) do not impinge equally on all children. Genetic data suggest, too, that on the whole these person-specific (i.e., nonshared) influences tend to have a greater effect than familywide (i.e., shared) ones (Plomin & Daniels, 1987). It is relevant, too, that temperamental differences do not have the same consequences in all circumstances. This is apparent, for example, in gender differences, where it seems that shyness tends to be associated with negative social interactions in boys but not girls (Stevenson-Hinde & Hinde, 1986), but high activity level tends to be accompanied by negative father–child interactions in girls but not boys (Buss, 1981). As Bates (1989) has pointed out, direct evidence of the impact of temperamental characteristics on interpersonal interactions is weak, but such effects are nevertheless likely to be important (Rutter, 1989).

In considering the possible operation of such effects, several facets need to be borne in mind. First, interpersonal effects are likely to be more important with some temperamental characteristics than others. The constellation of traits termed "difficult" focuses on those most likely to elicit negative responses from other people, and hence in Chess/Thomas terms, to provide a poor "fit" with environmental expectations and needs. Second, however, it is not to be expected that any trait, or group of traits, will always elicit the same responses or give rise to the same consequences. Thus, in a small sample, deVries (1984) found that during famine conditions in Africa, a "difficult" temperament was protective in leading to survival—presumably because infants with such characteristics were more successful in gaining the limited amounts of attention and food available. More generally, people are likely to differ in the temperamental features they view positively. What is "difficultness" for one parent may be "independence" for another; shyness may signal a need for support or provide a source of irritation. Moreover, acceptance of a behavior may be supportive of the individual or it may serve in an unhelpful fashion to accentuate a negative feature (Maccoby, Snow, & Jacklin, 1984). Third, it is quite likely that both interpersonal effects and psychiatric risks associated with temperamental features will be evident only, or mainly, at the extremes, with few consequences apparent in relation to variations within the normal range.

CONCLUSIONS

Since Alexander Thomas, Stella Chess, and Herbert Birch (Thomas et al., 1963) first emphasized the potential importance of behavioral individuality in childhood some 30 years ago, that message has come to be generally accepted. Also, we have gained a greater understanding of what is involved in the concept of temperament, together with a limited appreciation of how it operates. Already that knowledge provides useful leads for clinical practice (Thomas & Chess, 1980; Carey, 1989; Bates, 1989). Alex Thomas and Stella Chess have every reason to feel proud of both their accomplishments and those of their many disciples. However, as I have sought to bring out in this brief essay, there are many key questions still to be answered on the nature and role of temperamental differences, and the influence of Chess and Thomas on this important topic is going to continue to be evident for many years to come.

REFERENCES

Arnold, A. P., & Gorski, R. A. (1984). Gonadal steroid induction of structural sex differences in the central nervous system. *Annual Review of Neuroscience, 7,* 413–442.

Bates, J. E. (1989). Concepts and measures of temperament: Applications of temperament concepts. In G. A. Kohnstamm, J. E. Bates, & M. K. Rothbart (Eds.), *Temperament in childhood* (pp. 3–26; 321–355). Chichester, England: John Wiley.

Blakemore, C. (1991). Sensitive and vulnerable periods in the development of the visual system. In G. R. Bock & J. Whelan (Eds.), *The childhood environment and adult disease* (pp. 129–147). Ciba Foundation Symposium 156. Chichester, England: John Wiley.

Brunk, M. A., & Henggeler, S. W. (1984). Child influences on adult controls: An experimental investigation. *Developmental Psychology, 20,* 1074–1081.

Buss, D. M. (1981). Predicting parent-child interactions from children's activity level. *Developmental Psychology, 17,* 59–65.

Carey, W. B. (1989). Practical applications in pediatrics. In G. A. Kohnstamm, J. E. Bates, & M. K. Rothbart (Eds.), *Temperament in childhood* (pp. 405–419). Chichester, England: John Wiley.

Chess, S., & Thomas, A. (1984). *Origins and evolution of behavior disorders: From infancy to early adult life.* New York: Brunner/Mazel.

Chess, S., & Thomas, A. (1990). Continuities and discontinuities in temperament. In L. N. Robins & M. Rutter (Eds.), *Straight and devious pathways from childhood to adulthood* (pp. 205–220). Cambridge: Cambridge University Press.

deVries, M. W. (1984). Temperament and infant mortality among the Masai of East Africa. *American Journal of Psychiatry, 141,* 1189–1194.

Dodge, K. A. (1980). Social cognition and children's aggressive behavior. *Child Development, 51,* 162–172.

Garrison, W., & Earls, F. (1987). *Temperament and child psychopathology.* Newbury Park, CA: Sage.

Graham, P., Rutter, M., & George, S. (1973). Temperamental characteristics as predictors of behavior disorders in children. *American Journal of Orthopsychiatry, 43,* 328–339.

Hennessy, J. W., & Levine, S. (1979). Stress, arousal, and the pituitary-adrenal system: A psychoendocrine hypothesis. In J. M. Sprague & A. N. Epstein (Eds.), *Progress in psychobiology and physiological psychology.* New York: Academic Press.

Higley, J. D., & Suomi, S. J. (1989). Temperamental reactivity in non-human primates. In G. A. Kohnstamm, J. E. Bates, & M. K. Rothbart (Eds.), *Temperament in childhood* (pp. 153–167). Chichester, England: John Wiley.

Hunt, J. McV. (1979). Psychological development: Early experience. *Annual Review of Psychology, 30,* 103–143.

Kagan, J., Reznick, J. S., & Snidman, N. (1989). Issues in the study of temperament. In G. A. Kohnstamm, J. E. Bates, & M. K. Rothbart (Eds.), *Temperament in childhood* (pp. 133–144). Chichester, England: John Wiley.

Kohnstamm, G. A., Bates, J. E., & Rothbart, M. K. (Eds.). (1989). *Temperament in childhood.* Chichester, England: John Wiley.

Maccoby, E., Snow, M. E., & Jacklin, C. N. (1984). Children's dispositions and mother-child interaction at 12 and 18 months: A short-term longitudinal study. *Developmental Psychology, 20*, 459–472.

Magnusson, D. (Ed.). (1988). *Paths through life: A longitudinal research program.* Hillsdale, NJ: Lawrence Erlbaum.

Mayer-Bahlberg, H. F. L., Ehrhardt, A. A., & Feldman, J. F. (1986). Long-term implications of the prenatal endocrine milieu for sex-dimorphic behavior. In L. Erlenmeyer-Kimling & N. E. Miller (Eds.), *Life span research on the prediction of psychopathology* (pp. 17–30). Hillsdale, NJ: Lawrence Erlbaum.

Maziade, M. (1989). Should adverse temperament matter to the clinician? An empirically based answer. In G. A. Kohnstamm, J. E. Bates, & M. K. Rothbart (Eds.), *Temperament in childhood* (pp. 421–435). Chichester, England: John Wiley.

Maziade, M., Caron, C., Côté, R., Mérette, C., Bernier, H., Laplante, B., Boutin, P., & Thivierge, J. (1990). Psychiatric status of adolescents who had extreme temperaments at age 7. *American Journal of Psychiatry, 147*, 1531–1536.

Meyer, J. M., Eaves, L. J., Heath, A. C., & Martin, N. G. (1991). Estimating genetic influences on the age-at-menarche: A survival analysis approach. *American Journal of Medical Genetics, 39*, 148–154.

Mott, G. E., Lewis, D. S., & McGill, H. C., Jr. (1991). Programming of cholesterol metabolism by breast or formula feeding. In G. R. Bock & J. Whelan (Eds.), *The childhood environment and adult disease* (pp. 56–66). Ciba Foundation Symposium 156. Chichester, England: John Wiley.

Plomin, R., (1986). *Development, genetics and psychiatry.* Hillsdale, NJ: Lawrence Erlbaum.

Plomin, R., & Daniels, D. (1987). Why are children in the same family so different from one another? *Behavioral and Brain Sciences, 10*, 1–15.

Porter, R., & Collins, C. G. (Eds.). (1982). *Temperamental differences in infants and young children.* Ciba Foundation Symposium 89. London: Pitman.

Rutter, M. (1978). Family, area and school influences on the genesis of conduct disorders. In L. A. Hersov & M. Berger, with D. Shaffer (Eds.), *Aggression and antisocial behaviour in childhood and adolescence* (pp. 95–113) *Journal of Child Psychology and Psychiatry* (book suppl. 1). Oxford: Pergamon.

Rutter, M. (1982). Temperament: Concepts, issues and problems. In R. Porter & C. G. Collins (Eds.), *Temperamental differences in infants and young children* (pp. 1–19). Ciba Foundation Symposium 89. London: Pitman.

Rutter, M. (1986). Meyerian psychobiology, personality development and the role of life experience. *American Journal of Psychiatry, 143*, 1077–1087.

Rutter, M. (1987a). Temperament, personality and personality disorder. *British Journal of Psychiatry, 150*, 443–458.

Rutter, M. (1987b). The role of cognition in child development and disorder. *British Journal of Medical Psychology, 60*, 1–16.

Rutter, M. (1989). Temperament: Conceptual issues and clinical implications. In G. A. Kohnstamm, J. E. Bates, & M. K. Rothbart (Eds.), *Temperament in childhood* (pp. 463–479). Chichester, England: John Wiley.

Rutter, M. (1991). Nature, nurture, and psychopathology: A new look at an old topic. *Development and Psychopathology, 3*, 125–136.

Rutter, M. (1992). Adolescence as a transition period: Continuities and discontinuities in conduct disorder. *Journal of Adolescent Health, 13* 451–460

Rutter, M., Birch, H., Thomas, A., & Chess, S. (1964). Temperamental characteristics in infancy and the later development of behavioural disorders. *British Journal of Psychiatry, 110,* 651–661.

Rutter, M., & Pickles, A. (1990). Improving the quality of psychiatric data: Classification, cause and course. In D. Magnusson & L. Bergman (Eds.), *Data quality in longitudinal research* (pp. 32–57). Cambridge: Cambridge University Press.

Rutter, M., & Pickles, A. (1991). Person-environment interactions: Concepts, mechanisms, and implications for data analysis. In T. D. Wachs & R. Plomin (Eds.), *Conceptualization and measurement of organism-environment interaction* (pp. 105–141). Washington, DC: American Psychological Association.

Rutter, M. & Rutter, M. (1993). Developing minds: Challenge and continuity across the life span. *Harmondsworth, England: Penguin; New York: Basic Books.*

Rutter, M., Simonoff, E., & Silberg, J. (1993). How informative are twin studies of child psychopathology? In T.J. Bouchard, Jr. & P. Propping (Eds.) *Twins as a tool of behavioral genetics.* (pp. 179–194). Chichester, England: John Wiley.

Stevenson, J., & Graham, P. (1982). Temperament: A consideration of concepts and methods. In R. Porter & C. G. Collins (Eds.), *Temperamental differences in infants and young children.* (pp. 36–46) Ciba Foundation Symposium 89. London: Pitman.

Stevenson-Hinde, J., & Hinde, R. A. (1986). Changes in associations between characteristics. In R. Plomin & J. Dunn (Eds.), *The study of temperament: Changes, continuities and challenges* (pp. 115–129) Hillsdale, NJ: Lawrence Erlbaum.

Thomas, A., & Chess, S. (1977). *Temperament and development.* New York: Brunner/Mazel.

Thomas, A., & Chess, S. (1980). *The dynamics of psychological development.* New York: Brunner/Mazel.

Thomas, A., Chess, S., Birch, H., Hertzig, M., & Korn, S. (1963). *Behavioural individuality in early childhood.* New York: New York University Press.

Tyrer, P. (1988). *Personality disorders: Diagnosis, management and course.* London: Wright.

4

Inhibited and Uninhibited Temperaments

Jerome Kagan

It is usually the case that when inquiry surrounding a particular domain changes in both direction and pace, several historical factors are acting in concert. Less often, the work of a single investigator or research team is the critical catalyst for change. The renascence of interest in the temperamental qualities of children provides a clear example of the influence of the collaborative research team of Stella Chess and Alexander Thomas, for their work provided the impulse that led to a return of temperamental ideas to psychiatry, pediatrics, and developmental psychology. And like the fruitful concepts of the second-century physician Galen, many of the original Chess/Thomas constructs continue to be useful guides to the parsing of the variation in children's moods and behaviors (Thomas & Chess, 1977).

Thomas and Chess saw in the rich parental descriptions of infants and young children the small group that was consistently hesitant, timid, and shy when faced with unfamiliarity—slow to warm up—and a somewhat larger group that approached the same unfamiliar events quickly and with minimal restraint. Our laboratory, relying on behavioral observations of young children, has affirmed these Chess/Thomas discoveries. We believe, but have not yet proved, that the two groups, which we call inhibited and uninhibited, might be discrete categories and not physiological or psychological complements of each other. The remainder of this chapter summarizes what we have learned over the past 13 years of study of these two types.

This research was supported in part by a grant from the John D. and Catherine T. MacArthur Foundation and the Leon Lowenstein Foundation. The author thanks Nancy Snidman and Doreen Arcus for their collaborative efforts.

INHIBITED AND UNINHIBITED TYPES

We have observed over 800 children belonging to five independent cohorts of healthy white youngsters. One cohort has been followed from 2 weeks to 3 years of age; another, from 21 months to 7 years of age. Because four of these cohorts are still being studied, some conclusions remain tentative.

About 20% of healthy white infants, firstborn or later born, living with intact, two-parent families, show a distinct behavioral profile to unfamiliar visual, auditory, and olfactory stimuli at 4 months of age. The infants who are called *reactive* become extremely active motorically to about one third of the stimulus presentations, and especially to three-dimensional, moving, highly colored visual objects. Further, on some occasions when they are flexing and extending their limbs and arching their back, they fret or cry. The strong impression is that the distress is provoked by the increase in central arousal created by the stimulus events. When these reactive infants are observed in the laboratory at 14 months as they encounter unfamiliar events—strangers, wheels filled with noisy objects, an invitation to imitate unfamiliar acts, a request to taste a liquid through a dropper, an unexpected frown from an examiner—about two thirds are classed as inhibited because they show obvious fear in response to four or more of a total of 21 episodes.

Another group, about 35% of the same healthy population, is called *relaxed* at four months because the infants display very low levels of motor activity and little or no crying in reaction to the same stimuli. These children are uninhibited at 14 months; only 11% show four or more fears to the same battery of unfamiliar episodes while 60% show either no fears at all or only one fear across the battery of unfamiliar episodes (Kagan & Snidman, 1991).

Although we shall not describe in detail the other two profiles of behavior observed at 4 months, it is of interest to note that about 25% of the infants showed a combination of low motor activity but frequent fretting or crying in response to the same stimulus battery. The distress displayed by these infants appears to be due more often to a state of uncertainty about the discrepant events in the battery than to increased arousal. These infants show intermediate levels of fear at 14 months of age. The smallest group—about 10% of the population—showed high levels of motor activity, often as high as those of the reactive group, but these infants rarely fretted or cried. They, too, showed intermediate levels of fear. About 10% of the infants were difficult to classify into one of these four groups.

These results, which are summarized in Table 4-1, are based on the study of 440 infants from two different longitudinal cohorts observed at 4 and 14 months of age. These two temperamental styles appear to be heritable. Unpublished observations on over 150 same-sex monozygotic and dizygotic twin pairs seen at 14 and

TABLE 4.1
Proportion of Children with Low (0 or 1), Moderate (2 or 3), or
High Fear (4 or More Fears) at 14 Months Who Were Classified
as Reactive or Relaxed at 4 Months of Age

4 Month Profile	Low Fear	Moderate Fear	High Fear
Reactive ($N = 96$)	8	27	65
Relaxed ($N = 166$)	62	27	11

20 months at the Institute for Behavioral Genetics at the University of Colorado reveal heritabilities of 0.6 for inhibited behavior in response to unfamiliar laboratory procedures that include unfamiliar toys and adults. The inhibited children stayed closer to their mothers and waited a long time before playing. The uninhibited children rarely went to their mothers and played with the toys and approached the unfamiliar adult quickly. The correlation for inhibited behavior for monozygotic twins was 0.5 and for dizygotic twins was 0.2 (Robinson, Kagan, Reznick, & Corley, 1992; see, also, Matheny, 1989).

MECHANISMS

We believe, but cannot yet prove, that the excitability of the amygdala and its circuits to the corpus striatum, locus ceruleus, hypothalamus, central gray, and sympathetic nervous system participates in mediating the reactive and relaxed profiles we have described. Briefly, we believe that reactive infants inherit a neurochemistry within the amygdala and its circuits that leads to a very low threshold of activation to unfamiliar events. Hence, projections from the basal and lateral area of the amygdala to the ventral striatum and ventral pallidum, and from the central nucleus of the amygdala to the central gray, become activated easily when unfamiliar visual, auditory, and olfactory stimuli are presented to them. As a result, we see the profile of high motor activity and crying characteristic of reactive 4-month-olds. At 14 months of age, the low thresholds in the amygdala and its circuits mediate high levels of fear and avoidance of unfamiliar people and objects. The relaxed infants who become uninhibited children inherit a different neurochemistry, not the complement of the inhibited profile, which is associated with higher thresholds of excitability.

The evidence is insufficient to name a particular neurochemistry that renders the amygdala and its circuits excitable. Some candidates include norepinephrine, corticotropin-releasing hormone, GABA, and opioids, along with their appropriate receptors. The final answer is likely to surprise us.

Support for the claim that the amygdala and its projections are relevant comes from the consistent finding of larger rises in heart rate to mildly stressful events in inhibited than in uninhibited children, as well as early signs of a greater sympathetic influence on cardiovascular function in reactive infants (Kagan, Reznick, & Snidman, 1988). For example, the infants who were classified as reactive at 4 months had, as fetuses, higher heart rates during the last few weeks of pregnancy than did relaxed infants (mean of 422 vs. 433 msec). Moreover, the reactive infants had higher heart rates while sleeping in an erect posture when they were only 2 weeks old. Further, a spectral analysis of heart rate at 2 weeks of age while the infants were sleeping in an erect posture revealed that the reactive infants had significantly more power in the lower frequency band (from .01 Hz to the lower boundary of the respiratory peak representing vagal tone on the heart), suggesting greater sympathetic reactivity (Snidman & Kagan, 1992).

At 14 months of age, the reactive infants showed significantly larger heart rate accelerations than relaxed infants to a drop of dilute lemon juice on the tongue, implying greater reactivity in the circuit from the gustatory nucleus to the amygdala and sympathetic projections to the heart (Kagan & Snidman, 1991). Finally, reactive children with high fear scores showed an asymmetrical pattern of facial cooling to mild, cognitive stress at 21 months favoring greater cooling on the right than on the left side of the face. Relaxed infants with low fear scores showed greater cooling on the left side. This difference in direction of cooling—to the right for inhibited children and to the left for uninhibited ones—is in accord with the hypothesis of greater sympathetic reactivity for inhibited children. The sympathetic nervous system is usually more reactive on the right than on the left side of the body. Moreover, projections from the hypothalamus to the sympathetic nervous system are mainly ipsilateral. Because uncertainty and threat provoke vasoconstriction of the arteriovenous anastomoses serving the skin, mediated by α adrenergic receptors, the children who react to uncertainty with sympathetic discharge should show greater constriction and, therefore greater cooling, on the right side of the face (Kagan, Snidman, & Arcus, 1992).

ROLE OF THE ENVIRONMENT

No one claims that the temperamental characteristics we have described are deterministic and outside of the influence of experience. The environment acts on the phenotype created by the infant's temperament. Remember that some reactive infants are minimally fearful and some of the relaxed infants are highly fearful at 14 months of age. The environmental effect was more obvious at 21 months of age. When the subjects were observed at 21 months in a battery of unfamiliar procedures (including the placement of electrodes, blood pressure cuff; criticism from the examiner; presence of a clown, a robot; and being in a small room containing unfamiliar objects), about one third of the relaxed girls showed high fear scores compared with 6% of the relaxed boys. We interpret the increase in fear between 14 and 21 months among relaxed girls to mean that socialization experiences in and outside the home made some of these girls, perhaps temporarily, timid and restrained when they encountered unfamiliarity. However, even though these relaxed girls showed fear, they still retained frequent display of positive affect, in the form of talking and smiling, which is characteristic of uninhibited children. By contrast, the reactive, fearful girls continued to display a dour expression with minimal positive affect. Thus, even though some originally relaxed girls were fearful about the unfamiliar in the second year, they retained the positive affect characteristic of their temperamental group.

A second important difference between reactive and relaxed infants was in the type of fear displayed at 14 and 21 months. A child was given a fear score for crying in response to an unfamiliar event—like the application of electrodes or blood pressure cuff, or the appearance of the clown—or for refusing to approach an unfamiliar woman, a clown, or a metal robot, even though the child did not cry. Many more relaxed infants (65%) showed more of the latter category of avoidant fears than the former category of distress fears. By contrast, more reactive infants (78%) displayed more distress than avoidant fears.

Ordinal position is another potentially relevant experiential factor. Among reactive infants, firstborns are slightly more fearful than later borns in the second year, but there is no comparable ordinal position effect for the relaxed infants. We interpret that fact to mean that more mothers of firstborn than of later-born reactive infants may be protective of them and less likely than most parents to encourage them to cope with the minor stresses present in each day. As a result, many reactive firstborns are deprived of the opportunity to learn to handle uncertainty. The fact that ordinal position did not interact with temperament for relaxed infants illustrates the importance of both the child's temperament and home experience.

Although we believe that distinctive neurochemical profiles affecting the excitability of the limbic system define each temperamental type, it is possible that experience can modify these profiles of excitability. In one study, male rats were stressed by the unpredictability of living in unstable social groups because new males were introduced daily into the living area. Later, these stressed rats, along with those living under stable social conditions, were exposed to a novel event. Although all the animals, both the experimental and the controls, showed an increase in adrenal steroids in response to the novelty, the rats that had experienced prior stress showed a significantly greater increase in steroids, presumably because of the prior stress that altered the receptors, or increased the density of the receptors, for corticosteriods (Maccari et al., 1991). If stressful experience can alter neurochemistry for a period of time, perhaps reduction in stress has a complementary effect. If inhibited children develop coping reactions that permit them, over time, to experience less uncertainty, alterations in the excitability of the limbic circuits might occur, perhaps as a result of alterations in the density of particular receptors. We have seen some inhibited children who show over time a decrease in both fearful behavior and sympathetic reactivity, implying the absence of a fixed determinism in the early temperamental bias.

CLINICAL IMPLICATIONS

We suggest that a small proportion of inhibited children, perhaps a third, are at risk for extreme anxiety or social phobia in later childhood and adolescence and extreme introversion in adulthood. This estimate is based on earlier work at the Fels Institute (Kagan & Moss, 1962) and psychiatric interviews with parents of these children (Biederman et al., 1990). Not all parents are motivated to change their inhibited children. Inhibited children who are highly intelligent and motivated for academic mastery often select intellectual careers and become successful. I suggest that T. S. Eliot and Rita Levi-Montalcini are two examples. Parents who wish their children to be less timid find it useful to motivate them by titering their exposure to unfamiliarity and challenge in order to help them learn how to cope with uncertainty.

CONCLUSION

When the natural sciences were young, the first questions asked were about observable phenomena that appeared stable and were believed to be fundamental, like light, heat, the monthly phases of the moon, and the annual cycle of seasons. Although we have gained understanding of each of these original puzzles, it turned out that the investigations of light revealed discoveries that had the most powerful implications for our understanding of the essence of the atom. When 19th-century physicists discovered that the relations between light and heat could be explained in terms of frequency and energy, the stage was set for Max Planck's postulate of the energy quantum, Einstein's discovery of the photon, and soon after, with the help of elegant mathematics, Joseph Thomson's discovery of the electron, and Ernest Rutherford's positing of the atomic nucleus. It is less likely that such rapid progress would have been made if the talented scientists in this story had investigated more deeply the phases of the moon rather than light and heat. Only some roads lead to a pot of gold.

Psychology's list of fundamental phenomena include classical and instrumental conditioning of motor responses, acquisition of perceptual structures, memory, emotions, speech, language, and behavior to novelty—this list is not intended to be exhaustive. We are learning a great deal from active inquiry into all of these phenomena. But, as with the study of light, it may be that one of the above phenomena is more likely than others to lead to profound insights into human psychological functioning. At the moment, most psychologists are betting on the mechanisms of conditioning and memory as holding that prophetic power. Yet it is possible that because reactions to the unfamiliar involve all of the major brain systems—sensory, limbic, cortical, skeletal, and autonomic—understanding of behavioral reactions to novelty may provide a deep insight into the relations between basic brain circuits and behavior. And if this prediction is affirmed, Stella Chess and Alexander Thomas will have even more cause to enjoy the satisfaction of their extraordinarily creative careers.

REFERENCES

Biederman, J., Hirschfeld, D. R., Faraone, S. V., Bolduc, E. A., Gersten, M., Meminger, S. R., Kagan, J., Snidman, N., & Reznick, J. S. (1990). Psychiatric correlates of behavioral inhibition in young children of parents with and without psychiatric disorders. *Archives of General Psychiatry, 47,* 21–26.

Kagan, J., & Moss, H. A. (1962). *Birth to maturity.* New York: John Wiley.

Kagan, J., Reznick, J. S., & Snidman, N. (1988). Biological bases of childhood shyness. *Science, 240,* 167–173.

Kagan, J., & Snidman, N. (1991). Temperamental factors in human development. *American Psychologist, 46,* 856–862.

Kagan, J., Snidman, N., & Arcus, D. (1992). *Temperament and asymmetry in facial temperature.* Unpublished manuscript.

Maccari, S., Piazza, P. V., Deminiere, J. M., Lemaire, V., Moremede, P., Simon, H., Angelucci, L., & Le Moal, M. (1991). Life events-induced decrease of corticosteroid type 1 receptors is associated with reduced corticosterone feedback and enhanced vulnerability to amphetamine self-administration. *Brain Research, 547,* 7–12.

Matheny, A. P. (1989). Children's behavioral inhibition over age and across situations. *Journal of Personality, 57,* 215–235.

Robinson, J. L., Kagan, J., Reznick, J. S., & Corley, R. (1992). The heritability of inhibited and uninhibited behavior: A twin study. *Developmental Psychology, 28,* 1030–1037.

Snidman, N., & Kagan, J. (1992). *Cardiac function and fear during infancy.* Unpublished manuscript.

Thomas, A., & Chess, S. (1977). *Temperament and development.* New York: Brunner/Mazel.

5

Temperament Risk Factors for Type A Behavior Pattern in Adolescents

Jan Strelau* and Andrzej Eliasz

> Temperament research should keep in mind its responsibility to broaden our knowledge of the behavior of real human beings in real life. Otherwise, there is the danger that our research, no matter how elegant and sophisticated its design and execution may be, will become abstract and sterile. (Chess & Thomas, 1991, p. 28)

One of the central issues in temperament research is to show that temperament plays an important role in human adaptation to the environment and in regulating the individual's relationship with the external world, especially the social surroundings. The functional significance of temperamental traits in real human life is the best argument for devoting time and effort to studying the nature as well as other aspects of temperament.

The most extensive study, and the one in which the functional significance of temperament was displayed to the fullest extent, was conducted by Thomas and Chess (Thomas, Chess, & Birch, 1968; Thomas & Chess, 1977). Their New York Longitudinal Study (NYLS) showed that certain configurations of temperamental attributes in children are conducive to well-adapted behavior, whereas other clusters of temperament characteristics, known under the label "difficult child" (Thomas et al., 1968; Thomas & Chess, 1977), result often in behavior disorders

*The part of this chapter written by Jan Strelau was prepared during his 1-year tenure (1991–1992) as a Humboldt Research Award Winner at the University of Bielefeld.

in children. The concept of the difficult child has been the subject of empirical studies and theoretical considerations by many authors. It has to be stated, however, that in spite of Thomas and Chess's intention, the name difficult child, which refers to the child himself or herself, emphasize the significance of temperamental traits (the personological context) in determining difficulties (in behavior, education, etc.). Thomas and Chess (1977; Chess & Thomas, 1986) have shown many times that the patterns of temperament traits labeled difficult child result in behavior disorders *only* when in interaction with inappropriate caretaking or educational treatment or other inadequate social environments.

To clarify the role of reciprocal interaction between temperamental characteristics and the environment in determining a well-adapted or poorly-adapted individual, Thomas and Chess (1977; Chess & Thomas, 1986, 1991) have made use of the biological concept of "goodness of fit." Goodness of fit occurs when the person's temperament and other personological characteristics "are adequate to master the successive demands, expectations, and opportunities of the environment. If on the other hand, the individual cannot cope successfully with the environmental demands, then there is poorness of fit" (Chess & Thomas, 1991, p. 16).

Another concept, also developed in the context of studies on the functional significance of temperament, is that of the so-called temperament risk factors (TRF) introduced by Carey (1986, 1989).

> Temperament risk factors have been defined as any temperament characteristics predisposing a child to a poor fit (incompatible relationship) with his or her environment, to excessive interactional stress and conflict with the caretakers, and to secondary clinical problems in the child's physical health, development or behavior. (Carey, 1989, p. 16)

The concepts of difficult child and temperament risk factors are rooted in the interactional approach to the study of development of individuals. The first concept, however, suggests by the name itself that difficulties (in upbringing and education) result from the individual's temperamental traits. The notion of difficult child understood in this way suggests also evaluation of temperament characteristics (Strelau, 1989). The danger of such misunderstanding speaks in favor of the concept of temperament risk factors.

The thought behind the concepts of goodness or poorness of fit and TRF, especially the interactional approach represented by both concepts, is close to our understanding of the functional significance of temperament. To exemplify this importance by means of empirical data, a short presentation of selected theoretical issues is needed.

DEFINING TERMS

In spite of there being some differences between the authors of this article in their understanding and theories of temperament, we agree that the most crucial temperamental traits in human functioning are reactivity and activity. *Reactivity* refers to individual differences in intensity of responsive behavior and is determined by physiological mechanisms responsible for regulating the level of arousal. Reactivity, which resembles to some extent the Pavlovian concept of strength of excitation, codetermines the individual's sensitivity and endurance, the latter being expressed in the ability to react adequately to strong and/or long-lasting stimulation. This means, among other things, that high-reactive (HR) individuals, when confronted with situations of high stimulating value, behave in such a way as to reduce the level of stimulation. Under strong (extreme) stimulation, either the level of performance decreases in HR individuals or high psychophysiological costs (e.g., increased level of arousal, high level of anxiety) have to be paid by them in order to react adequately to the situation. Low-reactive (LR) individuals behave and react in a similar way to HR persons but in opposite situations, characterized by very low stimulative value (e.g., deprivation).

Activity refers mainly to operant (goal-directed) behavior and is defined by the range and amount of actions undertaken of a given stimulative value. Activity understood in this way is aimed at achieving and maintaining the stimulation need by a given individual. Thus the essence of activity consists in regulating the stimulative value of situations and behaviors in such a way as to satisfy the individual's need for optimal stimulation. The latter is assumed to be the standard for stimulation control (Eliasz, 1981.). There exists a relationship between reactivity and activity. High-reactivity individuals—characterized by low need for stimulation (because of their high sensitivity and low endurance)—in order to attain or maintain optimal level of arousal prefer activity of low stimulative value. Low-reactive individuals, who are known as having high need for stimulation (low sensitivity and high endurance), prefer activity of high stimulative value.

Since the temperament trait called activity develops in ontogenesis under the influence of social environment and educational treatment, it may happen that the stimulative value of the individual's activity does not correspond with his or her biologically determined level of reactivity. As has been shown in our studies (Eliasz, 1981; Strelau, 1983), a long-lasting discrepancy between level of reactivity and level of activity may cause disturbances in behavior. That brings us directly to the concept of *temperament risk factors*, slightly modified from Carey's (1986, 1989) definition. Since studies on temperament conducted in our laboratories refer mainly to adults and adolescents, the concept of TRF has been given a more universal meaning. Temperament risk factors are considered to be any temperamental trait or configuration of traits that in interaction with other factors acting persistently or recurrently (social environment, educational treatment, situations, the individual's characteristics, etc.) increases the probability of developing disorders or anomalies in behavior, or that favors the molding of a maladjusted personality. The development of disorders in behavior or maladjusted personality might have very broad negative consequences for both mental and physical health.

HIGH REACTIVITY AS TRF FOR CHILDREN UNDER SOCIAL PRESSURE: EMPIRICAL EVIDENCE

In two studies (Strelau, 1989) conducted on second-grade pupils, it has been shown that a highly demanding educational system when persistently acting in interaction with high level of reactivity leads in HR pupils to symptoms of hyperexcitation, which is not the case in LR individuals. Thus, high reactivity in interaction with an educational treatment of high stimulative value should be regarded in this very situation as a TRF.

Eliasz (1981) has shown that HR 14- to 15-year-old boys living in various urban areas adapt their life-style to social expectations with no differences between HR boys from the downtown and those from the outskirts of the city. In turn, LR boys from various areas differ significantly in how they spend their leisure time and do homework. High-reactive boys manifest submission to social influences as well as lack of adaptation to the physical environment. Low-reactive boys display relative independence from social stimuli and ability to adapt to ecological variables. Thus high reactivity can be a TRF if adolescents live in highly stimulative areas.

In this chapter we would like to present some data that illustrate the significance of the interaction between reactivity and upbringing methods in the shaping of Type A behavior pattern (TABP) and its psychological consequences in adolescents in terms of the TRF. The TABP is defined as "an action-emotion complex involving behavioral dispositions such as ambitiousness, aggressiveness, competitiveness, and impatience . . . and emotional responses such as irritation, hostility, and increased potential for anger" (Rosenman, 1990, p. 2). It is assumed that TABP is a risk factor for coronary heart disease (CHD) in adults, also called coronary artery disease (Friedman & Rosenman, 1974).

Studies reported in the literature indicate that TABP may be found also in children and adolescents and that parental and environmental influences are the main antecedents of TABP (see, for example, Matthews & Woodall, 1988). Steinberg (1985) has shown that to some extent early temperamental characteristics allow the prediction of TABP in young adulthood. High adaptability and negative mood are associated with achievement-striving, one of the crucial components of TABP.

A large-scale study conducted by Eliasz and Wrzesniewski (1986, 1988) on 1,040 trade- and high-school students of both sexes aged from 17 to 18 gives evidence that the shaping of TABP in adolescents is a complex process involving several variables. TABP results from, among other things, the interaction between social pressure on an adolescent to maximize achievement (at home and at school) and the individual's temperament. The results of this study show that TABP develops in both HR and LR individuals; thus there is no direct relation between temperamental characteristics, that is, level of reactivity, and TABP.

It came out, however, that there is an indirect relationship between both variables under discussion. The moulding of TABP develops in HR and LR adolescents under different psychophysiological costs. This finding is exemplified by data from 76 adolescent males representing extreme scores on TABP and trait anxiety. As may be seen in Table 5-1, more HR adolescents diagnosed as having high scores on TABP are characterized by high level of anxiety than are HR individuals with low scores of TABP. This finding does not take place when LR individuals are taken into account (see Table 5-2). In this study, which goes far beyond the problem raised in our chapter, reactivity was measured by means of the Strelau Temperament Inventory (STI, Strelau, 1983); trait anxiety, with the Three-Factor State and Trait Personality Inventory developed by Spielberger and adapted to the Polish population by Plonska (1983). The inventory for measuring the TABP in adolescents has been constructed by Wrzesniewski (Eliasz & Wrzesniewski, 1988).

On the basis of collected data, it might be concluded that in HR adolescents the development of TABP is mostly accompanied with high level of trait anxiety, whereas this is not the case in LR subjects. How can this finding be explained?

One of the constituents of TABP is high need for achievement (n-achievement). It motivates the individual toward highly stimulating forms of activity. It follows from the concepts of reactivity and activity that this need develops mainly in LR individuals, with a high need for stimulation. Activity typical for high

TABLE 5-1

Distributions for HR Adolescent Males with Low and
High Anxiety in Groups with Low and High TABP

	Anxiety		Total Number of Subjects
TABP	Low	High	
Low	23	19	42
High	9	25	34
Total Number of Subjects	32	44	76

Abbreviations: HR = high reactive; TABP = Type A behavior pattern.
$\chi^2 = 6.133$, $df = 1$, $p < .02$, $C = .273$, Ccor = .387.

TABLE 5-2
Distribution for LR Adolescent Males with Low and
High Anxiety in Groups with Low and High TABP

TABP	Anxiety		Total Number of Subjects
	Low	High	
Low	32	24	56
High	26	36	62
Total Number of Subjects	58	60	118

Abbreviations: LR = low reactive; TABP = Type A behavior pattern.
$\chi^2 = 2.754$, NS.

n-achievement is in LR individuals internally reinforced from the start through the fact that its stimulative value is consistent with the need for high stimulation. Thus the TABP present in LR individuals is consistent with their high level of need for stimulation. This is probably the case where TABP is not accompanied by a high risk of CHD.

In HR individuals the n-achievement is a result of external pressure—upbringing at home and education at school. Since the high stimulative value of n-achievement is in dissonance with the low need for stimulation typical of high reactives, submission to the social pressure that leads to the development of a TABP takes place at the cost of anxiety. Anxiety in HR adolescents with high scores of TABP should be regarded as the psychophysiological cost these individuals pay for performing activity whose stimulating value is beyond their temperamental capacity (level of reactivity). It was hypothesized that long-lasting dissonance between the TABP and high level of reactivity leads to the risk of CHD (Eliasz & Wrzesniewski, 1986). The hypothesis has been confirmed in two studies (Cofta, 1992; Eliasz & Cofta, 1992). It turned out that the discrepancy between low need for stimulation and highly stimulative TABP is associated with the risk of CHD and indexes of ill being. Thus, high level of reactivity when in interaction with social pressure that creates circumstances for the development of TABP should be regarded here as a TRF.

PREVENTION AND INTERVENTION

If we consider the dissonance between high reactivity and TABP as a precursor to risk of CHD, then both prevention and intervention programs should be undertaken. The prevention programs can be undertaken in order to reduce in HR adolescents the probability of development of TABP. These programs should be directed mainly at parents and teachers. They should be aware of the limited endurance of HR adolescents to long-lasting activity, participation in highly competitive groups, and so on. Parents and teachers should be instructed that an individual style of action can reduce emotional tension and the likelihood of overloading in children and adolescents (Strelau, 1983). The individual style of action can be acquired by children and adolescents when they have freedom in developing individual manners of achieving goals.

The intervention programs should be directed to HR adolescents with the first symptoms of TABP. These programs consist for example, in training adolescents in acquiring skills to organize work and to relax. This can reduce time pressure and attenuate the inability to relax typical of individuals with high TABP. The intervention programs might comprise some kind of therapy that can weaken hostility and limit competition to task situations at least.

SUMMARY

Incompatibility between temperament characteristics and environmental demands can result in some symptoms of disorders delineated here within the concept of temperament risk factors. Data have been presented that show that Type A behavior pattern, a predisposing factor in coronary heart disease, can be acquired by individuals quite different as to their temperament, that is, by high-reactive as well as by low-reactive adolescents. It turned out, however, that only in HR adolescents is TABP accompanied with high level of trait anxiety. In LR subjects TABP, which results from internal reinforcements, is adequate to their temperamentally determined endurance. In HR individuals TABP results from external reinforcements, that is, from strong social pressure to maximize educational goals, the latter being beyond their temperamentally determined capacity. It was hypothesized that a long-lasting incongruence between the TABP and high level of reactivity leads to the risk of CHD in HR adolescents as they move into adulthood. High levels of reactivity, when in interaction with social pressure that creates circumstances for the development of TABP, should be regarded here as a TRF. Prevention and early intervention programs are recommended in the case of HR adolescents living in highly demanding social surroundings.

REFERENCES

Carey, W. B. (1986). The difficult child. *Pediatrics in Review, 8*, 39–45.
Carey, W. B. (1989). Introduction—Basic issues. In W. B. Carey & S. C. McDevitt (Eds.), *Clinical and educational applications of temperament research* (pp. 11–20).

Amsterdam/Lisse, The Netherlands: Swets & Zeitlinger.

Chess, S., & Thomas, A. (1986). *Temperament in clinical practice*. New York: Guilford Press.

Chess, S., & Thomas, A. (1991). Temperament and the concept of goodness of fit. In J. Strelau & A. Angleitner (Eds.), *Explorations in temperament: International perspectives on theory and measurement* (pp. 15–28). New York: Plenum Press.

Cofta, L. (1992). *Zapotrzebowanie na stymulacje jako czynnik modyfikujacy wplyw wzoru zachowania A na zdrowie i jakosc zycia* [Need for stimulation as a modifier of the effect of the Type A behavior pattern on health and quality of life]. Unpublished doctoral dissertation, Institute of Psychology, Polish Academy of Sciences, Warsaw.

Eliasz, A. (1981). *Temperament a system regulacji stymulacji* [Temperament and the system of stimulation control.] Warszawa: Panstwowe Wydawnictwo Naukowe.

Eliasz, A., & Cofta, L. (1992). Temperament a sklonnosc do chorob [Temperament and proneness to illness]. In J. Strelau, W. Ciarkowska, & E. Necka (Eds.), *Roznice indywidualne: Mozliwosci i preference* [Individual differences: Capacities and preferences.] Warszawa-Wroclaw: Ossolineum.

Eliasz, A., & Wrzesniewski, K. (1986). Type A behavior resulting from internal or external reinforcements and temperament. *Polish Psychological Bulletin, 17*, 39–53.

Eliasz, A., & Wrzesniewski, K. (1988). *Ryzyko chorob psychosomatycznych: Srodowisko i temperament a Wzor zachowania A* [Psychosomatic disease risk: Environment, temperament and Type A behavior pattern]. Wroclaw: Ossolineum.

Friedman, M., & Rosenman, H. (1974). *Type A behavior pattern, stress, and coronary disease*. Hillsdale, NJ: Lawrence Erlbaum.

Matthews, K. A., & Woodall, K. L. (1988). Childhood origins of overt Type A behaviors and cardiovascular reactivity to behavioral stressors. *Annals of Behavioral Medicine, 10*, 71–77.

Plonska, Z. (1983). *Polska adaptacja Trojczynnikowego Inwentarza Stanow i Cech Osobowosci* [Polish adaptation of the Three-Factor State and Trait Personality Inventory]. Unpublished M.A. Thesis, University of Warsaw, Poland.

Rosenman, R. H. (1990). Type A behavior pattern: A personal overview. *Journal of Social Behavior and Personality, 5*, 1–24.

Steinberg, L. (1985). Early temperamental antecedents of adult Type A behaviors. *Developmental Psychology, 21*, 1171–1180.

Strelau, J. (1983). *Temperament, personality, activity*. London: Academic Press.

Strelau, J. (1989). Temperament risk factors in children and adolescents as studied in Eastern Europe. In W. B. Carey & S. C. McDevitt (Eds.), *Clinical and educational applications of temperament research* (pp. 65–77). Amsterdam/Lisse, The Netherlands: Swets & Zeitlinger.

Thomas, A., & Chess, S. (1977). *Temperament and development*. New York: Brunner/Mazel.

Thomas, A., Chess, S., & Birch, H. G. (1968). *Temperament and behavior disorders in children*. New York: New York University Press.

6

Temperament, Siblings, and the Development of Relationships

Judith Dunn

The publication of Alexander Thomas and Stella Chess's work on temperament played a key role in changing the way in which clinicians and developmental researchers viewed parent-child relationships—their development and their nature. The work on temperament has been of central importance in the shift toward a real recognition of the contribution of individual differences in children to the quality of their relationships with their parents. And the lessons to be learned from the work on temperament are relevant to *all* the relationships children form, including those with siblings, close friends, teachers, peers— relationships that are increasingly recognized as having potential influence on children's development (e.g., Berndt & Ladd, 1989; Boer & Dunn, 1992; Hartup, 1983). In this chapter some of these implications concerning broad developmental principles are discussed in the context of research on children's relationships with their siblings.

The relationship between siblings is distinctive in its emotional qualities, its competitiveness, ambivalence, and potential for support, provocation, rivalry, or aggression. It is also notable for the marked individual differences between sibling pairs in friendliness, hostility, dominance, and rivalry; this wide range of differences is found in siblings from infancy through middle childhood to adolescence (Abramovitch, Pepler, & Corter, 1982; Boer & Dunn, 1992; Furman & Buhrmester, 1985). The individual differences in conflict and aggression are of particular concern to clinicians and to parents, and the question of what factors contribute to such differences has become one of special significance. Why do some siblings quarrel unendingly and resort to violence, while others enjoy harmonious friendly relations?

This question gains in significance when the potential influence on young children's development of this intimate, powerful, and emotionally uninhibited relationship is recognized. Common sense suggests that the familiarity, intimacy, and frequency of interaction between siblings, and the emotional nature of the relationship, may be of developmental significance. And from a range of different theoretical backgrounds, the potential importance of this relationship has been emphasized: by those who argue, following Piaget (1965) and Sullivan (1953), that interaction between children has special developmental importance, by clinicians who see rivalry between siblings as long lasting in importance (Adler, 1959; Levy, 1937; Winnicott, 1977), by family systems theorists (Minuchin, 1985), and most recently by developmental behavior geneticists who focus on the within-family experiences that must explain the development of individual differences more generally (reviewed in Dunn & Plomin, 1990).

These arguments for links between sibling relationships and children's outcome are now supported by a considerable body of empirical evidence. There is now evidence that for siblings from toddlerhood to middle childhood, aggression shown by one sibling is correlated with aggression shown by the other (e.g., Beardsall, 1987; Brody, Stoneman, & Burke, 1987; Dunn & Munn, 1987), and that siblings play a shaping role in the development of aggressive behavior in both normal and clinic populations (Patterson, 1984, 1986). Furthermore, siblings who are very aggressive to their siblings are likely to have problems with peers outside the family (Dishion, 1986), and to develop other problems later (Richman, Stevenson, & Graham, 1982). It is not clear that poor sibling relationships play a *causal* role in the development of disturbance or are an index of more general disturbance—however, such findings alert us to the importance of understanding what factors contribute to poor sibling relationships.

There is also correlational evidence for associations between siblings' cooperative and empathetic behavior (Dunn & Munn, 1986) and for links between differences in sibling interaction and later sociocognitive abilities (Dunn, Brown, Slomkowski, Tesla, & Youngblade, 1991; Dunn & Munn, 1986; Light, 1979; Slomkowski & Dunn, 1992), and evidence that young children benefit cognitively from observing and imitating their older siblings (Hesser & Azmitia, 1989; Wishart, 1986). Again, this evidence heightens our interest in understanding the influences on the individual differences in sibling interaction that are associated with such outcome differences. Moreover, a novel set of findings links the development of children's adjustment problems in middle childhood to their responsiveness to the interaction between their siblings and parents and their sensitivity to relative differences in parental affection and interest in them and their siblings (Dunn, Stocker, & Plomin, 1990).

TEMPERAMENT AND INDIVIDUAL DIFFERENCES IN
SIBLING RELATIONSHIPS

What, then, accounts for the striking differences in types of interaction between siblings? A range of different possible contributing factors has been studied—parent-child relationships, differential treatment by parents, gender, age differences, life events, and so on (for review, see Dunn, 1992). Among these variables, the temperamental characteristics of the children stand out as important— and this is documented in a range of studies of siblings of different ages and varying backgrounds (Boer, 1990; Brody & Stoneman, 1987; Brody et al., 1987; Stocker, Dunn, & Plomin, 1989). The level of conflict between young siblings, for example, is higher in families with children who are active, intense in emotional response, negative in mood, or unadaptable in temperament. The developmental principle highlighted by Thomas and Chess—that individual differences in children's temperament contribute importantly to the quality of their close relationships—is strongly confirmed by the research on siblings. Two further issues of general significance in the study of relationships that studies of siblings and their temperamental characteristics have illuminated concern developmental change in relationships and changes in the relative contribution of the different partners in a dyadic relationship to the quality of that relationship.

TEMPERAMENT AND DEVELOPMENT CHANGE
IN RELATIONSHIPS

As children grow through infancy, toddlerhood, and the preschool period, their understanding of other people and their ability to communicate with those others are transformed (e.g., Astington, Harris, & Olson, 1988). It appears likely that such developments will affect importantly the nature of their relationships, yet although the contribution of developmental changes in early infancy to changes in the mother-child relationship has been discussed (Kaye, 1982; Trevarthen & Hubley, 1978), and attention drawn to these matters in theoretical discussions of relationships (Hinde, 1979, 1987), there is still little systematic empirical research that examines such developmental change in children's relationships as they grow up beyond infancy.

Studies of temperament and sibling interaction have, however, extended our understanding here: They have demonstrated the changing roles of older and younger siblings in their relationship through early childhood (Munn & Dunn, 1989). In a sample of siblings followed from the second year of the younger sibling, we found that at the early stage of the relationship (when the younger one was 24 months old) the older sibling was chiefly responsible for the frequency and duration of joint play, and shared fantasy play in the relationship, and that differences in the temperament of the older sibling were chiefly responsible for differences in these dyadic relationship measures. In families in which the older sibling was negative in mood, nonadaptable, and nondistractible, the sibling pairs engaged in less joint play. By the time that the younger sibling was 36 months, however, the temperamental characteristics of the younger sibling were also important in influencing the dyadic relationship. At this stage, the quality of the relationship was influenced by the temperament of *both* individuals—highlighting a notable change in the balance of the relationship.

Other findings of this study highlighted a further general principle concerning the significance of the *relative* contribution of the individual characteristics of two participants in a dyadic relationship: that the fit or "match" between two individuals in personality contributes to the quality of their relationship. The sibling pairs in the study differed notably in the duration and frequency of conflict between them. The nature of this conflict changed as the children grew up, and the significance of the individual differences in the temperament of the two children as contributors to the conflict in their relationship also changed. At the observations made when the younger siblings were 24 months, the extent of conflict in the relationship (which included considerable physical aggression) was related to the temperament of both older and younger sibling. A year later—when the nature of sibling conflict had changed from physical aggression to chiefly verbal hostility—differences in conflict between dyads were related not to the individual temperaments of older or younger sibling but to *the differences between the siblings in their temperamental characteristics.* That is, the conflict between the siblings was of greater duration in those families in which there was a "mismatch" between the two children in their temperamental characteristics than in families in which the children were similar in their temperament.

TEMPERAMENT AND CHILDREN'S ADJUSTMENT TO CHANGES IN FAMILY RELATIONSHIPS

Research on young children and their siblings has established a further point with far-reaching implications for our understanding of children's adjustment to stress and change—in which temperament again emerges as important. Thomas and Chess (1977) themselves documented the links between children's temperamental characteristics and their response to the arrival of a new sibling. Those children who readily adapted to new situations, and whose responses were typically positive, mild, and regular before the birth of a sibling, showed this same pattern of responses when their sibling was born. In a subsequent study, we found that the marked differences in how children reacted to this change in their family were related to their temperamental characteristics before the birth (Dunn & Kendrick, 1982). Thus children who were extremely negative in mood were especially likely to increase in withdrawal and in sleeping problems following the sibling birth, while those who were both negative in mood and extreme in their emotional reactions were likely to respond with increased clinging. The children who reacted with marked withdrawal were particularly unlikely to show positive interest in the baby. The significance of these findings, and the attention drawn to temperament by Thomas and Chess's original work, lies not only in what they tell us about young siblings and the alleviation of parental guilt about siblings' dislike for one another that they offer. The results have more general importance in what they suggest concerning the individual differences in children's responses to other potentially stressful changes, such as separation of parents and starting or changing school, all of which can involve for some children disturbance that is not trivial (Dunn, 1988).

Furthermore, children's temperamental makeup was also related to how these firstborns reacted to the interaction between their mothers and baby siblings as the months went by. Children who were relatively extreme on the traits of unmalleability and intensity of emotional response were especially likely to *protest* when their mothers engaged in interaction with the baby sibling, and they were less likely than other children to ignore such exchanges. Those who were extreme in emotional intensity more often watched the interaction between their mother and sibling, sucking their thumb or holding their comfort object, than did those who were average or below average in emotional intensity. These differences in responsiveness to other family members' interaction take on special importance in light of the new evidence for the salience of such within-family processes, and the comparisons that children make between self and sibling (Dunn & Plomin, 1990).

TEMPERAMENT AND SIBLINGS WITH HANDICAPPING CONDITIONS

As another illustration of the significance of temperament in understanding the development of children's problems, consider the question of whether growing up with a handicapped sibling has deleterious effects on children—affecting their adjustment and well-being—a question that is often raised by clinicians caring for families with sick or disabled children. Here, too, the work on temperament has proved illuminating. It should be noted that the research literature on the sibling relationships of children with disabilities or illness is very heterogeneous with respect to the severity and types of disability, and much of the research suffers from methodological limitations (for reviews, see Crnic & Leconte, 1986; Ogle & Powell, 1985; Schachter & Stone, 1987). When these caveats are borne in mind, two general points concerning the consequences of growing up with a handicapped sibling seem reasonably clear. The first is that most studies report that children with handicapped siblings suffer from more emotional and behavioral problems than do children with nonhandicapped siblings, but that there are considerable individual differences among children in the extent of these problems. The second point is that the nature and extent of the problems are related to characteristics of the handicapped child, such as the severity of the handicap or illness and the child's temperament, and to characteristics of the nonhandicapped sibling including temperament, as well as to characteristics of the parents, their marriage, and other aspects of family circumstances.

CONCLUSION

In 1986 Thomas and Chess commented that studies of temperament "may help to illuminate a number of basic issues in developmental psychology and psychiatry—genetic-environment interaction, developmental transitions and transformations, dynamics of family relationships, and the origins and evolution of behavior disorders" (Thomas & Chess, 1986, pp. 39–52). The one strand of research on children's relationships that we have discussed here—the work on early sibling relationships—has shown how a focus on individual differences in children's temperamental characteristics has indeed helped to clarify some fundamental topics in developmental psychology and psychiatry: the principles underlying the nature of relationships and developmental changes in relationships, and the varying significance of transitions in family structure for different children and their links with behavioral problems. We are a long way from understanding the processes that underlie the various patterns that have been described, but the importance of temperamental characteristics in contributing to children's relationships and adjustment and the fruitfulness of further work exploring continuities and changes in individual differences cannot now be questioned. And the implications for parents of this documentation of the significance of temperamental differences for children's relationships with siblings, parents, and peers must not be forgotten. The finger of blame for sibling conflict and disturbance cannot with justification now be pointed at parents as the sole source of influence. We should all—as parents, researchers, or clinicians—be grateful to Thomas and Chess for their pioneering work.

REFERENCES

Abramovitch, R., Pepler, D., & Corter, C. (1982). Patterns of sibling interaction among preschool-age children. In M. E. Lamb & B. Sutton-Smith (Eds.), *Sibling relationships across the lifespan* (pp. 61–86). Hillsdale, NJ: Lawrence Erlbaum.

Adler, A. (1959). *Understanding human nature.* New York: Premier.

Astington, J. W., Harris, P. L., & Olson, D. R. (1988). *Developing theories of mind.* Cambridge: Cambridge University Press.

Beardsall, L. (1987). *Sibling conflict in middle childhood.* Unpublished doctoral dissertation, University of Cambridge, England

Berndt, T. J., & Ladd, G. W. (1989). *Peer relationships in child development.* New York: John Wiley.

Boer, F. (1990). *Sibling relationships in middle childhood.* Leiden, The Netherlands: DSWO University of Leiden Press.

Boer, F., & Dunn, J. (1992). *Children's sibling relationships: Developmental and clinical implications.* Hillsdale, NJ: Lawrence Erlbaum.

Brody, G. H., & Stoneman, Z. (1987). Sibling conflict: Contributions of the siblings themselves, the parent-sibling relationship, and the broader family system. *Journal of Children in Contemporary Society, 19*, 39–53.

Brody, G. H., Stoneman, Z., & Burke, M. (1987). Child temperaments, maternal differential behavior, and sibling relationships. *Developmental Psychology, 23*, 354–362.

Crnic, K. A., & Leconte, J. M. (1986). Understanding sibling needs and influences. In R. R. Fewell & P. F. Vandasy (Eds.), *Families of handicapped children: Needs and supports across the life-span* (pp. 75–98). Austin, TX: PRO-ED, Inc.

Dishion, T. J. (1986, November). *Peer rejection.* Seminar at Oregon Learning Centre, Eugene, OR.

Dunn, J. (1988). Normative life events as risk factors in childhood. In M. Rutter (Ed.), *Risk and protective factors in psychosocial development.* Cambridge: Cambridge University Press.

Dunn, J. (1992). Sisters and brothers: Current issues in developmental research. In F. Boer & J. Dunn (Eds.), *Children's sibling relationships: Developmental and clinical implications.* Hillsdale, NJ: Lawrence Erlbaum.

Dunn, J., Brown, J. R., Slomkowski, C., Tesla, C., & Youngblade, L. (1991). Young children's understanding of other people's feelings and beliefs: Individual differences and their antecedents. *Child Development, 62*, 1352–1366.

Dunn, J., & Kendrick, C. (1982). *Siblings: Love, envy, and understanding.* Cambridge, MA: Harvard University Press.

Dunn, J., & Munn, P. (1986). Sibling quarrels and maternal intervention: Individual differences in understanding and aggression. *Journal of Child Psychology and Psychiatry, 27*, 583–595.

Dunn, J., & Munn, P. (1987). The development of justification in disputes with mother and sibling. *Developmental Psychology, 23*, 791–798.

Dunn, J., & Plomin, R. (1990). *Separate lives: Why siblings are so different.* New York: Basic Books.

Dunn, J., Stocker, C., & Plomin, R. (1990). Nonshared experiences within the family:

Correlates of behavioral problems in middle childhood. *Development and Psychopathology, 2,* 113–126.

Furman, W., & Buhrmester, D. (1985). Children's perceptions of the personal relationships in their social networks. *Developmental Psychology, 21,* 1016–1024.

Hartup, W. W. (1983). Peer relations. In P. H. Mussen (Ed.), *Handbook of child psychology, Vol. IV: Socialization, personality, and social development* (pp. 103–196). New York: John Wiley.

Hesser, J., & Azmitia, M. (1989, April). *The influence of siblings and non-siblings on children's observation and imitation.* Paper presented at the biennial meetings of the Society for Research in Child Development, Kansas, City, MO.

Hinde, R. A. (1979). *Towards understanding relationships.* New York: Academic Press.

Hinde, R. A. (1987). *Individuals, relationships, and culture.* Cambridge: Cambridge University Press.

Kaye, K. (1982). *The mental and social life of babies.* London: Methuen.

Levy, D. M. (1937). Studies in sibling rivalry. *American Orthopsychiatry Research Monograph,* No. 2.

Light, P. (1979). *The development of social sensitivity.* Cambridge: Cambridge University Press.

Minuchin, P. (1985). Families and individual development: Provocations from the field of family therapy. *Child Development, 56,* 289–302.

Munn, P., & Dunn, J. (1989). Temperament and the developing relationship between siblings. *International Journal of Behavioral Development, 12,* 433–451.

Ogle, P. A., & Powell, T. P. (1985). *Brothers and sisters: A special part of exceptional families.* Baltimore, MD: Paul H. Brooks.

Patterson, G. R. (1984). Siblings: Fellow travellers in coercive family processes. *Advances in the Study of Aggression, 1,* 173–214.

Patterson, G. R. (1986). The contribution of siblings to training for fighting: A microsocial analysis. In D. Olweus, J. Block, & M. Radke-Yarrow (Eds.), *Development of antisocial and prosocial behavior: Research, theories, and issues* (pp. 235–261). New York: Academic Press.

Piaget, J. (1965). *The moral judgement of the child.* New York: Free Press.

Richman, N., Stevenson, J. E., & Graham, P. (1982). *Preschool to school: A behavioral study.* London: Academic Press.

Schachter, F. F., & Stone, R. K. (1987). *Practical concerns about siblings: Bridging the research-practice gap.* New York: Haworth Press.

Slomkowski, C., & Dunn, J. (1992). Arguments and relationships within the family: Young children's disputes with mother and sibling. *Developmental Psychology, 28,* 919–924.

Stocker, C., Dunn, J., & Plomin, R. (1989). Sibling relationships: Links with child temperament, maternal behavior, and family structure. *Child Development, 60,* 715–727.

Sullivan, H. S. (1953). *The interpersonal theory of psychiatry.* New York: W.W. Norton.

Thomas, A., & Chess, S. (1977). *Temperament and development.* New York: Brunner/Mazel.

Thomas, A., & Chess, S. (1986). The New York Longitudinal Study: From infancy to early adult life. In R. Plomin & J. Dunn (Eds.), *The study of temperament: Changes, continuities and challenges* (pp. 39–52). Hillsdale, NJ: Lawrence Erlbaum.

Trevarthen, C., & Hubley, P. (1978). Secondary intersubjectivity: Confidence, confiding, and acts of meaning in the first year. In A. Lock (Ed.), *Action, gesture, and symbol: The emergence of language* (pp. 183–229). London: Academic Press.

Winnicott, D. W. (1977). *The Piggle.* London: Hogarth Press.

Wishart, J. G. (1986). Siblings as models in early infant learning. *Child Development, 57,* 1232–1240.

7

Is Temperament an Important Contributor to Schooling Outcomes in Elementary School? Modeling Effects of Temperament and Scholastic Ability on Academic Achievement

Roy P. Martin, Stephen Olejnik, and Lena Gaddis

The concept of temperament is an ancient one (Kohnstamm, 1989; Rutter, 1989). The concept has gone through cycles of prominence and neglect as a factor to be considered in explaining human behavior. Under the influence of the work of Alexander Thomas, Stella Chess, and colleagues (Thomas & Chess, 1977; Thomas, Chess, & Birch, 1968), the concept has again captured the imagination of educators, psychologists, physicians, and others interested in the development of children.

The senior author first came into contact with this concept through reading *Temperament and Development* (Thomas & Chess, 1977) during the late 1970s. He began to collect data using the Parent and Teacher Temperament

Questionnaires presented in that book, and by the early 1980s had begun work on the development of a measure of temperament that was directly based on the Thomas and Chess conception of temperament. With substantial professional support from Alex and Stella, we began a series of studies designed to predict educational processes and products from teacher ratings of temperament. One of these studies, a longitudinal study in which teacher ratings of temperament in first grade were used to predict achievement in both first and fifth grades, has only recently been thoroughly analyzed. It is with pleasure and humility that we dedicate this research to Alex and Stella, for without their research, mentoring, and friendship, it would certainly not have been possible.

Previous research on the relationship between teacher-rated temperament and educational achievement (see Martin, 1988b, 1989a, b, for reviews) has shown that the characteristics of activity level, distractibility, and task persistence (often referred to as the task orientation cluster of characteristics in classroom research) are typically the most strongly related to achievement of the temperament constructs (Martin, 1989a; Martin, Gaddis, Drew, & Moseley, 1988). Correlations with teacher-assigned grades and standardized achievement are typically in the .30 to .60 range, even when achievement is assessed up to 4 years later (Martin, 1989a).

This type of research also has revealed that the social adaptability cluster of characteristics (including the adaptability and approach/withdrawal characteristics) is related to reading and math achievement as assessed through teacher-assigned grades and standardized test scores, but these correlations are less consistent across studies, and are typically somewhat lower than those for the attentional cluster of variables (Martin & Holbrook, 1985; Pullis & Cadwell, 1982).

Finally, four other temperament characteristics assessed by researchers working in the Thomas and Chess tradition have not been found to be related in important or consistent ways to academic achievement. These include the intensity of expression of emotion, particularly negative emotion; the tendency to be in a negative or dark mood versus a happy, sunny mood over relatively lengthy periods of time; sensitivity to environmental stimulation such as light, or noise; and the tendency to be biologically rhythmic (to eat, sleep, eliminate, in a scheduled vs. unscheduled manner).

While the other contributors to this volume have presented reviews of research, I have prevailed upon the editors to allow us to present a small piece of original research that I believe serves a similar function; that is, it allows us to present a snapshot of the main point of our research, which is that temperament is an important predictor of achievement in schools, and may be as important in some contexts as cognitive ability. The current study attempts to model the effects of temperament and scholastic aptitude as assessed in first grade on achievement in the first and fifth grades. Modeling these effects through Linear Structural Relations (LISREL) analyses allows us to determine the relative effects of cognitive ability and temperamental characteristics on achievement. Specifically, the research was designed to answer three questions. First, is the proposed model adequate as judged against three statistical criteria? Second, does the model predict a sizable (practically meaningful) amount of variance in achievement? Third, what is the relative efficacy of scholastic ability and three temperament characteristics related to task orientation in the classroom (Activity Level, Distractibility, and Persistence) in the prediction of academic achievement?

METHOD

Subjects

During the initial assessment period, 104 children (49 males and 55 females) enrolled in six first-grade classrooms in one elementary school in northern Georgia participated in the research. They ranged in age from 76 to 94 months (mean = 81.4, SD = 4.26). Ninety-eight were white, six were African-Americans. The mean IQ on the Otis-Lennon Mental Abilities Test was 103.79 (SD = 14.5). The school from which the participants were selected was the only elementary school in a sparsely populated county in the foothills of the Appalachian Mountains. It was designated by the federal government as a low-income area, and the school received Title I funds.

Four years later, 93 of the subjects were found to still be in this school system. Sixteen had been retained and were in the fourth grade, while the remaining 77 were in the fifth grade. Only data from these 77 students (35 males, 42 females; all white) were analyzed in the current study.

Procedure

In the initial wave of assessment, temperament ratings were obtained using the Temperament Assessment Battery for Children—Teacher Form (TABC; Martin, 1988a). Teachers completed this questionnaire in late October and early November of the first-grade year. This 48-item measure was designed to assess six characteristics of children, 3 through 7 years of age, including activity level (gross motor vigor); adaptability (the ease and speed of adjustment to changing social circumstances); approach/withdrawal (the tendency to approach or withdraw in the initial interaction in a novel social situation); emotional intensity (the tendency to express emotions, particularly negative emotions, with greater or lesser vigor); distractibility (the tendency to have attention diverted by ambient stimulation);

and task persistence (a measure of attention span and the ability to keep working on a difficult learning task). Internal consistency reliabilities in the form of alpha coefficients range from .73 to .87 for the six scales. The temporal stability of the six scales of the teacher form has been studied in several samples (Martin et al., 1986). Six-month stabilities ranged from .69 to .85 when the same teacher made both ratings; the 12-month stability with different teachers making the ratings ranged from .41 to .67 for all scales except adaptability, for which the coefficient was not significantly different from zero. Martin (1988a) reports extensive validity data for this form of the TABC.

Academic achievement during the first grade was assessed by the American School Achievement Test (ASAT), Revised Edition (Primary Battery I, Form X), in the spring of the year. The ASAT is a group-administered achievement test designed to measure reading and mathematical computation and problem-solving skill. This is a well-standardized group-administered achievement test with strong psychometric properties and a sound validation history.

Scholastic aptitude (IQ) was assessed by the Otis-Lennon Mental Abilities Test (Elementary I Level, Form J) during the spring of the first-grade year. This is a group-administered instrument designed to yield a measure of general "g," the general factor of intelligence.

During the fifth-grade assessment, achievement data in the form of teacher-assigned grades (final year grades: A = 4.0, F = 0.0) for reading and mathematics and standardized achievement scores on the Metropolitan Achievement Test (MAT) were obtained. The MAT is a carefully developed and standardized series that was introduced in 1937.

RESULTS

Table 7-1 presents the correlations among temperament measures, the ability measure, and achievement measures obtained during first and fifth grades (values along the diagonal represent scale variance). Table 7-1 reveals that substantial relationships were observed between temperament characteristics and both first- and fifth-grade achievement. For example, Activity Level as rated by the first-grade teacher correlated in a range from $-.24$ to $-.42$ with achievement in the first grade, and between $-.24$ and $-.38$ with achievement in the fifth grade. Correlations for Distractibility and Task Persistence were even higher, ranging from $-.41$ to $-.55$ (Distractibility) and from .48 to .65 (Persistence) for first-grade achievement, and from -.31 to -.48 (Distractibility) and from .24 to .44 (Persistence) for fifth-grade achievement.

These correlations are somewhat difficult to interpret since scholastic ability (IQ) was related to both first- and fifth-grade reading and mathematics achieve-

TABLE 7.1

Correlations among Achievement Scores and Tempermental Characteristics
Assessed at Grade 1, and Achievement Scores Assessed at Grade 5

		1	2	3	4	5	6	7	8	9	10	11	12
Grade 1													
Reading	(1)		.80	.66	.51	.51	−.36	−.55	.65	.29	.53	.41	.24
Math	(2)		1.00	.64	.51	.43	−.31	−.51	.56	.31	.49	.42	.28
Achieve. R.	(3)			1.00	.54	−.24	−.41	.48	.40	.42	.56	.56	.48
Achieve. M.	(4)				1.00	.54	−.24	−.41	.48	.40	.42	.56	.48
IQ	(5)					1.00	−.19	−.31	.43	.39	.50	.53	.42
Activity	(6)						1.00	.41	−.38	−.27	−.24	−.27	−.38
Distract.	(7)							1.00	−.69	−.42	−48	−.40	−.31
Persist.	(8)								1.00	.44	.44	.41	.24
Grade 5													
Reading	(9)									1.00	.59	.64	.64
Math	(10)										1.00	.58	.53
Achieve. R.	(11)											1.00	.69
Achieve. M.	(12)												1.00

1-Grade 1, teacher-assigned reading grade.
2-Grade 1, teacher-assigned mathematics grade.
3-Grade 1, standardized achievement test score (ASAT) in reading.
4-Grade 1, standardized achievement test score (ASAT) in mathematics.
5-Grade 1, intelligence quotient on Otis-Lennon Mental Abilities Test.
6-Grade 1, teacher ratings of activity level.
7-Grade 1, teacher ratings of distractibility.
8-Grade 1, teacher ratings of task persistence.
9-Grade 5, teacher-assigned reading grade.
10-Grade 5, teacher-assigned mathematics grade.
11-Grade 5, standardized achievement test score (MAT) in reading.
12-Grade 1, standardized achievement test score (MAT) in mathematics.

ment (correlations were between .43 and .54 for first-grade achievement, and between .40 and .56 for fifth-grade achievement) and teacher temperament ratings (-.19 to .43). Thus, to determine the independent effects of academic ability and temperament on first and fifth grade, a model was created for reading and mathematics achievement separately that conceptualized Task Orientation, Scholastic Ability, First-Grade Achievement, and Fifth-Grade Achievement as latent variables, each of which was imperfectly measured through the variables listed in Figure 7-1 (for mathematics) and Figure 7-2 (for reading). The models were submitted to a structural equations evaluation using LISREL VI (Joreskog & Sorbom, 1984).

The numbers above the lines on Figures 7-1 and 7-2 are maximum likelihood estimates of path coefficients, and the numbers below the lines are the standard errors of that estimate. The variance–covariance matrix summarizing the interrelationships among the indicator variables was analyzed. We chose arbitrarily

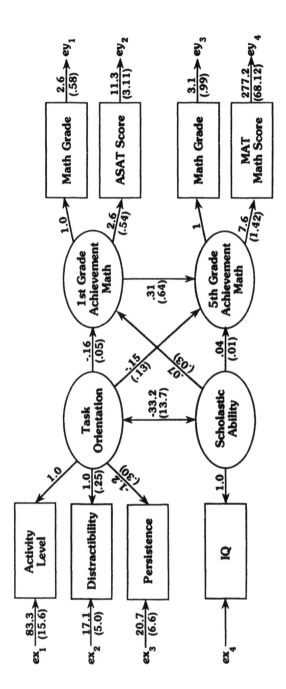

$\chi^2 = 9.74.$
$df = 13.$
$p = .715.$
Goodness-of-fit index = .946.
Note: Number above the line is the structural coefficient.
    Number below the line is the standard error of the structural coefficient.

Figure 7-1. Modeling Temperament and Scholastic Ability Effects on First- and Fifth-Grade Mathematics Achievement.

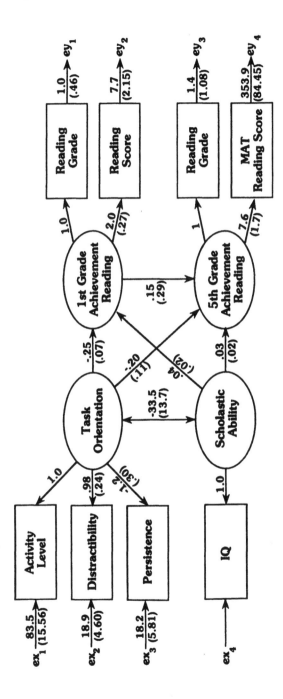

χ^2 = 20.96.
df = 13.
p = .074.
Goodness-of-fit index = .894.
Note: Number above the line is the structural coefficient.
Number below the line is the standard error of the structural coefficient.

Figure 7-2. Modeling Temperament and Scholastic Ability Effects on First- and Fifth-Grade Reading Achievement.

to set the scale for the Task Orientation indicators to be that of the Activity scale, and the first- and fifth-grade performance indicators were set to the scale of teacher grades.

The first issue addressed was, Is the model depicted adequate as judged by three criteria: (1) the chi-squared test, (2) the adjusted goodness-of-fit statistic, and (3) the standardized residuals? All three of the criteria used obtained supported the plausibility of the model. Chi-square and goodness-of-fit values are presented in Figures 7-1 and 7-2.

The second issue addressed was the proportion of variance explained by the model. For reading, over 89% of the observed variance and covariances could be explained by the proposed model; for mathematics, the percentage of variance explained was 94%. This was judged to be a very high level of prediction, and strongly supports the efficacy of the model.

The third question guiding this research was, Do teacher ratings of temperament (Activity Level, Distractibility, and Persistence) in first grade make a stronger unique contribution to the prediction of mathematics and reading grades than does cognitive ability? An examination of the total effects of Task Orientation and Ability on mathematics performance in first- and fifth-grade reading indicated that Task Orientation had over three times the impact of Ability at both grade levels. For reading, Task Orientation had over five times the impact of Ability for both first and fifth grades.

One of the most counterintuitive findings of this research is that there was a nonsignificant link between performance in first and fifth grades, using the *T*-value greater than 2.0 criteria suggested by Joreskog and Sorbom (1984). Thus, when IQ and temperament characteristics related to task orientation are controlled for, first-grade achievement did not significantly predict fifth-grade achievement.

DISCUSSION

This chapter has reported substantial correlations between one set of temperamental variables and academic achievement. These data support the findings of previous research (Martin 1988b, 1989a) that a moderate negative relationship exists between Activity Level and Distractibility (as assessed in early elementary school) and achievement in both reading and mathematics. A somewhat higher positive relationship exists between Task Persistence measured in first grade and academic achievement assessed in fifth grade.

The LISREL VI analyses indicated that when judged against three criteria, the model was a plausible model of the data. Further, the examination of total effects of Task Orientation and Ability on performance revealed that Task Orientation had a much stronger impact on mathematics and reading performance than did scholastic ability. This result is surprising; however, it seems likely that many factors contribute to the tendency to be active, distractible, and nonpersistent in the classroom, one of which is poor scholastic ability (Martin & Holbrook, 1985; Martin, 1988a). It may be that the temperament ratings of teachers inadvertently subsume some of the variance in cognitive ability scores that is predictive of achievement, thereby contributing more to the prediction of achievement than a simple IQ score. Another plausible explanation is that teachers ratings of temperament are contaminated by knowledge of achievement in the classroom. However, in this study temperamental characteristics were almost as predictive of fifth-grade achievement as first-grade achievement; thus, this explanation seems too simple to explain the obtained relationship.

A more complex interpretation of the data might utilize teacher expectations and behavior toward the child as a mediating variable. It is known that there is a relationship between teachers' estimates of academic ability and temperamental characteristics that is unexplained by measured academic ability (Martin & Holbrook, 1985). Thus, teachers have positive attitudes about children with characteristics that best fit the classroom environment (Keogh, 1982), and these positive attitudes undoubtedly affect the ratings of temperament. They may also affect teacher grading practices and teacher behavior toward the child. This, in turn, may affect future achievement of the child through effects on academic self-concept and achievement motivation.

Whatever the causal mechanism, this research indicates that one set of temperament characteristics makes a substantial contribution to the prediction of academic achievement on short- and long-term bases. In conjunction with measures of scholastic ability, high levels of prediction can be made over time spans ranging from 6 months to 4 years. If this kind of research is replicated, a place for temperament assessment in educational screening and assessment seems plausible.

Further, these data, if replicated, would logically create a press for educational programming designed to help the child control high activity level, high distractibility, and poor task persistence in preschool and the earliest grades of elementary school. One further implication of this research for the practice of psychology in the schools is that there has probably been far too much emphasis on the identification of children with a clinically significant attention deficit hyperactivity disorder to the exclusion of children who manifest subclinical problems of high activity and attention problems. Our data demonstrate that the relationship is a linear one throughout the sample studied. (None of the children in the sample were diagnosed as specifically having an attention deficit.) That is, attention problems and problems with control of activity have an important negative effect on schooling and achievement even in a "normal" population.

REFERENCES

Joreskog, K. G., & Sorbom, D. (1984). *LISREL VI: User's guide* (3rd ed.). Mooresville, IN: Scientific Software, Inc.

Keogh, B. (1982). Temperament: An individual difference of importance in intervention programs. *Topics in Early Childhood Special Education, 2*, 25–31.

Kohnstamm, G. A. (1989). Historical and international perspective. In G. A. Kohnstamm, J. E. Bates, & M. K. Rothbart (Eds.), *Temperament in childhood* (pp. 557–566). Chichester, England: John Wiley.

Martin, R. P. (1988a). *Temperament assessment battery for children—manual.* Brandon, VT: Clinical Psychology Publishing.

Martin, R. P. (1988b). Child temperament and educational outcomes. In A. D. Pellegrini (Ed.), *Psychological bases for early education* (pp. 185–205). Chichester, England: John Wiley.

Martin, R. P. (1989a). Activity level, distractibility, and persistence: Critical characteristics in early schooling. In G. A. Kohnstamm, J. E. Bates, & M. K. Rothbart (Eds.), *Temperament in childhood* (pp. 451–462). Chichester, England: John Wiley.

Martin, R. P. (1989b). Temperament and education: Implications for underachievement and learning disabilities. In W. Carey & S. McDevitt (Eds.), *Clinical and educational applications of temperament research.* Amsterdam/Lisse, The Netherlands: Swets & Zeitlinger.

Martin, R. P., Gaddis, L. R., Drew, K. D., & Moseley, M. (1988). Prediction of elementary school achievement from preschool temperament: Three studies. *School Psychology Review, 17*, 125–137.

Martin, R. P., & Holbrook, J. (1985). Relationship of temperament characteristics to the academic achievement of first grade children. *Journal of Psychoeducational Assessment, 3*, 131–140.

Martin, R. P., Wisenbaker, J., Matthews-Morgan, J., Holbrook, J., Hooper, S., & Spaulding, J. (1986). Stability of teacher temperament ratings over six and twelve months. *Journal of Abnormal Child Psychology, 14*, 167–179.

Pullis, M., & Cadwell, J. (1982). The influence of children's temperament characteristics on teachers' decision strategies. *American Educational Research Journal, 19*, 165–181.

Rutter, M. (1989). Temperament: Conceptual issues and clinical implications. In G. A. Kohnstamm, J. E. Bates, & M. K. Rothbart (Eds.), *Temperament in childhood* (pp. 463–482). Chichester, England: John Wiley.

Thomas, A., & Chess, S. (1977). *Temperament and development.* New York: Brunner/Mazel.

Thomas, A., Chess, S., & Birch, H. (1968). *Temperament and behavior disorders in children.* New York: New York University Press.

8

Temperament Research and Practical Implications for Clinicians

Michel Maziade

Almost all temperament researchers owe a tribute to the pioneering scientific work of Stella Chess and Alexander Thomas. In view of the dedication of this book, and thus this chapter, to Alex and Stella, my intention is: first, to share some thoughts about their influence on our own research program in child psychiatric epidemiology; second, to express some concerns about trends in the present evolution of child temperament research as a whole; third, to summarize the positive implications for clinical practice that can be derived from current temperament research; finally, consequent to these concerns, to discuss the directions we intend to take with our now 10-year-old temperament research program.

A CONTRASTING VIEW OF CHILD PSYCHOPATHOLOGY: INTUITION, COMMON SENSE, AND HUMILITY

A considerable number of the Québec epidemiological studies of children at risk of psychiatric disorders were influenced by Chess and Thomas's nondogmatic and eclectic view of child development and of the possible mechanisms involved in the appearance of psychopathology in children. As young child psychiatrists and researchers, we were struck by their humanistic moderation, their simplicity and humility in face of the complexity of human behavior and destiny. No doubt, their positions contrasted with those of other theoreticians and scientists of child psychiatry and psychology. This contrast came from their sticking to the facts based on their careful observations instead of elaborating premature and complex speculations about children's behavior, and also from the simplicity of their formulation of the role of temperament in the genesis of psychopathology and the common-sense and humility with which they professed it. Indeed, many times they stated that temperament was not a panacea (Thomas & Chess, 1977) but an additional and important parameter to consider both in the clinic and research, the aim of which is to shed light on the multifactorial causes of different childhood psychopathologies.

THE PAUCITY OF CLINICAL RESEARCH ON TEMPERAMENT

From the very beginning, our group was inspired by Thomas and Chess's contrasting view of child development; this reinforced our own proneness to gather solid data, based on simple hypotheses, rather than wasting time and energy in conceptualizing third- and fourth-degree hypotheses (which has been, for some time, the inclination of the second generation of temperament researchers) while first- and second-order theories remain unverified.

It is discouraging to see how few of the hundreds of valuable scientific reports published on temperament in the past 20 years have investigated the relationship of temperament (whatever the model in use) to the development of serious childhood psychopathology (Garrison & Earls, 1987a; Maziade, 1988, 1989; Rutter, 1989; Bates, 1989; Carey, 1989a; Carey & McDevitt, 1989; Keogh, 1989). We are still in need of controlled studies looking at the role of different temperament traits in the genesis of severe behavior deviancies and developmental delays, that is, those orienting a large proportion of our children to special education classes (7%–8% of the population in different countries) or those warranting treatment at a clinic (8%–15%) (Offord et al., 1987; Rutter, 1970). For instance, we are lacking controlled studies on the relationship of temperament to childhood and adolescent-onset schizophrenia and bipolar disorder, disruptive behavior disorders such as attention deficit hyperactivity disorder, opposition-conduct and antisocial disorders, and anxious and depressive disorders. Controlled studies of the use of temperament concepts in preventive and treatment strategies of these costly disorders are also very scarce.

The scientists in more basic sciences, the developmentalists and the theoreticians, gradually took over the temperament field during the past 20 years. As is the case in most other health fields, they found themselves to be in greater numbers than clinical researchers and epidemiologists. Therefore, the scientific course of the investigations in child temperament followed the "natural" course of research in other health fields, especially in child psychiatry and psychology. The science of temperament has become an almost unilateral science of the normal, average temperament in very young children, infants, and preschoolers. This "normalizing" or "developmentalistic" turn of temperament research is understandable and necessary. However, the temperament scientists, as a group, must avoid the pitfalls that a unilateral "normalizing" trend entails.

POSITIVE IMPLICATIONS OF TEMPERAMENT RESEARCH FOR CLINICAL PRACTICE AND SCHOOLING

Several good books have been published recently on the implications of temperament research for clinical practice and education (Carey & McDevitt, 1989; Chess & Thomas, 1986; Garrison & Earls, 1987b). There is a general agreement among most researchers that much research remains to be done on the use and role of temperament in clinical practice. Most also agree, however, that some general valuable implications of temperament research ought to be taken into consideration by clinicians and educators. If so, they can have some positive effects on the relationships between the counselor, the parent, and the problem child.

First, children are born different in terms of their temperamental styles. This cannot be ignored any more. Some children are born in the average range, but others come with extremely positive traits or extremely negative or socially undesirable temperament traits. In counseling for parents having a problem child this established fact cannot be ignored. The child's temperament may be as large a part of the problem as the parental attitudes. This concept in the mind of clinicians and educators can only have the positive effect of counteracting the still too frequent practice of automatically blaming the parents for the behavior problems of their children (Chess & Thomas, 1986; Carey, 1989b).

Second, since children of the same family are born different, the parents under counseling understand they can be relieved from some of their natural guilt toward the problem child, but, by the same token, they also understand they remain responsible for individualizing their attitudes to the temperamental differences of each of their children. No good and general principle of management can apply indiscriminately to every child. No school system can hope to apply valuable education rules and principles to all the children and ignore their duty to individualize some of their attitudes toward some temperamentally exceptional pupils (Keogh, 1989).

Third, most researchers are reluctant to suggest that enough scientific evidence exists on temperament for it to be used in a large-scale preventive setting in the population (Rutter, 1989; Maziade, 1989; Garrison & Earls, 1987b; Bates, 1989). To design efficient preventive interventions, we need to know the causative mechanisms leading to the clinical problem and the exact interactive role of temperament in the multifactorial mechanism. Since these are still unknown, we have no means to target the right factor(s) and to assess the efficiency (and cost-efficiency) of the preventive interventions. In ethical terms, the possible noxious effect of the identification, in the general population, of the children who present temperamental characteristics making them more vulnerable is not known. Large-scale screening of children's temperament must be done only in the context of an evaluative research program. In contrast, the clarification of the temperamental characteristics of a child who is already identified as problematic in the school or in the clinic is a very different issue, and by all means it should be encouraged in the context previously mentioned.

IMBALANCE BETWEEN BASIC-DEVELOPMENTAL AND CLINICAL-EPIDEMIOLOGICAL RESEARCH ON TEMPERAMENT

The original goal of Chess and Thomas in the New York Longitudinal Study (NYLS) was to determine the functional significance of temperament in the origins and evolution of clinical behavior disorders (Chess & Thomas, 1991). One of their motives was a desire to understand deviant behavior. Developmental and fundamental research on normal babies is certainly an avenue, but at some point, if the role of temperament in the development of severe psychopathology is to be understood, complementary temperament research on sick or seriously deviant and older children will be a necessity. We have argued, and a few others share this opinion (Kagan, Reznick, & Snidman, 1989; Rutter, 1989; Maziade, 1989), that temperament researchers must look at extreme temperament characteristics, and even at the combination of extreme (rather than average) features of temperament with particular environmental risk factors, to understand the mechanisms leading a child and family to cross a threshold beyond which a severe clinical problem arises, thus jeopardizing normal development and warranting a consultation. Researchers in other scientific fields are also accustomed to looking at natural phenomena in a qualitative way rather than only in a continuous or quantitative way. Einstein viewed a natural entity as a "bundle of qualities," two entities being the same if one could demonstrate that "their respective bundle of characteristics" did overlap or were similar (Einstein, 1979, pp. 51–52). Geologists investigate the extreme phenomenon of earthquakes to understand the natural movement of the earth's tectonic plates. Similarly, a clinical disorder can be viewed as a qualitatively separate entity on the basis of a specific set of biological and developmental causes. To demonstrate that temperament is involved in the causes of a serious disorder, researchers ought to conceptualize the study of a specific and severe disorder in children as a special combination of (1) extreme temperamental characteristics linked to an extreme innate physiological reaction and (2) discrete environmental risks interacting with the former in order to produce a special form of clinically disordered behavior or development.

Too large an imbalance of basic-developmental over clinical-epidemiological temperament research can only contribute to killing, with time or decades, this important field of investigation that inevitably remains largely in the field of health. To be seen by peers or outsiders as meaningful, health research must demonstrate an impact on the diagnosis or identification of significant or costly health problems and on their prevention or treatment. Otherwise, health practitioners and research administrators and organizations, especially during a time of tight budgets, may view the temperament research of the last two decades as a scientific ground of merely philosophical or theoretical importance, which is certainly not the case.

THE QUÉBEC STUDIES: A COUNTERCURRENT EPIDEMIOLOGICAL VIEW OF TEMPERAMENT

Relying on the existing body of data on child temperament, influenced by the intuition and findings of Chess and Thomas in the NYLS, and helped by our own background as clinicians, we became interested in temperament, especially extremely adverse traits of temperament, as a potential psychiatric risk factor in the population. Right from the beginning, this risk concept influenced the designs of our research program.

Therefore, our first interest in the late 1970s and early 1980s was not to build "our own" new temperament rating scales, as many were doing at the time; neither was it to compare babies on different scales and on observational protocol to consider whether these new scales were better than the existing ones; nor was it even to try to relate, in a first step, certain temperament dimensions with some kind of biological parameters in order to validate our own supposedly better Québec rating scales. We were just interested at that time, as is the mark of science, in borrowing the existing good data, the reliable and already tested instruments, and in going further to assess the potential vulnerability to psychiatric disorders associated with undesirable temperament traits and, in a second step, to analyze the mechanisms involved in this risk. After all, the temperament phenomenology in the early 1980s, whatever the model under study, had already shown up as moderately stable over time from infancy, and as influenced by genes (Matheny, Wilson, & Nuss, 1984; Matheny, 1984).

I remember very well how, in the first temperament conferences I attended in the early 1980s, the Québec work seemed to be viewed by the majority of temperament researchers as lacking originality and, let us say, showing a kind of "conceptual" backwardness. Probably our most "heretical" position at the time was that our group chose to look at "extreme" temperament features; this was totally contrary to the mind of the majority that the scientific gems to be discovered about temperament resided solely in "the continuum," or dimensional temperament—in other words, in average temperamental features.

Heresy can lead to something meaningful, and, in the following pages, I will summarize only our conclusive findings of the last decade about extremely difficult temperament on temperament Factor 1 (TF1) as a risk factor. A more detailed summary is provided elsewhere for the interested reader (Maziade, 1989; Maziade, Caron, Côté, Boutin, & Thivierge, 1990a).

A SUMMARY OF THE QUÉBEC TEMPERAMENT FINDINGS

This summary is based on a body of data coming out of several complementary epidemiological studies conducted over the past 10 years and involving more than 4,500 normal and clinical children: three cross-sectional studies of large random samples of the general population (Maziade, Boutin, Côté, & Thivierge, 1986), two longitudinal studies of extremely adverse or difficult temperament groups selected from these random samples, and two recent studies of large samples of children consecutively referred to a regional child and adolescent psychiatric clinic (Maziade et al., 1990a).

A child temperament profile, originating largely from the induction of Thomas, Chess, and Birch (1968) from the NYLS and composed of the traits of withdrawal in face of unfamiliar stimuli, of low adaptability, of high intensity in emotional expression, and of a general level of negative mood, has now been replicated several times in culturally different populations (see Matheny et al., 1984, and Maziade et al., 1986). We first consistently replicated this bipolar temperament cluster, very similar to the NYLS easy-difficult profile, through a first facto (Factor 1; TF1) derived from principal component analyses at different age levels in random samples of our general population (Maziade et al., 1984a,b, 1985; Maziade et al., 1986). This also provided us with normative temperament values based on the general population, thus allowing the definition of reliable and accurate extreme cut points on the temperament continuum.

Our prior longitudinal and cross-sectional studies indicated that extremely adverse traits on this temperament Factor 1 make children specifically at risk of developing externalizing disorders (i.e., DSM-III-R attention deficit hyperactivity disorder [ADHD] and opposition disorder) in the home associated with internalized symptoms outside the home (Maziade et al., 1989; Maziade, 1989; Maziade et al., 1990b). No other types of disorders such as developmental delays or severe isolated internalizing (anxiety, depression) disorders were found associated with TF1. This specific association was shown in our longitudinal studies in the general population at different age levels (Maziade, Côté, Boutin, Bernier, & Thivierge, 1987; Maziade, Côté, Thivierge, Boutin, & Bernier, 1989; Maziade et al., 1990b). This was also observed in a large sample of children referred to a regional child psychiatric clinic (Maziade et al., 1990a), in which an overproportion of extreme temperament on TF1 was observed, indicating again that TF1 is a risk factor bringing children to the clinic. Moreover, congruent with our findings in the general population, in the clinical sample these extreme TF1 children were referred particularly for oppositional or hyperactivity diagnoses (Maziade et al., 1990a). We also replicated several times findings that TF1, even extreme, was not by itself a risk in the population, and we circumscribed a precise risk interaction in which extremely adverse traits on TF1 predisposed longitudinally up to adolescence to externalizing (ADHD, opposition or conduct) disorders only when associated with a dysfunctional family discipline (Maziade, 1988; Maziade et al., 1990b). We have also found repeatedly a paradoxical association of externalizing disorder in the home and school and internalizing (anxious, depressive, emotional) symptoms, especially in school (Maziade, 1989). We showed that extreme temperament on TF1 was not equivalent to a clinical disorder since a large proportion of children do not develop behavior disorder and, conversely, a large proportion of children referred to the clinic do not present an extreme TF1 (Maziade et al., 1990a,b).

Concerning the mechanisms involved in the specific genesis of these children's externalizing disorders, we came to formulate a developmental hypothesis generated a few years ago (Maziade et al., 1989, 1990b) from these epidemiological findings. Why indeed are young children with an extremely adverse TF1 and living in a dysfunctional family, in terms of discipline, longitudinally predisposed to developing externalizing clinical disorder associated with internalizing symptoms, especially outside the home? We hypothesized that, if parental discipline is deficient, temperamentally extremely difficult children on TF1 (who have an innate tendency to withdraw from new situations, adapt poorly, are very intense, and have an overall negative mood) are more prone to develop clinical symptoms of opposition and overactivity in the family, that environment in which they are at ease and more adapted; however, outside the family, in novel or social situations that elicit more their lower adaptive abilities, these children are more likely to additionally display internalized clinical symptoms.

FUTURE DIRECTIONS

The findings of this 10-year epidemiological work on extreme temperament and childhood psychopathology led to a research protocol currently in progress. Before designing this new study, our group came to four methodological conclusions (Maziade, 1988, 1989) in order to further our knowledge about the mechanisms involved in the association between TF1 and externalized disorders (ADHD, opposition or conduct disorder), and ultimately to improve the nosology and lead to more efficient preventive and curative interventions for these clinical children. These conclusions are the following:

First, although at odds with the customary thinking of most temperament researchers who still prefer the investigation of dimensional or average-continuous traits of temperament, we decided to continue focusing on extreme temperamental features since we hoped to observe a replicable link with serious and socially costly childhood psychopathology and to understand the mechanisms. The view that the study of extremes is warranted is shared by a few researchers (Kagan et al., 1989; Rutter, 1989).

Second, we kept a multivariate risk design including the six or seven already well-replicated psychosocial risk factors associated with childhood disorders (Maziade, 1986; Rutter, 1983). Third, we continued our strategy of targeting the association between extreme temperament and serious childhood disorders by using representative clinical samplings. Over all, this strategy has paid off during the last decades of risk research on child temperament. The fourth conclusion, the most important in our view, is derived from our realization that the demonstrated predisposing relationship (or the specific longitudinal and transversal link between extreme temperament on TF1 and externalizing clinical disorders) was based solely on phenomenological definitions of both temperament traits, although found stable and consistent, and children's clinical disorders or diagnoses.

Consequently, we realized (Maziade et al., 1990a), for our subsequent studies, the need for adding biological variables to our usual multivariate designs. We tried to imagine what type of physiological markers, having sufficient empirical validity, could be specifically linked to phenomenological TF1 but not to the clinical externalizing symptomatology to which it predisposes. We also needed to target a marker that had a chance to be sufficiently independent of the environmental risk factors that we have been using in our prior longitudinal and cross-sectional designs (see Rutter, 1989).

Our attention was attracted by the established fact that a lower heart rate variability (HRV) was a valid index of a low excitatory threshold in the hypothalamic-pituitary-adrenal axis, in the reticular formation, and in the sympathetic system (Axelrod & Reisine, 1984). Heart rate variability could be easily assessed, in a nonintrusive way, in the clinical setting. Moreover, it has also been demonstrated that children and adults display a decreased HRV under moderately stressful situations that require attention (Obrist, Light, & Hastrup, 1982). Obrist and colleague (1982) have already shown considerable interindividual differences on HRV under various stressful conditions.

Another line of evidence comes from the brilliant work of Kagan and his colleagues (1988), clearly indicating that young children displaying inhibition and withdrawal reactions in novel or unfamiliar situations presented longitudinally a decreased HRV, substantiating the hypothesis that their cognitive state of uncertainty with novel or unfamiliar stimuli comes from a lower threshold of arousal (Reznick et al., 1986). Rhesus monkeys also vary in their response to novelty, the ones being slow to explore and avoidant showing higher heart rate in the face of novelty (Suomi, 1983, 1985, 1986).

APPROACH/WITHDRAWAL AND ADAPTABILITY: THE CORE OF TF1

Our frequently replicated observations (Maziade et al., 1984a,b, 1986) that withdrawal from novelty and low adaptability are the two traits having the highest explicative loadings on a first factor (Factor 1), coming out of principal component analyses, suggested that these two traits might constitute the core of TF1. With this possibility in mind, we hypothesized (Maziade et al., 1990a) on the basis of previously mentioned data that an adverse TF1 temperament could be specifically linked to a more stable heart rate under stressful conditions and, by deduction, to a lower threshold of arousal. This would render the difficult TF1 children phenomenologically more withdrawing from novelty, less adaptable, and secondarily, or as a reaction, with a more negative mood and high emotional intensity, and that would ultimately predispose them to externalizing disorder when the parental attitudes to discipline are dysfunctional.

TEARING DOWN THE BARRIER BETWEEN DEVELOPMENTAL AND CLINICAL RESEARCH

In conclusion, temperament researchers would find it beneficial to use and combine the complementary methodologies derived from developmental research on normal children, from biophysiological research, and from clinical-epidemiological research on deviant or seriously disturbed children, even though the latter is comparatively scarce. I have argued in this chapter that this combination of methods constitutes a promising, if not the only, way to elucidate the role of temperament in the development of severe childhood psychopathology.

Along the same line, in accord with the four methodological conclusions previously mentioned and with our prior findings, we are now testing a new hypothesis in a new sample of 150 children consecutively referred to the psychiatric clinic. We hypothesize that the children referred to the clinic for an externalizing disorder (ADHD, or opposition or conduct disorder) who present an adverse TF1 will display a more stable heart rate in the laboratory under moderately stressful conditions than those without an extremely adverse TF1, thus indicating a lower threshold of arousal for the former. Of course, by the same process, we want to validate a specific physiological marker for TF1 as a risk factor in the population, that is, a marker that would be linked to TF1 but not to the clinical symptomatology it predisposes to. In other words, our question is, Can we distinguish or classify different subgroups of clinically referred children, especially those with an externalizing diagnosis (ADHD, or opposition or conduct disorder) on the basis of their combined differences of physiological arousability, temperament Factor 1, and family functioning in terms of discipline? According to the data accumulated so far, we should find a significantly larger proportion of the referred externalizing disorders, especially ADHD, that are characterized by a combination of an extremely difficult temperament on TF1, a greater physiological arousability, and a dysfunctional family discipline. If this is verified, the practical implications for a developmental diagnosis, treatment for and prevention the numerous children presenting these disruptive behavior disorders will be of utmost value.

REFERENCES

Axelrod, J., & Reisine, T. D. (1984). Stress hormones: Their interaction and regulation. *Science, 224*, 452–459.

Bates, J. E. Applications of temperament concepts. In G. A. Kohnstamm, J. E. Bates, & M. K. Rothbart (Eds.), *Temperament in childhood* (pp. 321–355). New York: John Wiley.

Carey, W. B., McDevitt, S. C. (Eds.). (1989). *Clinical and educational applications of temperament research.* Amsterdam/Lisse, The Netherlands: Swets Zeitlinger.

Carey, W. B. (1989a). Practical applications in pediatrics. In G. A. Kohnstamm, J. E. Bates, & M. K. Rothbart (Eds.), *Temperament in childhood* (pp. 405–419). New York: John Wiley.

Carey, W. B. (1989b). Clinical use of temperament data in pediatrics. In W. B. Carey, & S. C. McDevitt (Eds.), *Clinical and educational applications of temperament research* (pp. 127–139). Amsterdam/Lisse, The Netherlands: Swets & Zeitlinger.

Chess, S., & Thomas, A. (1986). *Temperament in clinical practice.* New York: Guilford Press.

Chess, S., & Thomas, A. (1991). Temperament. In M. Lewis (Ed.), *Child and adolescent psychiatry* (pp. 145–159). Baltimore: Williams & Wilkins.

Einstein, A. (1979). *Comment je vois le monde.* Traduit de l'allemand par Régis Hanrion (pp. 44–52). France: Flammarion.

Garrison, W. T., & Earls, F. J. (1987a). Relationship between temperament and psychopathology. In W. T. Garrison & F. J. Earls (Eds.), *Temperament and child psychopathology* (pp. 50–65). Newbury Park, CA: Sage.

Garrison, W. T., & Earls, F. J. (1987b). *Temperament and child psychopathology.* Newbury Park, CA: Sage.

Kagan, J., Reznick, J. S., & Snidman, N. (1988). Biological bases of childhood shyness. *Science, 240,* 167–171.

Kagan, J., Reznick, J. S., & Snidman, N. (1989). Issues in the study of temperament. In G. A. Kohnstamm, J. E. Bates, & M. K. Rothbart (Eds.), *Temperament in childhood* (pp. 133–144). New York: John Wiley.

Keogh, B. K. (1989). Applying temperament research to school. In G. A. Kohnstamm, J. E. Bates, & M. K. Rothbart (Eds.), *Temperament in childhood* (pp. 437–450). New York: John Wiley.

Matheny, A. (1984). Twin similarity in the developmental transformations of infant temperament as measured in a multi-method, longitudinal study. *Acta Geneticae Medicae et Gemellologiae, 33,* 181–189.

Matheny, A., Wilson, R. S., & Nuss, S. M. (1984). Toddler temperament: Stability across settings and over ages. *Child Development, 55,* 1200–1211.

Maziade, M (1986). Etudes sur le tempérament: Contribution à l'étude des facteurs de risques psychosociaux de l'enfant. *Neuropsychiatrie de l'Enfance et de l'Adolescence, 34*(8–9), 371–382.

Maziade, M. (1988). Child temperament as a developmental or an epidemiological concept: A methodological point of view. *Psychiatric Developments, 6*(3), 195–211.

Maziade, M. (1989). Should adverse temperament matter to the clinician? An empirically based answer. In G. A. Kohnstamm, J. E. Bates, & M. K. Rothbart (Eds.), *Temperament in childhood* (pp. 421–435), New York: John Wiley.

Maziade, M., Boudreault, M., Thivierge, J., & Capéraà, P. & Côté, R. (1984a). Infant temperament: SES and gender differences and reliability of measurement in a large Quebec sample. *Merrill-Palmer Quarterly, 30*(2), 213–226.

Maziade, M., Côté, R., Boudreault, M., Thivierge, & J. Capéraà, P. (1984b). The New York Longitudinal Studies model of temperament: Gender differences and demographic correlates in a French-speaking population. *Journal of the American Academy of Child Psychiatry, 23*(5), 582–587.

Maziade, M., Capéraà, P., Laplante, B., Boudreault, M., Thivierge, J., Côté, R., & Boutin, P. (1985). Value of difficult temperament among 7-year-olds in the general population for predicting psychiatric diagnosis at age 12. *American Journal of Psychiatry, 142*(8), 943–946.

Maziade, M., Boutin, P., Côté, R., & Thivierge, J. (1986). Empirical characteristics of the NYLS temperament in middle childhood: Congruities and incongruities with other studies. *Child Psychiatry and Human Development, 17*(1), 38–52.

Maziade, M., Côté, R., Boutin, P., Bernier, H., & Thivierge, J. (1987). Temperament and intellectual development: A longitudinal study from infancy to 4 years. *American Journal of Psychiatry, 144*(2), 144–150.

Maziade, M., Côté, R., Thivierge, J., Boutin, P., & Bernier, H. (1989). Significance of extreme temperament in infancy for clinical status in preschool years: I. Value of extreme temperament at 4–8 months for predicting diagnosis at 4.7 years. *British Journal of Psychiatry, 154,* 535–543.

Maziade, M., Caron, C., Côté, R., Boutin, P., & Thivierge, J. (1990a). Extreme temperament and diagnosis: A study in a psychiatric sample of consecutive children. *Archives of General Psychiatry, 47,* 477–484.

Maziade, M., Caron, C., Côté, R., Mérette, C., Bernier, H., Laplante, B., Boutin, P., & Thivierge, J. (1990b). Psychiatric status of adolescents who had extreme temperaments at age 7. *American Journal of Psychiatry, 147*(11), 1531–1536.

Obrist, P. A., Light, K. C., & Hastrup, J. L. (1982). Emotion and the cardiovascular system: A critical perspective. In C. E. Izard (Ed.), *Measuring emotions in infants and children* (pp. 299–316). Cambridge: Cambridge University Press.

Offord, D. R., Boyle, M. H., Szatmari, P., Rae-Grant, N. I., Links, P. S., Cadman, D. T., Byles, J. A., Crawford, J. W., Munroe Blum, H., Byrne, C., Thomas, H., & Woodward, C. A. (1987). Ontario child health study: II. Six-month prevalence of disorder and rates of service utilization. *Archives of General Psychiatry, 44,* 832–836.

Reznick, J. S., Kagan, J., Snidman, N., Gersten, M., Baak, K., & Rosenberg, A. (1986). Inhibited and uninhibited children: A follow-up study. *Child Development, 57,* 660–680.

Rutter, M. (1970). *Education, health and behavior.* London: Longman.

Rutter, M. (1983). Stress, coping, and development: Some issues and some questions. In N. Garmezy & M. Rutter (Eds.), *Stress, coping, and development in children* (pp. 1–41). New York: McGraw-Hill.

Rutter, M. (1989). Temperament: Conceptual issues and clinical implications. In G. A. Kohnstamm, J. E. Bates, & M. K. Rothbart (Eds.), *Temperament in childhood* (pp. 463–479). New York: John Wiley.

Suomi, S. J. (1983). Social development in rhesus monkeys: Consideration of individual differences. In A. Oliverio (Ed.), *The behavior of human infants* (pp. 71–92). New York: Plenum Press.

Suomi, S. J. (1985). Biologic response styles: Experiential effects. In H. Klar (Ed.), *Biologic response styles: Clinical implications* (pp. 1–17). Washington, DC: American Psychiatric Press.

Suomi, S. J. (1986). Anxiety-like disorders in young nonhuman primates. In R. Gittelman (Ed.), *Anxiety disorders of childhood* (pp. 1–23). New York: Guilford Press.

Thomas, A., & Chess, S. (1977). *Temperament and development.* New York: Brunner/Mazel.

Thomas, A., Chess, S., & Birch, H. G. (1968). *Temperament and behavior disorders in children.* New York: New York University Press.

PART III

INDIVIDUAL DIFFERENCES AS RISK FACTORS: DEVELOPMENT, BIRTH WEIGHT, AND CHRONIC ILLNESS

9

Variations, Deviations, Risks, and Uncertainties in Human Development

Ann M. Clarke and A. D. B. Clarke

From the moment of conception, the human organism is potentially or actually at risk for a variety of problems. These include chromosome aberrations; single gene or polygenic effects; toxic, infective, or traumatic factors; and psychosocial influences that may well interact with the former, and may themselves be of pervasive significance. Risk itself can range from unlikely through probable to, at the extreme, almost certain.

Our growing understanding of development suggests complex relationships within the individual between four major factors. In a simplified sketch, there is, first, the *biological trajectory,* incorporating both the intrauterine and later physical environmental factors and the genetic program. The latter is unlikely to be linear across time. Nor do genes normally dictate a precise outcome but offer a range of possible reaction with other factors. Second, there is the *psychosocial trajectory,* which changes over time, especially at periods of life transitions. Third, we know that there are *transactions* during development. Individual characteristics may prompt their possessor to choose or be chosen by, or indeed create, particular environments that, in a feedback manner, reinforce or modify those behaviors. Fourth, *chance events or encounters* can sometimes exert powerful effects, deflecting the life path. To call these four agents and their interactions complex would be an understatement. Even an armchair consideration implies variability in individual and thus in group outcome. Moreover, individual predictions from the early years to adulthood are precarious and group predictions must be *actu-*

arial. Both must be based on extensive knowledge of the parents and the children's micro- and macroenvironmental settings; moreover, predictions will vary according to domain: IQ scores are easier to forecast, within reason, than academic achievement; temperament is difficult to predict over long time periods, except at the extremes (e.g., unusually "inhibited" or "difficult" early behavior); need achievement and motivation, which are so important in development, arise out of transactions between the individual and significant others throughout the life span.

This chapter will provide examples illustrative of its theme, namely, that many interactive factors influence human development, normal or abnormal, throughout life. Moreover, a given deviant condition, justifying a particular classification, can present in a range of forms. Outcome, too, can exhibit a variety of possibilities, and even the most potent risk factors, singly or in combination, allow at least some individuals to escape their common consequences. Indeed, the very notion of risk implies uncertainty.

It is important to emphasize not only that biological and social processes interact over time but that to view the more cognitive domains of personality development separately from the orectic may be misleading; nevertheless, it may be convenient to divide our territory into the predominantly cognitive and the predominantly social and emotional.

VARIATIONS IN IQ

The IQ, which stands proxy for general intellectual ability, is probably the most thoroughly studied index in psychology, and appears to be strongly canalized. Over the years a variety of twin and adoption studies have shown intellectual variations in the general population to be rather highly heritable; these issues will be discussed elsewhere in this book.

Across time there are commonly changes in ordinal position, and, depending on the sample, in level. Constancies will of course depend on a number of variables, for example, the particular process being studied, the age at which the assessments are made, the accuracy of the measuring device, the maturational pathway for the individual, and so on.

There is a long-established rule that the longer the time interval, the greater the likelihood of change in ordinal position in IQ, leading to diminishing correlations. However, recently there have been several studies showing rather high correlations across the childhood years (see Clarke & Clarke, 1984). Furthermore, the substantial concurrent and predictive validity of intelligence tests for academic attainment during the years up to adolescence indicates that for cognitive abilities there appears to be a considerable interrelationship and also a fair degree of stability of test scores and their correlations over time.

Carr (1992) has pointed out that in her prospective longitudinal study of a birth cohort of Down's syndrome (DS) persons from infancy the distribution of IQ scores at 21 years showed a range of 60 points around a mean of 42, similar to that covering virtually the entire normal population from 70 to 130, around a mean of 100. Moreover, during the life span, individual DS children showed the same fluctuations in IQ over time as would be demonstrated in a sample of normal youngsters, although, as with normal populations, there were high correlations for the group from one test occasion to another. So, even among DS cases, prediction of adult outcome from childhood status may be hazardous, except to predict that such persons never reach above average status. However, there was on the whole a strong tendency, as implied by the high test–retest correlations, for children with high or very low scores to remain roughly in their positions, as would be expected in a normal population, and there were significant correlations between early childhood IQs and scholastic achievement at 21. There was, of course, a decrement in average IQ after the first 4 years, as in other longitudinal studies of DS youngsters.

Since there is little evidence implicating environmental events in developmental changes in IQ, except in very unusual circumstances (Clarke & Clarke, 1976), and since developmentally retarded children show the same pattern of change over time as do normal persons, we conclude that these alterations are mainly due to a combination of maturational processes and test "errors." The latter includes differences in content and standardization and also motivational fluctuations.

SCHOLASTIC PROBLEMS

Scholastic attainment is probably the prime behavioral mediator in fulfillment of potential. Hence some attention will be paid to risks of educational failure as posing severe problems for those affected.

In an overview of the National Child Development Study, Fogelman (1983) indicates that for school attainment "only about 40 per cent of children were in the same broad band (i.e. the top, middle or bottom third of the total distribution) at 7 and 16, and about one-quarter of those in the top third at 16 had not been there at 11" (p. 353). Dividing a range of attainments into thirds represents a very broad criterion against which constancy or change could be evaluated. Even so, a substantial group showed relative change. The same cohort contained a small number of seriously disadvantaged children who not only did not show the normal scholastic gain over time but demonstrated some evidence of "cumulative deficit" in attainment as age increased, confirming the findings of a number of other studies.

Reading Difficulties

Of all the educational problems that may befall individual children during their schooldays, difficulty in acquiring reading skills is probably the most serious, since literacy underlies progress in so many subjects, and thus in adult life. The extent of the problem is debatable, depending upon definitions, age, and other variables, but probably includes up to 15% of pupils in an advanced nation. These of course comprise a very heterogeneous group, ranging from the seriously mentally retarded to children whose domestic circumstances provide neither the motivation, nor role models, nor the peace and active support to acquire literacy. In addition, there are a few youngsters of above average ability who may exhibit a specific reading retardation, sometimes of severe degree.

In a classic English study Rutter and Yule (1975), using data from a total population of children in a rural area, sought to elucidate the concept of dyslexia or specific reading retardation in comparison with general reading backwardness. They showed that when reading ability was regressed onto age and IQ, the distribution of residuals departed from normality. Superimposed on the normal curve was a "hump" of children obtaining significantly lower reading scores than would be expected from age and IQ. Although the paper provoked controversy, the findings have been replicated. Specific reading retardation was shown to differ significantly from reading below average for age in terms of a number of external criteria.

Experimental studies of reading and spelling in younger and older children and also several comparisons of mono- and dizygotic twins have revealed that difficulty with phonological coding is a feature of *both* specific reading retardation and reading backwardness. There is significant heritability for reading disability and highly significant heritability for spelling after controlling for IQ (Pennington, 1990).

The importance of phonological disability has been stressed by Bryant and his colleagues, who suggest that separate contributions to literacy come from processes based on phonemic awareness and from ability to detect rhyme. Many ingenious experiments over the years underline this conclusion, including an intervention study in which prereaders benefited significantly in later establishing reading skills (see Bryant & Bradley, 1985; Goswami & Bryant, 1990). As an aid to greater literacy, there is a case for a substantial focus on rhyming and alliteration games as part of the preschool and kindergarten curriculum.

PERSONALITY DEVELOPMENT AND DEVIATIONS

There are great problems in assessing the extent of consistency and variability in personal and social characteristics over time. These range from differences in assessment methods to situational effects. Interesting and important research has been reviewed in Brim and Kagan's (1980) edited book and by Clarke and Clarke (1984). Kagan summarizes a position similar to the one we have held for many years:

> The view that emerges from this work is that humans have a capacity for change across the whole life span. It questions the traditional idea that the experiences of the early years, which have a demonstrated contemporaneous effect, necessarily constrain the characteristics of adolescence and adulthood. . . ." (Brim & Kagan, 1980, p. 1).

Magnusson (1991) offers an overview of his longitudinal study, which began in 1965 and in which he has been concerned with the ways in which individual and environmental factors interact. He cites the common finding that certain environments pose a developmental risk. However, he points out, "most people from a particular environment do not become criminals or abusers of alcohol. In fact, many of the people who make constructive, highly useful contributions to society are from the very environments believed to predestine social maladjustment" (pp. 1–2).

It has long been assumed on the basis of clinical evidence that conduct disorders tend to be relatively persistent, and the results of several contemporary prospective studies bear this out. For example, Esser, Schmidt, and Woerner (1990) followed a *random* sample of 356 eight-year-old children in West Germany up until the age of 13, finding that although the overall prevalence rate of 16% for all psychiatric disorders remained constant across the two ages, the persistence of conduct disorders in individual cases was very much greater than that for those with emotional disorders, which more often than not had cleared up, and other children with newly arising disorders had replaced them.

Farrington and West's well-known British prospective longitudinal study (West, 1982) also showed the frequent persistence of conduct disorders that started early in life. Their earliest contact with a total sample of indigenous boys from six inner-city primary schools was at age 8 to 9, and they later noted that the factor that best predicted future delinquency was a measure of "troublesomeness" derived from observations of teachers and classmates at primary school. The German study, in similar vein, indicated that conduct disorders were related to prior learning disabilities and domestic stresses (Esser et al., 1990). It appears that failure *at* school and failure *of* schools are among several factors that are probably causally linked to persistent conduct disorder.

Other correlates repeatedly identified are low family income, large family size, parental conflict and unsatisfactory child-rearing practices, parental criminality, and low IQ in the child.

Even in an economically very favorable environment, the developing individual is not immune to risk. The exemplary New York Longitudinal Study (Chess & Thomas, 1984) has provided the fullest and most reliable account of problems that may befall youngsters born into privileged homes, and it is a pleasure to pay tribute to these outstanding scientists. The subjects were 133 infants from 84 families, followed into adulthood. There was only one person with mild mental retardation (and additional diagnosis of organic personality disorder), one of three cases of brain damage. The other two cases of brain damage showed difficult behavior during the course of development, but this was mitigated by average IQs; although these two persons were emotionally vulnerable, they were reasonably successful adults. As would be predicted in a sample of this kind, the risk of conduct disorders was virtually nil, and, when occurring, they were nonpersistent; one case of mild conduct problems had improved by adult life, while the other, diagnosed in childhood as moderate, had completely recovered by young adulthood. One child had a recurrent major depression that on follow-up was unchanged, while of 40 children exhibiting adjustment disorders, mostly mild, 29 had recovered by early adulthood, 5 had improved, 2 were unchanged, 2 were mildly to moderately worse, with 2 markedly worse. In addition, to exemplify the hazards of early prediction, 12 persons exhibited fairly severe disturbances commencing in adolescence. Of these, 6 were completely recovered in adult life, including 3 with severe problems, 2 had improved, and 4 were unimproved or worse.

Although certain risk factors, childhood difficult temperament and severe parental conflict, predicted an unfavorable outcome for early adult adjustment, there were individual subjects with either difficult temperament or severe parental conflict who maintained a healthy developmental course throughout childhood, adolescence, and the adult years. Moreover, the 5 children who at 3 years had both a difficult temperament and exposure to parental conflict, although showing a specially high incidence of severe behavior disorder during childhood (4 out of the 5), had by adulthood completely recovered. Of course, the results must be seen in the context of very skilled professional help from birth onward.

RISKS, RESILIENCE, AND VULNERABILITY

The social correlates of a large number of pathologies, varying from severe to mild, are well known. The most dire forms of social adversity for children are being reared in conditions of isolation, cruelty, and almost total neglect, including chronic and severe malnutrition. Skuse (1984) reviewed nine such cases and points to rapid progress made after discovery as an important prognostic indicator. It appears that Waddington's (1957) self-righting tendency is a powerful agent in most humans. This is a genetic mechanism that tends to restore the individual to a normal life path if improved circumstances allow this.

The most robust correlates of childhood problems are the educational attainments and general intelligence of the parents, which may of course be interpreted as caused either biologically or socially. Single mothers in poverty are, however, particularly vulnerable to both biological and social risks.

There is known to be a natural escape rate from even extreme disadvantage. For example, in one British study from age 5 to the early thirties, Kolvin, Miller, Scott, Gatzanis, and Fleeting (1990) indicate that "change is the dominant feature" (p. 167). While only 44% of those multiply deprived at age 5 remained as adults in the same category, the remainder shifted to lesser degrees of adversity, but almost 13% escaped completely and functioned as normal citizens. This study, which was concluded in the 1980s, did not include ethnic minorities.

The precise mechanisms of resilience and of vulnerability have not yet been fully delineated, but numerous studies indicate some pointers, outlined in Clarke and Clarke (1992).

Protective factors seem to be: (1) Constitutional dispositions that will render some children attractive even to the most depraved parents and probably to other members of the family and to a wider community. These include sociability, problem-solving ability, and planning ability, leading gradually to an internal locus of control. These children are likely to attract the positive attention of teachers in school, to acquire a sense of self-esteem and self-confidence and a belief in their own ability to adapt to changing circumstances, and themselves to change them. (2) Some network of affectional support, which may be absent even in the best institutions, but may be present in very disadvantaged homes. (3) Schools in which children are valued and encouraged to learn. There are by now massive amounts of research data in support of the view that schools may differentially enhance both achievement and adjustment. (4) A peer group, probably based on school, which will be prosocial. This means that individual children will need to be sufficiently attractive in positive ways to be chosen as friends. (5) An ability to plan purposefully that will, according to Rutter (1989), make a big difference to choice of career and/or choice of continuing education, as well as to delaying marriage and childbearing until an appropriate time.

In large-scale studies based on ordinary communities, all these have been found to be protective of children in seriously disadvantaged circumstances. In addition, there are accounts of rare intervention programs starting in the preschool period and either continuing or initiating a sequence of positive, ongoing consequences.

Factors rendering persons vulnerable to adversity seem to be the following: (1) Temperamental irritability and lack of sociability, often combined with some degree of mental retardation. Infants growing up in large, chaotic, discordant families may not have the opportunity to gain an understanding of social cause and effect, nor to develop planning ability, or knowledge of the desirability of delayed gratification and an internal locus of control. (2) Lack of emotional security and strong affectional ties with any one person, be it a sibling, grandmother, neighbor, or other significant individual. Children who lack these supports are likely to be rated *troublesome* by teachers and later by peers in school, to be unpopular with peers, and to seek attention and emotional support in socially undesirable ways. (3) Attendance at schools in which the tranquillity and academic press necessary to enable children to learn are lacking, and being part of large, affectionless families that are unable to exercise firm but kind control. (4) Growing up in a social situation characterized by poverty and lack of hope, from which they lack the personal resources to attempt an escape.

Intervention for those most at risk is fraught with difficulties, and the objectives of early intervention have changed over the years (for excellent reviews, see Meisels & Shonkoff, 1990). Preschool intervention typically yields short-term advantages, both for children and for parents, effects that should not be undervalued. Longer-term benefits will depend on the intervention initiating a chain of ongoing, positive consequences, which may be difficult to achieve (Clarke & Clarke, 1989) except in adoptive families. In the latter, intervention is total and continues through the major developmental period.

SUMMARY

In this chapter we have outlined some findings from a few major areas in human development, emphasizing that even in normal growth, psychological characteristics that dictate or reflect the life path show both individual constancies and changes. To some extent development can be open-ended. This view, originating in our own work more than 30 years ago, appears to have some generality. However, conditions such as severe mental retardation or autism are exceptions.

Risks by definition constitute probabilities, both of occurrence and outcome, not certainties. They may vary from significant but weak (e.g., the birth of a handicapped child to a 37-year-old mother) to strong (e.g., conduct disorder at age 8 leading in many cases to adult problems).

Studies of those who succumb to risks in comparison with those who escape their probable destiny have already begun to identify relevant psychological qualities. In turn this may lead to better intervention strategies. As we indicated in *Early Experience: Myth and Evidence* (Clarke & Clarke, 1976), "What emerges very strongly from our evidence is the need for a greater recognition of the possibility of personal change following misfortune" (p. 271) either through the accumulation of positive influences or through a radical change in circumstances.

REFERENCES

Brim, O., & Kagan, J. (Eds.). (1980). *Constancy and change in human development.* Cambridge, MA: Harvard Educational Press.

Bryant, P. E., & Bradley, L. (1985). *Children's reading problems.* Oxford: Blackwell Scientific Publications.

Carr, J. (1992). Longitudinal research in Down syndrome. In N. W. Bray (Ed.), *International review of research in mental retardation* (Vol. 18, pp. 197–223). New York: Academic Press.

Chess, S., & Thomas, A. (1984). *Origins and evolution of behavior disorders.* New York: Brunner/Mazel.

Clarke, A. D. B., & Clarke, A. M. (1984). Constancy and change in the growth of human characteristics. *Journal of Child Psychology and Psychiatry, 25,* 191–210.

Clarke, A. M., & Clarke, A. D. B. (Eds.). (1976). *Early experience: Myth and evidence.* London: Open Books; New York: Free Press.

Clarke, A. M., & Clarke, A. D. B. (1989). The later cognitive effects of early intervention. *Intelligence, 13,* 289–297.

Clarke, A. M., & Clarke, A. D. B. (1992). How modifiable is the human life path? In N. W. Bray (Ed.), *International review of research in mental retardation* (Vol. 18, pp. 137–157). New York: Academic Press.

Esser, G., Schmidt, M. H., & Woerner, W. (1990). Epidemiology and course of psychiatric disorder in school-age children—results of a longitudinal study. *Journal of Child Psychology and Psychiatry, 31,* 243–263.

Fogelman, K. (Ed.). (1983). *Growing up in Great Britain.* London: Macmillan.

Goswami, U., & Bryant, P. E. (1990). *Phonological skills and learning to read.* London: Lawrence Erlbaum.

Kolvin, I., Miller, F. J. W., Scott, D. Mcl., Gatzanis, S. R. M., & Fleeting, M. (1990). *Continuities of deprivation? The Newcastle Thousand Family Study.* Aldershot, England: Gower House Publishing.

Magnusson, D. (1991). Individual development in a longitudinal perspective. *Reports from the Department of Psychology, Stockholm University,* No. 773.

Meisels, S. J., & Shonkoff, J. P. (Eds.). (1990). *Handbook of early childhood intervention.* New York: Cambridge University Press.

Pennington, B. F. (1990). The genetics of dyslexia. *Journal of Child Psychology and Psychiatry, 31,* 193–201.

Rutter, M. (1989). Pathways from childhood to adult life. *Journal of Child Psychology and Psychiatry, 30,* 25–51.

Rutter, M., & Yule, W. (1975). The concept of specific reading retardation. *Journal of Child Psychology and Psychiatry, 16,* 181–197.

Skuse, D. (1984). Extreme deprivation in childhood: II. Theoretical issues and a comparative review. *Journal of Child Psychology and Psychiatry, 25,* 543–572.

Waddington, C. H. (1957). *The strategy of genes.* London: Allen & Unwin.

West, D. J. (1982). *Deliquency: Its roots, careers and prospects.* London: Heinemann.

10

Conditions of Risk for Maldevelopment: Prematurity

Margaret E. Hertzig

Alexander Thomas and Stella Chess have had a lifelong professional interest in the study of individual differences in development. My own association with them coincided with the inception of the centerpiece of this interest, the New York Longitudinal Study (NYLS). As a medical student moonlighting as a research assistant, I had the great good fortune to participate, together with their collaborators, Herbert Birch and Sam Korn, in the development of methods of data collection and analysis that permitted the definition of individual differences in temperament. One of the most robust findings of this ongoing investigation of the developmental course of temperament organization in a sample of 133 children born to middle-class parents living in New York City and its surrounding suburbs during the mid-1950s is the association between the constellation of "difficult" temperamental attributes and the emergence of behavior disorder. The identification of "difficult" temperament as a condition of risk has had far-reaching implications for the understanding of the pathogenesis and treatment, as well as for the prevention, of psychopathology during childhood. Clinicians and researchers alike have sought to further clarify mechanisms that operate to enhance the deleterious consequences of "difficult temperament" or diminish its impact. Children born prematurely are also at increased risk of delayed, deviant, or disordered development—and it is particularly fitting that a selected review of factors involved in individual differences among low-birth-weight children be included in a collection of papers honoring Chess and Thomas's contributions to child development and child psychiatry.

BACKGROUND

The association between low birth weight and a myriad of neurological, cognitive, and behavioral disorders is well established, as is the association between prematurity and social disadvantage. However, the negative consequences of low birth weight are neither uniform nor inevitable. While the physical and mental handicaps of some prematurely born children may be profound, others exhibit no discernible disability. Thus, prematurity has come to been identified as a model system within which to examine the potential influence of both biological and social factors on the development of children. A focus on the biological side of the equation led Pasaminick and Knobloch (1966) to propose a "continuum of reproductive casualty" to account for the varied negative outcomes retrospectively identified as linked to low birth weight. Alternatively, Sameroff and Chandler (1975) have suggested a "continuum of caretaking casualty" to incorporate the environmental risk factors contributing toward the poor developmental and behavioral outcomes of many prematurely born children.

The importance of the concept of "caretaking casualty" has been amply confirmed by the findings of epidemiologically based studies. Werner and Smith (1977) have reported that children from advantaged homes with the most severe of perinatal complications—if free from obvious physical defect—had mean IQ scores that were closely similar to those of children with no perinatal complications who grew and developed in disadvantaged social circumstances. By 18 years of age, 10 times as many children had problems that could be related to the effects of poor early environment as had problems that could be related to the effects of perinatal conditions of risk. Data such as these are consistent with the view that the impact of the reproductive casualty does indeed pale in comparison with that of the environment (Sameroff & Chandler, 1975), and underscore the importance of exploring the developmental consequences of low birth weight in children who are socially and economically well situated.

NEW YORK LONGITUDINAL STUDY OF LOW BIRTHWEIGHT CHILDREN

In the early 1960s, Birch and Thomas directed attention to the development of socially advantaged low-birth-weight children when they elected to apply the methods of the New York Longitudinal Study to the anterospective investigation of a group low-birth-weight children whose families were intact, and whose parents were middle-class as defined by education and occupation. My familiarity with the NYLS was invaluable when I assumed responsibility for the conduct of this investigation in 1973.

Sample and Methods

The sample consisted of 66 children in 63 families, born between 1962 and 1965, who weighed between 1,000 and 1,750 gm at birth. Details of complications of pregnancy, delivery, and neonatal course, as well as estimates of gestational age and intrauterine growth, were abstracted from obstetrical and neonatal records. In addition to data on temperament, full reports of medical and/or psychiatric consultation and treatment and progress in school were obtained. Wechsler Intelligence Scale for Children (WISC) IQ's as well as Wide-Range Achievement Test (WRAT) scores in reading and arithmetic were ascertained in the eighth year of life. At this time as well, all children were assessed neurologically in the course of a clinical examination designed to detect both localizing and nonfocal neurological signs (Hertzig, 1974, 1981, 1983; Hertzig & Mittleman, 1984). These bodies of data made it possible to examine associations between variation in neurological handicap and perinatal factors in addition to low birth weight, as well as to educational and behavioral outcome. Similarities and differences in temperamental organization between low-birth-weight children and the normal weight subjects of the NYLS were examined, and relations between neurological status, temperament, and behavior described.

Neurological Status

Thirteen children (20%) had localizing neurological findings, clinically describable as one or another variant of cerebral palsy. Among the remainder, none of whom suffered from discernible motor handicap, 20 (30%) were found to have two or more nonlocalizing signs of CNS dysfunction. The clinical neurological examination was considered to be within normal limits for age in only one half of the sample. Children with both localizing and nonlocalizing neurological abnormalities were significantly more likely to have sustained perinatal complications additional to low birth weight than were those whose neurological examinations were normal. However, a history of prenatal complications was significantly more frequent among children who subsequently were found to have nonfocal signs, while children with localizing findings were significantly more likely to have experienced postnatal complications. This pattern of findings provided construct validity for the clinical neurological assessment, permitting comparisons between neurologically defined subgroups.

Behavior and Temperament

No significant differences in IQ or reading and arithmetic achievement test-score levels were found between those with nonlocalizing neurological signs and those who were neurologically normal, but those with nonlocalizing findings were significantly more likely to have exhibited educational and/or behavioral difficulties than were those who were neurologically normal. Forty-five percent of the children with nonlocalizing findings as compared with 12% of those who were neurologically normal were receiving special educational interventions ($\chi^2 = 7.2719$, $df = 1$, $p < .01$). Fifty percent of those with nonfocal signs and only 15% of those who had no evidence of neurological abnormality on clinical examination had been referred for psychiatric consultation ($\chi^2 = 7.4527$, $df = 1$, $p < .01$).

Differences in temperament between the low-birth weight children and the full-term subjects of the NYLS, as well as between neurologically defined subgroups of prematurely born children, were examined by means of multivariate techniques that permitted the comparison of weighted scores for each temperamental dimension. Multivariate techniques were also employed to examine differences in overall "difficulty" as determined by an index constructed by summing weighted scores for the following five temperamental attributes: rhythmicity, adaptability, approach-withdrawal, intensity, and mood. As a group, during the first 3 years of life, the low-birth-weight children were significantly less distractible, exhibited higher sensory thresholds, and were more intense and less adaptable than were the normal-weight subjects of the NYLS. However the low-birth-weight children were no more likely to exhibit their intensity and nonadaptability in combination with irregularity, negative mood, and withdrawal to new situations (the "difficult child" constellation) than were their full-term counterparts. Both children with localizing findings and those with nonfocal neurological signs were significantly more "difficult" than were those who were neurologically normal. Children who came to psychiatric notice were significantly more likely to be both neurologically impaired and temperamentally "difficult," but difficult temperament did not appear to increase the risk of behavior difficulty beyond that already conferred by the presence of neurological dysfunction. Among children with clinical evidence of neurological abnormality, those who came to psychiatric notice were not significantly more "difficult" than those whose parents did not seek psychiatric consultation. In summary, prematurity imposes a significant burden on the development of even socially advantaged children of low-birth-weight, mediated by the integrity of the central nervous system, so that children who exhibit clinical evidence of neurological dysfunction in the absence of visible physical handicap are at greater risk of behavioral and educational disability than children of similar birth weight who clinically appear neurologically intact.

THE EFFECTS OF ADVANCES IN NEONATAL CARE

The subjects of the New York Longitudinal Study of Low Birthweight Children were born before the revolution in neonatal care. What has been the impact of mechanical ventilation, parenteral nutrition, extracorporeal membrane oxygenators and artificial surfactant, introduced during the past 25 years, on the mortality and morbidity of low-birth-weight infants? Over the past quarter of a century, survival, particularly for very low-birth-weight (VLBW) (< 1,500 gm) infants has improved markedly. While mortality for newborns weighing less than 750 gm continues to be high, with two thirds dying, the neonatal death rate (i.e., within the first 28 days of life) for infants with birth weights of 1,000 to 1,500 gm has fallen from more than 50% in 1960 to less than 10% in 1985. In 1960 more than 90% of all infants weighing less than 1,000 gm died; currently, more than 70% of those between 750 and 1,000 gm survive. Interestingly enough, the proportion of neonatal intensive care unit (NICU) survivors who have serious mental and physical handicaps has not changed significantly since the introduction of modern neonatal intensive care practices. Of course, the increased likelihood of survival of the low-birth-weight and most particularly the VLBW infant has resulted in a larger absolute number of seriously handicapped children. Moreover, as the rate of serious long-term disability increases with decreasing birth weight, the smallest of survivors remain at particularly high risk despite improved medical interventions. Specific medical complications common among LBW and VLBW infants including intraperiventricular hemorrhage, bronchopulmonary dysplasia,and nutritional deficits are associated with increased risk of serious neurodevelopmental and cognitive deficits. Increasing grades of intracranial hemorrhage, as detected by ultrasound during the neonatal period, are associated with increasing incidence of significant motor and cognitive abnormalities. But even this measure of the integrity of the CNS is not uniformly accurate, as some children with evidence of intraperiventricular hemorrhage are spared (Blackman, 1991).

The findings of studies that have addressed the stability of an infant's developmental and neurological status over time suggest a general continuity in developmental level at least during the first 4 years of life. Children who appear cognitively and motorically normal tend to continue to display an absence of handicap in these areas during the preschool period (Ross, Lipper, & Auld, 1985). However, there is increasing evidence suggesting that many VLBW infants who appear motorically and cognitively normal prior to school entrance develop more subtle problems when faced with formal educational demands. Many VLBW children require supplemental speech and language or other remedial services, as well as placement in special education classes. Poor visual-motor skills, visual integrative problems, and impaired performance on tasks assessing spatial relations and memory have been reported to occur with increased frequency among VLBW children in comparison to matched control groups composed of full-term classmates (Bauchner, Brown, & Peskin, 1988).

PSYCHOSOCIAL FACTORS AFFECTING THE OUTCOME OF PREMATURELY BORN CHILDREN

It is clear that modern methods of care and treatment have contributed to a significant reduction in the mortality of LBW and VLBW infants and that this reduction in mortality has resulted in an absolute, although not proportionate, increase in the number of seriously motorically and cognitively impaired children. Unfortunately, advances in neonatal care have not been accompanied by concomitant changes in factors affecting the health of poor women and their babies. While the fundamental causes of low birth weight are, as yet, only partially understood, many associated conditions including poor nutrition, small stature, obstetrical complications, and less than adequate maternal health are all more common among poor women, as is reduced access to prenatal care. Prematurity remains disproportionately a problem of the poor with the incidence of low birth weight some two to three times higher among women who are socially disadvantaged (Wise & Meyers, 1988). Thus, an increasing focus on the medical aspects of the care of the VLBW infant directs attention once again to the role of social/environmental factors in determining the quality of long-term outcome among those VLBW infants who are free of visible handicap.

Social Class

While social class is a time-honored marker of potential psychosocial risk, it is only a summary variable, incorporating in a single designation a number of different factors that may interfere with a given family's ability to provide a nurturant context for a developing child. The concept of cumulative risk has emerged as a consequence of attempts to specify more precisely components of psychosocial risk. For example, Sameroff and colleagues (1987) have assessed 10 risk factors, maternal mental health, anxiety, quality of mother-child interaction, level of education, parental perspectives, occupation of head of household, minority group status, family social support, family size, and stressful life events, in a study of the cognitive and behavioral characteristics of 215 full-term 4-year-old children. Regardless of socioeconomic status, significantly greater impairments were found among children with four or more risk factors than among those who were exposed to no more than one factor. Escalona (1982) has suggested that infants who are born prematurely may be even more vulnerable to environmental insufficiencies than full-term babies.

Temperament and Attachment

Goldberg, Corter, Lojkasek, and Minde (1990) have attempted to define pathways of influence of four factors (neonatal medical complications, infant temperament, mother-child relationships, and family environment) on mother and teacher reports of behavior problems in VLBW children who were free of significant motor or cognitive impairment at 4 years of age. The two outcome measures, mother-reported problems and teacher-reported problems, were not correlated, raising the possibility that behaviors of which home-based caretakers may be unaware that interfere with successful adjustment to preschool may also contribute to the increased educational difficulty experienced by many VLBW children. Maternal reports of behavior problems were predicted only by prior maternal reports of temperamental difficulty. Teacher reports of behavior problems were predicted by measures of maternal responsiveness and maternal well-being as well as by maternal descriptions of difficult temperament. Medical complications, beyond that of VLBW, were not related to outcome as described by either teachers or parents. However, results of ultrasound studies were not available to these investigators, making it impossible to assess the influence of documented neonatal hemorrhage on later behavioral organizations.

Assessment of the quality of mother-child attachment at year 1 was also unrelated to either mother or teacher reports of behavioral disturbance. The discrepancy between this finding and the widely held tenet that disturbances in the mother-child relationship are a source of psychopathology is noteworthy. While the original Ainsworth classification scheme has been shown to be a good predictor of a variety of social competencies in preschool children (Main, Kaplan, & Cassidy, 1985; Sroufe, 1983), its utility as a predictor of behavior disorder in full-term preschool children has been previously questioned (Bates & Bales, 1988). It is of particular interest that none of the measures in this multimeasure study were directly related to social class, a finding that underscores the limitations that attach to assumptions of a one-to-one correspondence between inadequacies in caretaking environment and social and economic disadvantage.

Protective Factors

Some children, even some both born prematurely and reared in impoverished and discordant homes, emerge as adults with all of the hallmarks of competence—stable personalities, good peer relations, academic achievement, commitment to education and to purposive life goals, and a remarkable degree of resilience in the face of life's adversities. In recent years increased attention has come to be directed toward the study of factors that facilitate "escape from risk." One of the most comprehensive of these efforts has been the investigation—now spanning some 30 years—of the children of Kauai (Werner, 1989). Some one third of the initial sample of 698 infants were considered "at risk" because they had experienced both moderate to severe degrees of perinatal stress and reared in poor homes troubled by discord, desertion, divorce, or parental alcoholism or mental illness, by mothers with little formal education. Although two of three of these at-risk children developed serious behavior or learning problems during childhood and adolescence, by the age of 18 one in three developed instead into a competent, confident, and caring young adult.

Comparisons between these two groups of individuals exposed to comparable levels of initial risk permitted the identification of characteristics within the individuals, within their families, and outside the family circle that contributed to resiliency. As infants, the resilient subjects were temperamentally easier, good-natured, and affectionate, with fewer eating and sleeping difficulties, than were the high-risk infants who later developed serious behavior problems. As toddlers the resilient children were described as more alert, autonomous, socially orientated, and advanced in communication and self-help skills. Though not especially gifted in school, these children tended to use whatever skills they had effectively. They had many interests and engaged in activities and hobbies that provided solace in adversity and a reason for pride.

Resilient children tended to grow up in families with four or fewer children, with a space of at least 2 years between themselves and their next sibling. Few had experienced prolonged separations from primary caretakers during the first year of life, and all had established a close bond with at least one care-giving person during the toddler and preschool years. Nurturance, however, could have come from substitute parents, including grandparents, older siblings, neighbors, or regular babysitters, who played important roles as positive models for identification.

As they grew older, resilient children tended to have at least one and usually several close friends. They relied on an informal network of kin, neighbors, and peers for counsel and support in times of crisis. Some had a favorite teacher who became a role model, friend, and confidant. Participation in extracurricular activities played an important part in the lives of resilient youth, especially those that were cooperative enterprises. As the number of stressful life events accumulated over time, more of such protective factors were needed as counterbalance to ensure continued positive adaptation.

INTERVENTION STRATEGIES

In reviewing data from this study and others Rutter (1987) has characterized a number of different protective processes as follows: those that reduce the impact of risk through alterations of exposure to or involvement in risk situations, those that reduce the likelihood of negative chain reactions stemming from risk encounters, those that promote self-esteem and self-efficacy through the availability of secure and supportive personal relationships or successful task accomplishments, and, finally, those that open up new opportunities.

Clearly, developmental interventions during the early years of life seek to optimize development in all of these ways. Given the complexity of factors affecting the outcome of at-risk children over time, it is unreasonable to expect that a single approach to intervention will be uniformly effective. Preventive interventions for infants and children at increased biomedical risk can be divided into those that are provided before and after discharge from the neonatal intensive care unit. Initial approaches to neonatal intervention tended to consist of one or more types of very early environmental manipulations including tactile stimulation (sucking, massaging, flexing, positioning); vestibular-kinesthetic stimulation (rocking, oscillating waterbeds); auditory stimulation (singing, music boxes, recorded mother's voice, recorded heartbeat); and visual stimulation (decoration of surroundings, mobiles). Although short-term benefits on growth, development, and medical status have been reported, variability in both methods and results is considered too great to permit generalized programmatic recommendations. Moreover, these types of interventions are not risk free. Excessive handling may exacerbate autonomic nervous system instability, and be associated with hypoxia, apnea, and bradycardia in premature infants. Increasingly, it is recommended that interventions during the neonatal period be individualized, functional, modifiable, and sensitive to the autonomic and neurodevelopmental status of individual infants (Bennett & Guralnick, 1991; Gorski, Hole, Leonard, et al., 1983; see also the chapter by Medoff Cooper in this volume).

These considerations have led to attention being redirected toward the development of individualized care plans designed to reduce excessive environmental light, noise, and traffic and to minimize intrusive handling, as well as to help both hospital staff and parents interpret the readiness cues of the immature infant with the goal of enhancing the quality of early parent-infant interactions. Preliminary outcome data suggest that infants who receive personalized care have reduced requirements for oxygen, shorter hospital stay, and improved performance on tests of infant development (Bennett & Guralnick, 1991). However, it has proved to be particularly difficult to involve many poor women in programs designed to facilitate interaction with their hospitalized infants because of lack of transportation, need to care for older children at home, and other crises of daily living (Brown, LaRossa, Aylward, et al., 1980).

Most successful programs designed to optimize the development of low-birthweight infants following discharge from the NICU have utilized a comprehensive combination of family support, parent education, and child development approaches. Infant-focused interventions are designed to stimulate and enhance developmental skills, while more parent-focused interventions are directed toward improving the quality of parent-child interactions. The results through 3 years of age of a large multicenter intervention study that assessed cognitive, behavioral, and health outcomes indicate that intervention group children performed significantly better on the Stanford-Binet Intelligence Scale than did children in comparison groups. The effect of intervention varied significantly with birth weight, with the heaviest infants making the greatest gains. Mothers of intervention group children reported significantly fewer behavioral problems than did mothers of controls, but no differences were found in measures of growth, scales of health status, or incidence of serious health conditions (Bennett & Guralnick, 1991). Although it is virtually impossible in most programs to specifically relate positive outcome effects to individual components of the overall intervention plan, it is reasonable to expect that broad complex approaches should result in more significant and more persistent improvements than approaches that are more simplistic and narrowly based.

Although intervention during infancy and the preschool years is of undeniable importance, it must be recognized as well that protection lies less in the psychological chemistry of the moment or short term than in the ways in which people of all ages deal with life changes and what they do about their stressful or disadvantageous life circumstances (Rutter, 1987). Attention needs to be directed beyond early childhood toward the identification of later potential turning points in people's lives—school entrance with its opportunities for peer relationships and systematic task mastery; the termination of formal education and accompanying prepartions for work, intimate relationships, and parenting; geographic moves and the like—when risk trajectories may also be amenable to redirection onto a more adaptive path. Alexander Thomas and Stella Chess have assumed such an open-ended approach in tracing the progress of the original NYLS sample from early infancy to adulthood. The results of their efforts clearly demonstrate that the course of development can be affected for good or for ill by events occurring well beyond infancy and the preschool years. Efforts to understand and ameliorate the potentially deleterious effects of exposure to conditions of biological and social risk must also continue over the life span.

REFERENCES

Bates, J. E., & Bales, K. (1988). Attachment and development of behavior problems. In J. Belsky & T. Nezworski (Eds.), *Clinical implications of attachment.* Hillsdale, NJ: Lawrence Erlbaum.

Bauchner, H., Brown, E., & Peskin, J. (1988). Premature graduates of the newborn intensive care unit: A guide to follow-up. *Pediatric Clinics of North America, 35,* 1207–1226.

Blackman, J. A. (1991). Neonatal intensive care: Is it worth it? Developmental sequelae of very low birthweight. *Pediatric Clinics of North America, 38,* 1497–1511.

Bennett, F. C., & Guralnick, M. J. (1991). Effectiveness of developmental intervention in the first five years of life. *Pediatric Clinics of North America, 38,* 1513–1528.

Brown, J., LaRossa, M., Aylward, G., et al. (1980). Nursery-based intervention with prematurely born babies and their mothers. Are there effects? *Journal of Pediatrics, 97,* 487–492.

Escalona, S. K. (1982). Babies as double hazard: Early development of infants at biologic and social risk. *Pediatrics, 70,* 670–676.

Goldberg, S., Corter, C., Lojkasek, M., & Minde, K. (1990). Prediction of behavior problems in four-year-olds born prematurely. *Development and Psychopathology, 2,* 15–130.

Gorski, P. A., Hole, W. T., Leonard, C. L., et al. (1983). Direct computer recording of premature infants and nursery care: Distress following two interventions. *Pediatrics, 72,* 198–204.

Hertzig, M. E. (1974). Neurologic findings in prematurely born children at school age. In M. Rolf & A. Thomas (Eds.), *Proceedings of the Fifth Conference of the Society for Life History Research.* Minneapolis: University of Minnesota Press.

Hertzig, M. E. (1981). Neurologic "soft" signs in low birthweight children. *Developmental Medicine and Child Neurology, 23,* 778–791.

Hertzig, M. E. (1983). Temperament and neurologic status. In M. Rutter (Ed.), *Developmental neuropsychiatry.* New York: Guilford Press.

Hertzig, M. E., & Mittleman, M. (1984). Temperament in low birthweight children. *Merrill-Palmer Quarterly, 30,* 201–211.

Main, M., Kaplan, N., & Cassidy, J. (1985). Security in infancy, childhood, and adulthood: A move to the level of representation. In I. Bretherton & E. Waters (Eds.), *Growing points of attachment theory and research.* Monographs of the Society for Research in Child Development 50 (1-2, Serial no. 209).

Pasaminick, B., & Knobloch, H. (1966). Retrospective studies in the epidemiology of reproductive casualty: Old and new. *Merrill-Palmer Quarterly, 12,* 2–26.

Ross, G., Lipper, E. G., & Auld, P. A. M. (1985). Constancy and change in the development of premature infants weighing less than 1501 grams at birth. *Pediatrics, 76,* 885–891.

Rutter, M. (1987). Psychosocial resilience and protective mechanisms. *American Journal of Orthopsychiatry, 57,* 316–331.

Sameroff, A., & Chandler, M. (1975). Reproductive risk and the continuum of caretaking casualty. In F. Horowitz, M. Hetherington, S. Scarr-Salapatek, & S. G. Siegel (Eds.), *Review of child development research* (Vol. 4). Chicago: University of Chicago Press.

Sameroff, A., Seifer, R., Barocas, R., et al. (1987). Intelligence quotient scores of 4 year old children: Social environmental risk factors. *Pediatrics, 79,* 343–350.

Sroufe, L. A. (1983). Individual patterns of adaptation from infancy to preschool. In M. Perlmutter (Ed), *Minnesota symposium on child psychiatry* (Vol. 16, pp. 41–81). Hillsdale, NJ: Lawrence Erlbaum.

Werner, E. E. (1989). High risk children in young adulthood: A longitudinal study from birth to 32 years. *American Journal of Orthopsychiatry, 89,* 72–81.

Werner, E. E., & Smith, R. S. (1977). *Kauai's children come of age.* Honolulu: University of Hawaii Press.

Wise, P. H., & Meyers, A. (1988). Poverty and child health. *Pediatric Clinics of North America, 35,* 1169–1186.

11

Chronic Illness as a Psychological Risk Factor in Children

Melvin Lewis

Approximately one child in 10 experiences a chronic physical illness by age 15 (Pless, Roghmann, & Haggerty, 1972). In 1988 three million children in the United States were estimated to suffer from chronic illness (Schoenborn & Marano, 1988). Twelve percent to 13% of children with chronic illness in one study were found to have emotional problems (Rutter, Tizard, & Whitmore, 1970). In a population study of 3,000 children, Walker, Gortmaker, and Weitzman (1981) found that about 30% had a chronic illness, and that the children with a chronic illness were 2.5 times more likely to have behavioral and social problems than were the healthy children in the study. In another controlled, general population interview study of 3,294 children aged 4 to 16 years, Cadman, Boyle, Szatmari, and Offord (1987) found that children with both chronic medical conditions and associated disability had a threefold or more risk for psychiatric disorders (attention deficit hyperactivity disorder [ADHD], overanxious disorder, depression, conduct disorder) and were at considerable risk for social adjustment problems compared to their healthy peers. Children with chronic medical conditions but no disability had about a twofold increase in psychiatric disorders but not very much increased risk for social adjustment difficulties.

Thus, although the *risk* for maladjustment is increased in children with chronic illness, the majority of children with chronic health problems do *not* have mental health problems or social or school adjustment problems. Put positively, most children with chronic illness seem to overcome their adversity. What, then, are the stress and risk factors in children with chronic illness, both general and illness specific, that may help or hinder the child's and the family's coping capacities?

GENERAL FACTORS AFFECTING OUTCOME

Numerous general factors operate in children with chronic illness as they do with other children. Such factors include the adaptive capacities of the parents, the sociocultural context of hospitalization, and the nature of particular hospital experiences, including the degree and duration of discomfort and pain. The child's internal abilities to cope with stress also vary in relation to the child's developmental stage (O'Dougherty & Brown, 1990) and temperament (Chess & Thomas, 1986). Disordered parenting, abuse, divorce, and poverty are serious adverse factors.

In some chronic illnesses certain general psychosocial factors are often prominent, although they may not be causative. Thus lower socioeconomic status (SES), poor diet, poverty, unhygienic living conditions, or living in an environment of violence may contribute to the debilitating effects of chronic illnesses as disparate as failure to thrive, chronic otitis media, various chronic eating disorders, and brain damage. In almost every condition, such factors may have at least some effect on the etiology and outcome of that condition for a particular child. Every illness has a psychosocial component.

The child's cognitive level and intelligence will also have an impact in terms of the child's general understanding of his or her body and the child's changing concepts of the nature of illness (Schonfeld, 1991). The most striking change in the child's understanding of both body function and illness causality occurs during the cognitive stage of concrete operations (age 7 to 11 years). Young children often resort to the concept of "immanent justice" to understand illness. Young children believe the illness is a justified punishment for some misdeed they think or fantasize they have committed and for which they subsequently feel guilt and shame. (Children may try to avoid reporting symptoms to avoid such "punishment.") With experience, explanations, and cognitive development through the stages of concrete and formal operations, the concept of immanent justice gives way to the concept of contagion. Children here develop a germ ("bug") theory, often elaborated from a television commercial. When children are in the cognitive stage of formal operations (11 or 12 years of age onward), they can comprehend the notion of multiple symptoms being caused by one illness, and begin to have a more rational idea of the relationship among organ functions, symptoms, and treatment methods. At all ages, children will benefit from truthful, educational explanations of how illness in fact comes about and what goals the treatment is to accomplish, all at a level the child can comprehend and with words the child can understand. This educational approach is the basis for appropriate preparation of the child for treatment and, in the end, for the prevention of undue anxiety and for the enhancement of coping skills in the child.

Children's concepts about chronic illness also vary in part with their experience of the illness. For example, children who experience a chronic orthopedic condition or a seizure disorder in general show less sophisticated concepts about illness than do normal children, although children with other kinds of chronic illness have somewhat more sophisticated concepts about bodily function than do normal children (Perrin, Sayer, & Willett, 1991).

Chronic illness often involves chronic or recurrent hospitalization, which may add to the risk of emotional upset (Breslau, Staruch, & Mortimer, 1982; Shanow, Ferguson, & Diamond, 1984). Cumulative risk may arise from such stresses as loss of autonomy, relative immobilization, impaired function, and disfigurement. The parents may experience fatigue, guilt, depression, and anxiety, as well as marital stress and financial drain. Both child and parents feel a loss of control as they increasingly have to adapt to the hospital staff, and they may then begin to lose their feeling of competence. The whole family, including siblings, may become isolated. Recurrent illness and hospitalization during the first 5 years may impair the child's attachments (Mrazek, Anderson, & Strunk, 1985). Parents have an especially formidable task in helping their child with a chronic illness believe he or she is a valued human being (McCollum, 1981).

Within the hospital, the staff may gradually feel discouraged by the slowness or absence of progress; or worse, by the deterioration that may steadily be taking place. Feelings of frustration and anger may be displaced from staff to parents, and vice versa. Denial and avoidance may set in. For example, hospital staff may assume that because a child has been previously hospitalized, the parents and child are therefore automatically familiar with and prepared for the procedures that will be performed; further preparation is then deemed unnecessary. In truth, each hospitalization is a unique experience for the child and parents, requiring still again preparation and maintenance as far as possible of familiar routines and playthings, as well as living-in for younger children, visiting, special nursing, child life care and school programs, surrogate parenting when necessary, a receptive ward environment, and an ongoing dialogue between parents and staff, with opportunities for counseling and therapy if indicated.

The class or category of causes of the illness, including genetic and traumatic categories, may have its own implications (guilt is a common reaction), as may an undue delay in making the diagnosis. Specific illnesses are often accompanied or followed by specific psychological reactions. Anxiety and fears about anticipated acute episodes, pain, major surgery, disfigurement, and death, as well as progressive loss of function and energy, often accompanied by depression, despair, and withdrawal, may be present in a wide range of chronic illnesses, including congenital heart defects, juvenile rheumatoid arthritis, ulcerative colitis, muscular dystrophy, leukemia, asthma, diabetes, epilepsy, cystic fibrosis, and brain damage. Virtually every category of disorder—congenital, traumatic, infective, neoplastic, degenerative, hormonal—in every physiological system or organ, can exhibit a chronic illness. A description of the specific psychological reactions commonly found in each such chronic condition could well be a component of the description of each disorder described in pediatric texts. A few child psychiatry texts have attempted to describe some of the salient psychiatric features of some of the more frequently occurring disorders (Graham, 1986; Lewis, 1991). The psychosocial literature on many of these conditions is very extensive (e.g., Hobbs & Perrin, 1985; Routh, 1988; Arnold, 1990). Some representative specific illness stressors and possible psychological effects are shown in Table 11-1.

Children and their families who are devastated and overwhelmed by a particular chronic illness in the child may experience hopelessness, helplessness, disorganization, and numbness. Frightening aspects of the illness may be repeatedly

TABLE 11-1
Specific Illness Stressors and Possible Psychological Effects

Illness	Stressful Medical Interventions	Possible Effects
Epilepsy: A condition in which there is continuing proclivity to have seizures	Adverse anticonvulsant medication drug effects Regular blood tests Hospitalization for status epilepticus Brain surgery	Anxiety and fear of unconsciousness Sense of control and autonomy severely affected Social stigmatization, rejection, and discrimination Parental overprotection or rejection Heightened dependency on parents
Asthma: A respiratory disorder characterized by intermittent and reversible attacks of difficulty in breathing	Repeated hospitalizations Allergy shots Bronchodilators Mist inhalation Corticosteroids Antibiotics for infection Beta-agonists	Fear of dying by suffocation Fear of abandonment Maladaptive use of wheezing to express conflicts Physical and social restrictions Family disruption (sleep interruption, dietary and housekeeping problems) Growth retardation secondary to steroids

Illness	Stressful Medical Interventions	Possible Effects
Diabetes: A metabolic disease in which there is a lack of insulin or impairment in the insulin mechanism	Insulin injections Diet restrictions Blood and urine testing Hospitalizations for acute episodes	Parent–child control struggle over insulin-food-exercise regimen Adolescent rebellion Pain of daily injections Fear of coma or insulin shock Anxiety over long-term complications
Chronic Otitis Media: Infection of the middle ear with chronic discharge through a perforation of the tympanic membrane	Repeated ear examinations Ear drops Surgical intervention	Hearing loss, with possible subsequent educational disadvantage, learning disability, and reading difficulty Social isolation Developmental delay
Heart Defects: Congenital abnormalities of the heart structure	Catheterization for diagnosis and treatment Corrective surgery Palliative surgeries Antibiotics Digitalis for heart failure	Parental guilt and depression over defect Coping with a life-threatening illness Extensive painful procedures Prolonged separation during infancy Difficulty disciplining child (fear of precipitating symptoms) Child's fear of pain, mutilation, death Activity restrictions
Irritable Bowel Syndrome: A functional bowel disorder characterized by alternating diarrhea and constipation	Dietary restrictions Stool softeners Antispasmodic medication Exercise program Antidepressant medication Treatment of fecal impaction	Fear of loss of control Feelings of shame and inadequacy Emotional tension, anxiety, and depression Physical response to life stress Conflicts over holding back vs. letting go Difficulty dealing with anger and aggressive feelings

Continued on next page

Continued from previous page

Illness	Stressful Medical Interventions	Possible Effects
Juvenile Rheumatoid Arthritis: An inflammatory process affecting the joints	Aspirin Physical therapy Steroids Gold therapy injections Orthopedic intervention (splints and surgery)	Pain and feelings of maltreatment, punishment, and persecution Activity limitation Deformity and crippling Depression and mood alteration
Muscular Dystrophy: A neuromuscular disorder in which striated muscle progressively deteriorates	Physical therapy Surgery for contractures Caloric-restricted diet Correction of spinal deformity Postural drainage exercises Orthopedic prosthesis and motorized equipment	Anguish and guilt over diagnosis Coping with knowledge of early crippling and death Chronic physical and mental exhaustion Progressive helplessness and dependency due to loss of strength Isolation and rejection by peers Great difficulty managing anger and aggressive feelings Sacrifices required by other family members Need for respite for parents and siblings
CNS Infection and Its Sequelae (Bacterial Meningitis): An inflammation of the membranes surrounding the brain resulting from bacterial infection, which may give rise to chronic brain dysfunction	Lumbar puncture Blood culture Spinal fluid culture Antibiotic therapy Respiratory isolation Treatment of increased intracranial pressure	Fear of child's death Fear of residual brain damage Coping with possible residual deficits: Mental retardation Seizures Hydrocephalus Hemiparesis Learning disability Hearing impairment

Note. From an original table by M. O'Dougherty and R. T. Brown in *Childhood Stress* (pp. 327–329), edited by L. E. Arnold, 1990. Adapted and reprinted by permission of John Wiley & Sons, Inc.

reexperienced, bad dreams may occur frequently, and there may be withdrawal and isolation; the child may become fearful of any possible future repetition of the acute episode, feel insecure, and begin to exhibit intensified attachment behaviors, sleep disturbances, and school difficulties. One could well think of this set of reactions as a chronic or recurrent type of post-traumatic stress disorder from which the child cannot easily escape.

Children who undergo bone marrow transplantation for such conditions as relapsing acute lymphocytic leukemia, neuroblastoma, and severe combined immunodeficiency syndrome are particularly at risk for post-traumatic stress disorder (Stuber, Nader, Yasuda, Pynoos, & Cohen, 1991). The combined stress of life-threatening illness and intensive medical treatment poses a stress that is nearly overwhelming to these children, who then exhibit post-traumatic stress symptoms, including denial and avoidance.

Other specific reactions may also occur. For example, children who are HIV positive (or even unaffected children) who are exposed to other family members (including a parent or sibling) who are dying or have died of AIDS may react to the overwhelming loss with protest, despair, and detachment, as well as helplessness and hopelessness. There is often a need to keep the diagnosis a secret. Projection of feelings of anxiety and anger may also occur. Survivors may experience survivor guilt.

PSYCHOSOCIAL APPROACHES TO PREVENTION AND INTERVENTION

Given this array of risk factors and stressors, assessment is a prerequisite for psychosocial treatment (Pless & Roghmann, 1971; Pless, 1984). Models for assessing the dimensions of causation and dysfunction associated with any chronic illness may include adaptations of models used to understand the child's responses to stress in general. For example, the following constructs relating to stress responses have been proposed:

1. Competence and coping in relation to the locus of control along an internal-external dimension (Rutter, 1966)
2. Proneness to helplessness or hopelessness (Schmale, 1972)
3. The role of the family as a support system (Caplan, 1976)
4. The adaptive and prophylactic aspects of denial (Koocher et al., 1980; Goldberg, 1983)

Psychological help in communication among family members should be an integral part of the care of the child and family. Children need to have some comprehensible understanding of their illness and the unwanted aspects of the treatment. Children and their parents also need to have some feeling of control over the disease and the treatment, and some feeling of hope. Such psychological help may be offered through support groups for child and parents, child life specialists' activities, special nurse assignments, ward meetings, and specialized therapies offered by mental health staff. Special therapies may include psychotherapy and behavioral approaches to pain management.

The pediatric staff too need support—at ward rounds, staff meetings, and on an ad hoc basis. When the stress of fear, separation, and pain in children with chronic illness causes symptoms of anxiety and behavioral problems, the pediatric staff may seek psychiatric consultation and liaison to understand and deal with these problems. Often the reactions among the staff members is an indication that attention must be paid to the staff members' needs as well as those of the child and parents.

Parents of children with chronic illness usually feel that the child's teachers should be informed and that they, the parents, should be the informants, although the physician should also be involved, particularly about medication issues and emergencies (Andrews, 1991). Likewise, the physician's care of the child can benefit from information from the school about difficult behavior and learning problems (Liptak, & Revell, 1989). On the other hand, only 45% of adolescents with cancer believed it would be helpful to them if more information about their illness were given to friends and teachers (Levenson, Pfefferbaum, Copeland, & Silberberg, 1982). Care should therefore be taken that the question of imparting information to the school should first be discussed with the adolescent. In any event, schools vary in how much information they want to or can comprehend. The services of a school nurse are usually helpful.

The family as a support system is a vital factor in the management of children and their families in these circumstances. The model of "goodness of fit" may be particularly appropriate in offering help to such families (Chess & Thomas, 1986). The reactions of the child and family are often the resultant of several interacting factors, including (1) the cognitive and emotional developmental level of the child; (2) the child's strengths and vulnerabilities, including temperament, intelligence, and degree of central nervous system intactness; (3) the presence of special risk factors, which may include previous stresses, parental dysfunction, pain, and lethality; (4) the dose and duration of the stressful experiences, which may be frighteningly severe, repetitive, and/or prolonged; and (5) the quality and endurance of support among family and friends and in the hospital, school, and community. In a sense, the goodness-of-fit model might be extended beyond the family to include the broader environment encountered by the child with a chronic illness, that is, the interactions among the child, family, hospital staff, school, community, and state. To achieve successful interaction and the best level of comprehensive care for the child with a chronic illness, a high level of collaboration, coordination, continuity, and leadership is often required to support and help these children and their families, and a multitheoretical as well as multimodal approach is almost always necessary.

REFERENCES

Andrews, S. G. (1991). Informing schools about children's chronic illnesses: Parents' opinions. *Pediatrics, 88*, 306–311.

Arnold, L. E. (Ed.). (1990). *Childhood stress.* New York: John Wiley.

Breslau, N., Staruch, K., & Mortimer, E. (1982). Psychological distress in mothers of disabled children. *American Journal of Diseases of Children, 136*, 682–686.

Cadman, D., Boyle, M., Szatmari, P., & Offord, D. (1987). Chronic illness, disability, and mental and social well-being: Findings of the Ontario Child Health Study. *Pediatrics, 79*, 805–813.

Caplan, G. (1976). The family as a support system. In G. Kaplan & M. Kallilea (Eds.), *Support systems and mutual help: Multidisciplinary explorations* (pp. 19–36). New York: Grune & Stratton.

Chess, S., & Thomas, A. (1986). *Temperament in clinical practice.* New York: Guilford Press.

Goldberger, L. (1983). The concept and mechanisms of denial: A selective review. In S. Brezwitz (Ed.), *The denial of stress* (pp. 83–102). New York: International Universities Press.

Graham, P. (1986). *Child psychiatry: A developmental approach.* Oxford: Oxford University Press.

Hobbs, N., & Perrin, J. M. (Eds.). (1985). *Issues in the care of children with chronic illness.* San Francisco: Jossey-Bass.

Koocher, G. P., O'Malley, J. E., Grogan, J. L., et al. (1980). Psychological adjustment among pediatric cancer survivors. *Journal of Child Psychology and Psychiatry and Allied Disciplines, 21*, 163.

Levenson, P. M., Pfefferbaum, B. J., Copeland, D. R., & Silberberg, Y. (1982). Information preferences of cancer patients age 11–20 years. *Journal of Adolescent Health Care, 3*, 9–13.

Lewis, M. (Ed.). (1991). *Child and adolescent psychiatry: A comprehensive textbook.* Baltimore: Williams & Wilkins.

Liptak, G. S., & Revell, G. M. (1989). Community physician's role in case management of children with chronic illness. *Pediatrics, 39*, 465–471.

McCollum, A. T. (1981). *The chronically ill child: A guide for parents and professionals.* New Haven: Yale University Press.

Mrazek, D. A., Anderson, I. S., & Strunk, R. C. (1985). Disturbed emotional development of severely asthmatic preschool children. *Journal of Child Psychology and Psychiatry and Allied Disciplines, 26*(Suppl 4), 81–94.

O'Dougherty, M., & Brown, R. J. (1990). The stress of childhood illness. In L. E. Arnold (Ed.), *Childhood stress* (pp. 326–349). New York: John Wiley.

Perrin, E. C., Sayer, A. G., & Willett, J. B. (1991). Sticks and stones may break my bones . . . . Reasoning about illness causality and body functioning in children who have a chronic illness. *Pediatrics, 88*, 608–619.

Pless, I. B., & Roghmann, K. J. (1971). Chronic illness and its consequences: Observations based on three epidemiological surveys. *Journal of Pediatrics, 79*, 351–359.

Pless, I. B., Roghmann, K. J., & Haggerty, R. J. (1972). Chronic illness, family functioning, and psychological adjustment: A model for the allocation of preventive mental health services. *International Journal of Epidemiology, 1*, 271–277.

Pless, I. B., & Roghmann, K. J. (1984). Clinical assessment: Physical and psychological functioning. *Pediatric Clinics of North America, 31*, 33–45.

Routh, D. K. (Ed.). (1988). *Handbook of pediatric psychology.* New York: Guilford Press.

Rutter, J. B. (1966). Generalized expectancies for internal versus external control of reinforcement. *Psychological Monographs, 80*, 609.

Rutter, M., Tizard, J., & Whitmore, K. (Eds.). (1970). *Education, health and behavior.* London: Longmans.

Schmale, A. H. (1972). Giving up as a final common pathway to change in health. *Advances in Psychosomatic Medicine, 8*, 20–40.

Schoenborn, C. A., & Marans, M. (1988). *Current estimates from the National Health Interview Survey: United States, 1987* (Vital and Health Statistics, Series 10, No. 166, DHHS Publication No. PHS 88–1594). Washington, DC: U.S. Government Printing Office.

Schonfeld, D. (1991). The child's cognitive understanding of illness. In M. Lewis (Ed.), *Child and adolescent psychiatry: A comprehensive textbook* (pp. 949–953). Baltimore: Williams & Wilkins.

Shanow, P. T., Ferguson, D. M., & Diamond, M. E. (1984). Early hospital admissions and subsequent behavioral problems in six-year-olds. *Archives of Disease in Childhood, 59*, 815–819.

Stuber, M. L., Nader, K., Yasuda, P., Pynoos, R. N., & Cohen, S. (1991). Stress responses after pediatric bone marrow transplantation: Preliminary results of a prospective longitudinal study. *Journal of the American Academy of Child and Adolescent Psychiatry, 30*(6), 952–957.

Walker, D. K., Gortmaker, S. L., & Weitzman, M. (1981). Chronic illness and psychosocial problems among children in Genesee county. *Community Child Health Studies.* Cambridge, MA: Harvard School of Public Health.

PART IV

ENVIRONMENTAL SETTINGS AND THEIR INTERACTIONS WITH INDIVIDUAL DIFFERENCES

12

Temperament and the Developmental Niche

Charles M. Super and Sara Harkness

The flowering of temperament theory over the last quarter century has asserted and elaborated an important perspective on individual behavior. In the process it has also contributed to a uniquely productive dialectic with our understanding of children's environments. Within the framework of Thomas and Chess's New York Longitudinal Study (NYLS), the initial focus on individual dispositions grew into an emphasis on the interplay of temperament and environment. For scientists concerned with the role of environmental factors in development, this emphasis stimulated a reexamination of earlier assumptions. In this chapter we will describe a theoretical framework—the developmental niche—that was developed in part to accommodate the lessons of temperament theory. We will illustrate its utility in cross-cultural research, and finally, returning to the clinical origins of Chess and Thomas's work, we will consider how the niche perspective can be applied to the task of parent guidance.

FROM DIFFICULT INFANT TO GOODNESS OF FIT

Recognition that some individual variations in behavior are related to biologically based differences in temperament was, when it came, a landmark change in developmental theory. As formulated by Thomas, Chess, and their associates (e.g., Thomas, Chess, Birch, Hertzig, & Korn, 1963), temperament theory was

The preparation of this chapter was supported in part by a grant from the Spencer Foundation. All statements made and views expressed are the sole responsibility of the authors.

originally intended as a corrective to the overly environmental zeitgeist of the late 1950s, as an objection in particular to the then dominant psychoanalytic and social-learning assumptions about the experiential basis of such differences (see Chess & Thomas, 1984, p. 14). The voluminous amount research that followed, not only from the NYLS investigators but also from others, has documented the importance of constitutional differences and has given them a prominent place in many textbooks on human development. Debates continue, to be sure, about the particular dimensions of temperamental variation, their stability over time and across situations, and the most effective way to measure such dispositions. That all these debates take place within a general assumption of the existence of temperamental variation in infancy and childhood, however, is testimony to a profound shift over the past decades in views on socialization and the emergence of psychopathology.

Of particular interest to many psychologists and psychiatrists has been the confluence of temperamental characteristics identified by the NYLS researchers as the "difficult infant" syndrome. In the original formulation, for a group of middle-class New Yorkers, the syndrome centered on an infant who was negative in mood, irregular in biological rhythms, intense in response, withdrawing from new experiences, and slow to adapt (Chess & Thomas, 1984). Infants and young children with these characteristics were particularly problematic for their families, disrupting daily functioning, depriving parents of sleep, and creating interpersonal stresses. Over time, young children with high ratings on this constellation of traits were found in the New York study to have poorer ratings of behavioral adjustment than those who did not fit the "difficult" picture.

The NYLS researchers were insightful in quickly following up their early work with a contrast sample, one of working-class families of Puerto Rican background. In these families there was much less demand for the early establishment of regular sleep and feeding schedules, for the early acquisition of self-feeding and self-dressing skills, and for quick adaptation to new situations and new people— the very demands that proved stressful for children with a "difficult temperament." The pattern of environmental demands was different, and hence the functional characteristics of the syndrome were different. Correspondingly, it was found that early ratings of difficult temperament did not predict poor adjustment prior to school age in this group of Puerto Rican children (Korn & Gannon, 1983). Other characteristics, however, did present an opportunity for a poor match between the child and the environment. Activity level, for example, was a contributor to half of the clinical referrals that emerged from the Puerto Rican study, while this was not true in the original middle-class sample, who lived in more spacious and less densely populated apartments.

This early cultural comparison highlighted an observation that was also evident from examination of individual case studies in the NYLS: Although temperamental dispositions are present early in life, their functional significance for development is evident only in the context of particular family expectations and demands. Goodness of fit between individual temperament and specific environment, not either one alone, has become the more robust construct for developmental theory. The evolution of a powerful model of temperamental individuality, in short, necessarily turned attention to the nature of the environment as well. The first postulate contributed by temperament theory to this reexamination of the environment is that different kinds of environments find various temperament constellations differentially acceptable.

A second postulate is presented in Bell's (1968) landmark reinterpretation of the socialization literature, in which he suggested that individual variations in behavior (such as those related to temperament) differentially elicit responses from caretakers. The environment is not an unyielding mold, pressing uniformly on all children. Fussy and calm children, fearful and bold ones, do not call forth the same reactions from parents, peers, siblings, and teachers. Children contribute to the construction of their own social space, and thus to the direction of their own development. Empirical research on this proposition has been slow to accumulate, but the principle of innate dispositions differentially eliciting environmental responses is now widely accepted, and new elaborations have added to the strength of this position (e.g., Plomin, Loehlin, & DeFries, 1985).

From these two postulates—that different kinds of environments find various temperaments differentially suitable, and that within any type of environment various temperaments elicit different responses—it is but a small step to realize that different environments have different patterns of responding to individuals from across the spectra of temperament. Behind the patterns, one can imagine, there must be systematic regulation of the environment incorporating structural features beyond the immediate interface with the child. Further, one might ask in what other ways such environmental regulation structures the course of development. To accommodate the two postulates concerning the interaction of temperament and environment, in other words, one is led to a new set of perceptions and questions about the dynamic organization of children's environments.

THE DEVELOPMENTAL NICHE AND THE
PATTERNING OF ENVIRONMENTAL RESPONSIVENESS

It is a central tenet of social anthropology that elements of the human environment are connected in an orderly manner. Economic production, kinship structures, political organization, moral values, patterns of child rearing, and all other features of human culture are recognized to be systematically interrelated. Culture, in short, is a system in the formal sense, an open system with self-regulating subsystems that are constantly adjusting to external forces as well as internal dynamics. Relating this principle to developmental issues has been a continuing challenge in psychological anthropology (e.g., LeVine, 1973; Whiting & Edwards, 1988; Whiting & Whiting, 1975). A framework we have found useful in examining the interaction of culture and development, drawing on these traditions, is to take a child's-eye view, looking outward to see the impact of cultural reality on the "developmental niche" (Harkness & Super, 1983, 1985; Super & Harkness, 1986).

In brief, the child's developmental niche has three subsystems: (1) the physical and social settings in which the child lives; (2) the customs of child care and child rearing provided and promoted by the community; and (3) the psychology of the caretakers, including their affective orientation and their beliefs and values about children and the nature of growth. Homeostatic mechanisms tend to keep the three subsystems in harmony with each other and appropriate to the developmental level and individual characteristics of the child (including temperament). Nevertheless, the three components have different relationships to other features of the larger environment and thus constitute somewhat independent sources of disequilibrium. Regularities within and among the subsystems and thematic continuities and progressions across the niches of infancy and childhood provide material from which the child abstracts the social, affective, and cognitive rules of the culture.

Our comparative research in Kenya and the United States demonstrates how the three components of the developmental niche operate to define what temperamental characteristics are difficult for most families in the two settings, and also how they structure the pattern of familial responses to children with different dispositions. In Kokwet, a small farming community of Kipsigis people in the Western Highlands of Kenya, where we lived in the early 1970s, daily life for infants was set in the homestead, in and around the family's cluster of thatched- or tin-roof huts. For infants over 4 months old, much of the immediate caretaking was the responsibility of an older sister, a customary arrangement in many East African communities (Harkness & Super, 1991). The mother was usually available if needed, for she would be doing household or farm chores nearby, such as food preparation, cleaning, or weeding in the fields. However, it was the sister who tended to most of the baby's immediate needs, holding, entertaining, and putting to rest, or taking the baby to the mother for nursing when distraction, soothing, body contact, and rocking would no longer satisfy a fussy child. A variety of beliefs about the nature of infant needs and child capabilities supported this arrangement (see Super & Harkness, 1992).

In Kokwet, as in the original New York study and in a middle-class sample of our own in suburban Boston, there was a constellation of infant characteristics that was particularly troublesome, unpleasantly demanding on family members and disruptive of the preferred routines for efficient household functioning. The particular behaviors that made up this constellation, however, were somewhat different from those of the NYLS's difficult infant syndrome. Rather than the intense, arrhythmic, and negative infant who was difficult in the U.S., study, in Kokwet the troublesome baby was one who was easily upset, could not be comforted by back-carrying, and thus required intervention on the part of the already busy mother rather than the older sister.

Beyond this static difference in what constellation of infant characteristics proved most disruptive in the two groups, one can also find a more dynamic illustration of how families adapt to their infants, or of how the pattern of responses elicited by the same characteristic varies between cultural groups. Rhythmicity, to use the strongest example, correlates strongly with the amount of caretaking by the mother (compared to others) in both samples—but in opposite directions. American infants *low* on Rhythmicity spent more of their time interacting with their mothers. Those who were more predictable apparently facilitated an efficient distribution of time by their mothers away from them, tending to other tasks and projects, while those who scored lower on Rhythmicity either could not so easily be left, or required the mother's renewed attention sooner. In Kokwet, in contrast, it was the infants *high* in Rhythmicity who spent more time interacting with their mothers. Presumably, the mother who could depend on some kind of schedule from her baby could more easily arrange to be available for feeding and socialization when the baby was likely to be awake and need her. But if that was not possible (and it would be less possible as the infant was more unpredictable in timing), it was not of such importance as to require a major adjustment of the mother's tasks. This appears to be the central difference between the two cultural systems. In Kokwet the older sister would be in charge of entertaining the baby and coming to find the mother when necessary. Contrastingly, a reliance on secondary caretakers was discouraged in metropolitan Boston by the logistics of maternal activities, as well as beliefs about the importance of responsive maternal care for the establishment of emotional attachment.

ACADEMIC PERSPECTIVES

In each locale, the combination of physical and social settings, customary methods of care, and caretakers' beliefs about infant development jointly determined the pattern of environmental responses to the baby's individual characteristics. From the point of view of anthropological theory, this observation helps resolve longstanding problems with understanding both the divergence of behavioral development across cultures and the diversity of behavior within each group (LeVine, 1973; Wallace, 1961). Without a theory of temperament, psychological anthropology would have difficulty moving beyond the now abandoned notion of a prototypical personality shaped by each culture. With such a theoretical companion, anthropology is able to continue its traditional interest in how common meanings and thematic behaviors come to be salient within cultural groups, while at the same time accommodating the diversity of personalities and performance. In a single community, there will be shared customs, socially based beliefs about development, and an array of daily settings. The interplay of these subsystems and the patterns of meaning abstracted from them by children will bear strong similarity across families. But individual differences in personality and temperament will still flourish, and the available adaptations to infant characteristics will contribute further to the organization of individual diversity.

From the perspective of psychology, the pairing of temperament theory and the developmental niche elaborates recent developmental insights concerning the nature of the environment and its coevolutionary relationship with the individual (e.g., Sameroff & Chandler, 1975). It adds to the postulate of mutual responsivity a framework for understanding how that responsivity is organized, that is, for understanding the nature of environmental constraints on the coevolution of individual and context. Not all accommodations to a child are equally easy in any particular case; hence, some constellations of temperament will be more conducive to health or dysfunction than others.

CLINICAL PERSPECTIVES

Clinical recognition of child temperament as a central aspect of a presenting problem necessarily shifts attention to altering the environment. Chess and Thomas (1984) are explicit:

> The goodness of fit conceptualization of the origins and evolution of behavior disorders in children . . . provides a useful theoretical guide for implementing a parent guidance procedure in individual cases. The diagnosis of a behavior disorder in a child is assumed to result from a poorness of fit between the child's capacities, motivations, and/or behavioral style and the expectations and demands of the environment. An analysis can then be made which identifies the specific features of the child and environment which, in interaction with each other, are producing the poorness of fit and consequent psychopathological development. Once these specific features are identified, a program can then be formulated which will relieve the excessive stress . . . and ameliorate the symptoms. . . . This program can be spelled out with the parents, and their understanding and implemen-

tation of the specific changes to be made can be monitored in follow-up sessions. (pp. 252ff.)

Two aspects of this approach warrant highlighting: first, the way in which the clinician's attention is directed toward "specific features" of the child's immediate environment and, second, the central role accorded to parents as thoughtful ("understanding") mediators of the program for change. In both regards it is notable from the clinical perspective that the developmental niche is in part an individualist construct. Whatever commonality one child's niche shares with those of other children in the same family, community, or culture, the systematic environment for that child is unique, reflecting the particular family structure, history, and membership, as well as the peculiarities of coincidence. The clinical task of "relieving the stress" of poor fit through altering parental understanding addresses this issue directly.

The developmental niche perspective emphasizes homeostatic forces that bias against successful introduction of single, discordant elements; profound change occurs instead when the coordination of elements transforms the whole. Many a good program for stimulating behavioral change in children fails because it is never adequately implemented, and hindsight often suggests that failure occurs because of resistance to change in other aspects of the niche. In contrast, an intervention that recruits and coordinates support from all subsystems is more promising.

This can be illustrated with the case of the Papadopoulos family (a pseudonym), who consulted with one of us (CMS). The distractible, energetic, nonadaptable, and intense 8-year-old son was generally noncomplaint with parental requests, especially those involving any kind of family chores. His apparent inability to carry out even simple responsibilities was a source of considerable frustration to the mother, embarrassment to the father, and discord between the parents. The mother attributed much of the problem to the father's nearly complete absence from the boy's life—working two jobs, the father left early in the morning and came home after midnight, 6 days a week. Her weekday threats regarding the boy's behavior were usually forgotten by the time Sunday arrived. The father, on the other hand, saw at the core of the problem the mother's disorganization and her inability to define and execute household rules; she was, in his eyes, a failure as mother and manager of the home.

The initial intervention, a straightforward approach to behavior management, was devised with the parents and the boy after a brief course of group instruction for parents in behavior modification (four evenings). Two specific chores were selected: to clear the table after dinner and to feed the family pet, in each case to be done with no more than one reminder from the mother. Each evening the boy reviewed a task list with his mother, checked the completions and failures, and awarded himself gold stars for success, building toward a coveted prize. In the first 2 weeks of this plan, success was low (about 30% completion) and showed no promising trends. After another diagnostic session with the family, one small but essential change was made to the intervention. Instead of the gold stars being awarded each evening by the mother and boy together, a hierarchy of authorization was required. The boy signed the chart to indicate completion of his chores, the mother signed to indicate the accuracy of the chart, and the chart then was left on a hall table for the father to review and provide a final signature upon his midnight return home. Only then could the stars be given, usually the following day. With this single change—a complicated, unwieldy one from some perspectives—success in the chores came immediately, and the family moved ahead to address several underlying issues.

A variety of paradigms could be used to understand the dramatic results, including most obviously family systems theory (e.g., McGoldrick, Pearce, & Giordano, 1982). But if one focuses on the individual boy and the niche he inhabited, the essential aspect of the second intervention was its invocation of the customary authority relations for this very traditional Greek Orthodox family. In a symbolic way, the father was brought back into the daily setting of the boy's life. Previously, external forces had drawn the father out of the family's evening routines, and the custom of paternal authority was no longer mutually supportive with the social setting of family chores. In addition, the psychological expectations of the parents for each other's role were incompatible with the boy's noncompliance. It is noteworthy that had the child been of a different disposition—less distractible, more adaptable, and less intensely negative in his response to maternal reminders—the inconsistencies in the niche would not have been called forth to such salience. But provoked by the boy's behavior, the niche was unable to respond adaptively. Even though the parents understood the discrete behaviorist intervention and their motivation appeared sincere, implementation proved ineffective given the family's reliance on the authority of a father who was not actually present on a daily basis. The present perspective, in sum, brings to attention two sets of relationships. One concerns how the existing subsystems of the developmental niche have failed to respond constructively to the temperamental demands of the child. The second concerns how the proposed therapeutic elements will shift the coordination of the subsystems. To diagnose the behavior disorder and to envision the possible responses of the niche to intervention one must understand the meaningful subsystem relations in the particular family, which requires a sensitive clinical eye and an ethnographic posture (Harkness, Super, & Keefer, 1992a).

The method of parental guidance developed by Chess with an appreciation of temperament is explicit in the use of parental understanding to implement change. The psychological effect of explaining about temperament and goodness of fit to desperate parents is evident to anyone, clinician or neighbor, who has had occasion to do so: The parent is enormously relieved that "I didn't cause this whole thing" and has renewed energy to focus on changes in daily behavior. The nature of the problem is reframed, expectations for child behavior are altered, and attention is directed toward environmental management. Clinical recommendations often include alteration of the settings of daily life for the child, such as less TV, more supervision during peer play, scheduled time for homework, or outside, high-energy activity. Although social customs are not altered at the clinical level, the way parents use customs is an avenue of intervention. In a society as diverse as contemporary America, and in a domain as complex as child rearing, the perceptive clinician can often direct the parents to previously ignored customs (such as an infant-carrying pouch), or to common practices (such as use of rewards to build compliance) that diverge from "proper" prescriptions that are assumed but not strongly defended by the parents. In all these cases, the clinical task is to alter the conceptual model used by parents in directing their own behavior.

Curiously, we have little systematic knowledge about how such interventions are received by parents and incorporated into their thinking or actions. There is, to be sure, a substantial literature on theories and tactics in the treatment of the *child* for behavior disorders, and also a wealth of handbooks and programs for parent training, including some evaluations of patterns of success and failure. Parental belief systems, however, have only recently come under study in their own right (e.g., Goodnow & Collins, 1990; Harkness, Super, & Keefer, 1992b; Sigel, 1992). They can play a singularly potent role in clinical practice, as the Chess and Thomas model of parental guidance demonstrates. A systematic understanding of the child's environment, as facilitated by the developmental niche framework, can help the practitioner to work more effectively with parents to achieve the power that comes from coherence.

There is a pleasing symmetry to the broad sweep of effects induced by Thomas and Chess's insistence that behavioral individuality is present from the beginnings of infancy. Their work, and that of others inspired by them, has established a new domain of scientific understanding about the individual. It has also prompted theoretical reexamination of the environmental perspectives against which their work was a reaction. The synthesis of these two perspectives—individual and environmental—contributes to the resolution of theoretical and practical issues in both academic and clinical contexts.

REFERENCES

Bell, R. Q. (1968). A reinterpretation of the direction of effects in studies of socialization. *Psychological Review, 75*, 81–95.

Chess, S., & Thomas, A. (1984). *Origins and evolution of behavior disorders.* New York: Brunner/Mazel.

Goodnow, J. J., & Collins, W. A. (1990). *Development according to parents: The nature, sources, and consequences of parents' ideas.* Hove, England: Lawrence Erlbaum.

Harkness, S., & Super, C. M. (1983). The cultural construction of child development: A framework for the socialization of affect. *Ethos, 11*(4), 221–231.

Harkness, S., & Super, C. M. (1985). Child-environment interactions in the socialization of affect. In M. Lewis & C. Saarni (Eds.), *The socialization of emotions* (pp. 21–36). New York: Plenum Press.

Harkness, S., & Super, C. M. (1991). East Africa. In R. Hiner & J. M. Hawes (Eds.), *Children in comparative and historical perspective: An international handbook and research guide* (pp. 217–240). Westport, CT: Greenwood Press.

Harkness, S., Super, C. M., & Keefer, C. H. (1991, April). *Ask the doctor: The role of the pediatrician in the development of American parental ethnotheories.* Paper presented at biannual meeting of the Society for Research in Child Development, Seattle.

Harkness, S., Super, C. M., & Keefer, C. H. (1992a). Culture and ethnicity. In M. D. Levine, W. B. Carey, & A. C. Crocker (Eds.), *Developmental-behavioral pediatrics* (2nd ed., pp. 103–108). Philadelphia: W.B. Saunders.

Harkness, S., Super, C. M., & Keefer, C. H. (1992b). Learning to be an American parent: How cultural models gain directive force. In R. G. D'Andrade & C. Strauss (Eds.), *Cultural models and motivation.* (pp. 163–178). Cambridge: Cambridge University Press.

Korn, S., & Gannon, S. (1983). Temperament, culture variation, and behavior disorders in preschool children. *Child Psychiatry and Human Development, 13*, 203–212.

LeVine, R. A. (1973). *Culture, behavior, and personality.* Chicago: Aldine.

McGoldrick, M., Pearce, J. K., & Giordano, J. (Eds.). (1982). *Ethnicity and family therapy.* New York: Guilford Press.

Plomin, R., Loehlin, J. C., & DeFries, J. C. (1985). Genetic and environmental components of "environmental" influences. *Developmental Psychology, 21*, 391–402.

Sameroff, A. J., & Chandler, M. J. (1975). Reproductive risk and the continuum of care-taking casualty. In F. D. Horowitz (Ed.), *Review of child development research* (Vol. 4). Chicago: University of Chicago Press.

Sigel, I. (Ed.). (1992). *Parental belief systems: The psychological consequences for children and families* (rev. ed.). Hillsdale, NJ: Lawrence Erlbaum.

Super, C. M., & Harkness, S. (1981). Figure, ground, and gestalt: The cultural context of the active individual. In R. M. Lerner & N. A. Busch-Rossnagel (Eds.), *Individuals as producers of their development: A life-span perspective* (pp. 69–86). New York: Academic Press.

Super, C. M., & Harkness, S. (1982). The infant's niche in rural Kenya and metropolitan America. In L. L. Adler (Ed.), *Cross-cultural research at issue* (pp. 47–55). New York: Academic Press.

Super, C. M., & Harkness, S. (1986). The developmental niche: A conceptualization at the interface of child and culture. *International Journal of Behavioral Development*, *9*, 545–570.

Super, C. M., & Harkness, S. H. (1992). *The cultural regulation of temperament-environment interactions.* Unpublished manuscript.

Thomas, A., Chess, S., Birch, H. G., Hertzig, M., & Korn, S. (1963). *Behavioral individuality in early childhood.* New York: New York University Press.

Wallace, A. F. C. (1961). *Culture and personality.* New York: Random House.

Whiting, B. B., & Edwards, C. P. (1988). *Children of different worlds: The formation of social behavior.* Cambridge, MA: Harvard University Press.

Whiting, B. B., & Whiting, J. W. M. (1975). *Children of six cultures: A psycho-cultural analysis.* Cambridge, MA: Harvard University Press.

13

Kids in Context: Temperament in Cross-Cultural Perspective

Marten W. deVries

Child growing so big
Weighing heavy on your mama's back
Kicking your stocky feet
Careless on your mama's tursh
Child boy and buck skin
Firmly pressing mama's breasts
Child boy with kinky hair
terraces on your round head
What will you grow to be like
Off your mother's back
Off the grass matres
Away from the bleating goats by the river
Will you grow up to be. . . .

—WALTER BGOYA
Ngora, Tanzania, 1967

It was a brisk sunny morning in a Kikuyu settlement in the Kenya Highlands. Florence, a 34-year-old mother of three children, was pregnant and working in her field of cassava and corn. Her husband was at work, her sister lived a mile away, and her children were in school or playing at a homestead nearby.

126

Florence had felt contractions since 4:00 A.M. and had prepared her bedside table with a sharp, clean knife, some string to tie the cord, and a number of cloths and blankets before going to farm. Feeling the contractions quickening, she retired to her bed, and alone delivered an active, male infant without complications. After a brief rest, she announced the birth to the neighbors and sent word to her husband and family.

Five days later, as part of a comparative infant development and temperament study among Kikuyu, Masai, and Digo infants, I examined the boy at her home using the Brazelton Neonatal Behavioral Assessment Scale (NBAS). The baby was extraordinarily alert and active. In fact, he turned out to be the most active, well-organized, and stable infant of all the Kikuyu babies I examined. In general, infants examined at home were better organized and stable than those born in the hospital (deVries & Super, 1978). Moreover, the group of mothers who delivered alone at home, in contrast to those at home with family or doctors present, gave birth to the most competent infants. As Florence's son illustrates, these babies were the most stable, organized, interactional, and active. Although many factors could account for such findings, including birth order, testing conditions, and the circumstances that lead to the seeking of hospital attention for delivery (deVries & Super, 1978), at least some aspects of family structure or maternal behavior or control of delivery may have played a beneficial role in the infant's performance during the first weeks of life (deVries, 1987a). This vignette is one of many that illustrate that even at the beginning of life, a multiplicity of influences affect developmental outcome.

Infant temperament, when examined through the lens of cross-cultural research, tends naturally to bring into focus the power of social and environmental influences on development. Cross-cultural studies provide the opportunity for distinguishing the multiple environmental forces that affect development from the child's own contribution, a central concern in the work of Alexander Thomas and Stella Chess. Thirty years of study have made it clear that children's developmental options are created or removed by the interplay of sociocultural and personal factors at the outset of their lives, and that these factors strongly influence the remainder of their development.

Cases in this chapter that illustrate this interplay are drawn from a study inspired by the New York Longitudinal Study (Thomas, Chess, Birch, Hertzig, & Korn, 1963). The cross-cultural study was designed to investigate the role that temperament played in developmental outcome within the first year of life and assess the different familial and cultural reactions to infant "difficulty" in three East African societies. A mix of ethnographic and quantitative techniques was used to gather systematic information on child-rearing practices and maternal and family expectations, as well as infant characteristics. The infant temperament questionnaire (ITQ) developed by Carey (1970) provided a useful tool for describing infants in different sociocultural settings. Although there has been some controversy (Bates, 1980), temperament and the "difficulty" concept have proved developmentally important and, perhaps most importantly, clinically relevant (Thomas & Chess, 1980). Whether the difficult temperament concept was measurable across cultures and to what extent culturally guided infant care practices influenced temperament and development were examined (deVries, 1989). To do this a brief longitudinal design, beginning with neonatal measurements such as the Brazelton NBAS (deVries & Super, 1978), cognitive and psychomotor measures appropriate to the first months of life, ITQ-temperament evaluations at 4 to 8 months, spot observations, and interviews about child-rearing patterns were used. A follow-up of most of the children took place later during their first year. A subgroup of difficult and easy Digo and Masai children has been visited every 4 to 5 years since the initial study. The variables collected in this way were placed within a model of four categories of influence on infant development: the child's fit with the mother and family, the impact of cultural child-rearing practices, the physical environment, and infant characteristics. The model argues for increasing the scope of variables when evaluating temperament outcomes. Although much of the data in the study is quantitative at the group level (deVries & Sameroff, 1984; deVries, 1984), the model and clinical utility of temperament are best brought into perspective by means of examining representative cases.

The cases are drawn from a study of 178 infants from three Kenyan societies that differ on a number of environmental dimensions. The study explored which aspects of the environment interacted with temperament characteristics. Strong associations were found for cultural child-rearing patterns, the degree of modernization, cultural and maternal expectations, ecological setting, and specific early life events (deVries & Sameroff, 1984). These factors were related to measures of temperament and influenced developmental course. The portraits that follow demonstrate a diversity of developmental outcome and highlight the nonlinearity of development over a period of 17 years. Such information underscores the need for flexible clinical responses and for assessing risk and infant difficulty using more complex models that include sociocultural and environmental factors. The temperament concept not only brings the infant's contribution to the surface but also renders visible other factors that impinge on development. Infant temperament then brings into relief the environment in which the infant is embedded.

TEMPERAMENT AND GOODNESS OF FIT

Hamadi was a shy, often frightened, and distressed secondary school student of 18. In 1991, these traits were evident on both temperament tests and in interviews. At the age of 3 months, however, it was a different story. Hamadi could sit, was bowel and bladder trained, and had a normal temperament with strong approach tendencies. He was active and motorically competent. In 1974, he was the most advanced infant in the Kikuyu, Digo, and Masai sample on the Bayley motor and mental tests. Moreover, his mother was caring and warm, and his father interested and supportive. Hamadi was a Digo boy, who lived with his family of four siblings in a fishing and agrarian community of approximately 3,000 people on the tropical Kenyan coast, in a family that had sufficient resources. During the first 4 years of his life, Hamadi was seen as an extraordinarily skilled and socially active young boy. In school, he did not live up to expectations. During this time, he experienced himself as shy and others noted that he had become withdrawn. At the same time, his activity level increased over previous temperament measures (2 SD above other Digo children of the same age). How was Hamadi's early energetic, intellectual capacity transformed to withdrawal, shyness, and gradually to fear, anger, and overactivity? In interviews, his teachers and parents stated that they could not accommodate Hamadi's energetic style sufficiently. They implied that his active curiosity did not "fit" with Digo ideas of what a young boy should be like and that this had led to continual friction and conflict, which further contributed to his behavior. The poor "fit" between Hamadi and his cultural environment, of course, is not the only contribution to his behavior, although other environmental psychosocial and functional risk factors were not found. The case does illustrate how a child at low risk and with strong adaptive capacity, in a culture that has other goals, such as "leveling" and not rewarding excellence, developed a poor behavioral adjustment, becoming a withdrawn, shy and overactive, chaotic young man.

Enkeri was born in Masai land in early 1974. He, like Hamadi, was behaviorally competent, but Enkeri on temperament evaluation scored "difficult" (deVries, 1984). He was more intense, persistent, and active, while less distractible and rhythmic in daily behavior. In general, Enkeri cried and fussed more and was less "adaptive" than his age mates. These are all characteristics that place children at risk for behavioral problems and trauma in Western cultures (Thomas et al., 1963; Carey, 1970). Characteristics of this kind, however, are valued and admired in Masai infants and children. The Masai live a pastoral life-style, herding cattle and goats within the East African Rift Valley that straddles the Kenyan Tanzanian–frontier. They subsist at the edge of the semiarid savannah's capacity to sustain human life, in an environment where infant characteristics like Enkeri's may be useful for survival.

At 4 months, Enkeri was normal in height and weight for Kenyan infants (Vogel, Muller, Odingo, Onyango, & de Geus, 1974). This was unusual during the middle of 1974, a period when the drought took hold of Masai land with a vengance. Grazing land, already reduced by the dry season a year before, disappeared, and 80% of Enkeri's father's herd was lost. Under normal circumstances, much of Masai infants' supplemental diet is derived from cattle and goat's milk. Many infants died during this period as a result of maternal and infant malnutrition and secondary causes such as measles and illness related to disturbances of breast feeding and poorly prepared substitute dry milk. As the drought worsened, Enkeri lost substantial weight, but survived, as did most infants with similar "difficult" temperament characteristics. That the difficult infants survived was a surprise, since this "difficult" group was assumed to be at risk like those vulnerable in the West. Among the Masai, a Western urban "poor fit" became "good fit." The cultural expectation that Masai babies should be active and assertive had provided a survival advantage for Enkeri as did demand breast feeding of "fussy" babies. Under these circumstances, instead of being a risk factor, difficult temperament proved to be protective in this period of drought and the high mortality of his peers. Some children with "easy" temperaments in the study did not survive. The interaction of temperament, culturally maintained expectations of "what an infant is," and associated child-rearing and feeding techniques helped transform this potential high-risk infant into a survivor (deVries, 1987b, 1989). This mechanism holds up to a number of alternative explanations such as the influence of prior health status and family variables. In the total Kenyan study, difficult infants were also larger than the easy ones, perhaps from nursing more frequently. Rapid weight gain among "difficult" children in the West (Carey, 1985) and ethnographic observations among the hunter-gatherers (Konner & Worthman, 1980), in shanty towns in Brazil (Scheper-Hughes, 1987), and of aboriginal infants (Chisholm, 1983) also support this finding. In all these settings infant crying is responded to with breast feeding and subsequent growth. If the infant does not cry, he or she is assumed not to be hungry. Breast feeding in the West is elective for mothers, while in Africa it may be a matter of life and death. In the West the "distance" from environmental pressure is large, but in Africa, Brazil, and the Australian bush land, environmental pressure such as drought and infectious diseases is an omnipresent aspect of the environment. In the lives of the infants studied these selective pressures were palpable. Such environmental conditions highlight adaptive processes often obscured by the well-developed social security and economic system in Western societies. The subsistence economies studied are just that. They exist at the edge of the carrying capacity of the environment, and both child and culture must adjust to survive in this reality.

At 13 Enkeri became a warrior with his age-mates. Some years later he ambivalently entered primary school after much discussion with his family. His father had been able to replenish his herd since 1974, and sell cattle for school fees. Then Enkeri was caught between school and warrior activities. At school, with its authoritarian orientation, his temperament style of high activity and low adaptability, coupled with his tendency to get angry in relation to authoritarian instruction, often got him into disciplinary problems. These troubles had him long for the easier and freer life of a warrior. Earlier, when Enkeri's temperament had fit nicely with the Masai expectation of infancy and warriorhood, these difficult characteristics were socially reinforced and maintained throughout early development. Later, in the school situation, the temperament characteristics that contributed to his survival as a baby and his competence as a warrior created problems. In his new niche of schoolboy in a developing Kenya, these characteristics were of little use.

In the cases of Hamadi and Enkeri, the fit or clash of cultural expectations and individual characteristics contributed to developmental outcomes such as school performance, health, and psychological well-being. Growth and survival could be facilitated at one stage while behavioral difficulty was fostered at another. Such nonlinearity of development is complex. Description of the development of Digo twins during the first year of life illustrates the complex way culture places its stamp in attempting to assure continuity in the characteristics of its members.

ASSURING SURVIVAL: DIGO TWINS

Fatuma, who did not expect or want twins, or the cesarian section required to bear them, sat listless, almost mute, staring into the distance on the fourth day after delivery. One of the twins was considerably smaller and scored poorly on the NBAS. The small infant had decreased alertness and visual following and poor defensive movements and was almost incapable of the pull-to-sit maneuver. During the early postpartum period, Fatuma shunned both infants, but eventually, on the eighth day, she began caring for the larger active infant while ignoring the smaller one. On the tenth day, when it was time to leave the hospital, Fatuma was still not caring for the smaller infant in spite of the best efforts of the hospital staff and other mothers. The smaller infant was at extreme risk, given the negative maternal attitude, poor neonatal competence, harsh perinatal experience, and the stress that the twins would create in this economically marginal family.

At a 2 to 3 month follow-up visit Fatuma still expressed negative feelings toward the smaller infant. The grandmother and sister had assumed much of the caretaking. Both infants were obviously ill, and the smaller one seemed irritable and lethargic. A traditional doctor was called who shrewdly diagnosed a "depression" caused by a complex of social and witchcraft factors resulting from the surgical intervention that had left her vulnerable to spirit possession. This amounted to a rationale for maternal "neglect." Accordingly, he based his intervention on the Digo belief that infants have increased social needs and capacities at 3 months of age and prescribed that Fatuma attend more directly to her infant's communications. Fatuma's mother should teach her how to do this. Moreover, the spirit possession could be ameliorated by a ritual healing dance, thereby essentially activating a Digo ad hoc aid group. All prescriptions were carried out.

At the 4 to 6 month follow-up, tests showed that the now only slightly smaller infant performed better on both social and coordination items of the Bayley test. The temperament profile gathered from Fatuma and her mother showed a more active, intense, negative, withdrawn, and persistent infant who was less distractible and rhythmic. The mother still reported not liking the infant and carried out only minimal caretaking, but the child's demanding style was a strong solicitor of care from the mother and other female kin. At 4 months, the "at-risk" infant with numerous predisposing risk factors scored "difficult" on her temperament evaluation but had surpassed her more able twin. I think this transformation highlights the influence of the traditional social security system—starting with Fatuma's form of marriage. She paid a low bride price that provided maximal freedom of choice and economic power. This gave her the freedom to elicit care from distant kin and to move her homestead closer to a supportive maternal uncle. Her well-to-do uncle, her mother's brother, was capable of financing the healing ritual and providing prescribed support. Digo ideas about "what a baby is" and the expected sequence of infant development with rapid increases in motoric and social competence during the first year (deVries & deVries, 1977) guided specific training intervention of both the grandmother and the traditional healer. The Digo notion of the causality in pediatric illness held that the child's problems resulted from maternal resource depletion, created in this case by postoperative vulnerability to spirit possession. The problem could thus be defined as a social one, spirit possession, enabling society to interfere directly by means of healing rituals to limit the threat to the infant. A second factor was the availability of competent female kin, who, because of their early child care experience as young girls, had been trained in specific Digo infant care practices that facilitated the transfer of maternal care. These factors embedded the care of the twins (twins are also valued by the Digo, in contrast to many other societies) in society at large, supplementing maternal infant care deficits. This influx of multiple levels of support from society and maternal kin enabled the at-risk twin to pull up and surpass her sibling. Which factor directly contributed to the smaller twin's better performance—her release from maternal depression, her temperament characteristics, the superior rearing skills of other women, or better supplementary feeding—cannot be completely ascertained, but the response of the group certainly played a role in this developmental outcome.

The twins' story also points out the vulnerability of babies in changing social systems when new methods are inadequately available and old ones no longer viable. In contrast to then, the case of Fatuma's twins in disrupted Digo society of the 1990s might have resulted in a situation where the traditional healer was not active enough, or a marriage residence pattern in which the wife and husband moved away from supportive kin, either of which would have tended to maintain the high-risk level. If the idea of "what a baby is" had been westernized, the child would not have been expected to act socially at 2 to 3 months. In short, a more passive approach to the smaller infant would likely have resulted in mortality. As in Enkeri's story, "difficult" temperament traits resulted in the survival of "fussy" babies; a similar mechanism may be at work here. "Difficulty" may be conceptualized as the baby's contribution to the rearing environment under harsh conditions that assures that he or she will not be ignored.

MULTIPLE-INFLUENCE TRANSACTION MODEL

A simple model is required to organize the multiplicity of influences on the developing child so that our conception of risk and protective factors may be accommodated clinically and include both individual and environmental realities. Since problems and solutions come from a variety of sources that differ in their impact during different stages of development, there is no simple prediction of risk possible; instead, a multiplicity of potential factors need to be taken into account. The Masai cases are particularly instructive; a risk in Western cities becomes a survival advantage on the equatorial savannah, convincingly demonstrating that development can be understood only in context. Context then needs to be included in our analysis of infant characteristics.

Models for viewing infant development as transactions with the environment (Sameroff, 1975; Sameroff & Chandler, 1975) and the mechanism for how cultural child-rearing practices are tuned to specific environmental challenges that guide development and protect against environmental risk have been described (LeVine, 1974; Super & Harkness, 1986; Whiting & Whiting, 1973). In this model, the above processes and descriptions are included and categorized into four domains of influence on infant development: the infants' own contribution, the mother and family, the physical-environmental contribution, and the sociocultural contribution. Today, these four elements may be quantitatively defined by means of field research and psychometric strategies. The first contribution is the developing individual's own characteristics over time. These include the temperamental and life historical characteristics that make up the core of individuals' personal experience. Second, is the important role of the mother or significant other caretaker. Her function is contingent on a series of internal mental states and social pressures often quite removed from the input of the infant. Further, we may include here the absence or presence of siblings and the availability of a limited or extended kin network. In certain cultures the father, ritual leaders, or mother's brother may play an important role in providing protection. The third aspect is the physical environment, the adaptive niche, whether it is the carpeted, furnished living room of a New York or Paris apartment, or a mud and dung wattle dwelling on the Masai plain. This includes the availability of physical resources, economic means, and concrete physical aspects of the environment (which, for example, could include alkaline soil, which keeps urine from putrifying on the hut floor, thereby rendering biological toilet training slips tolerable, in comparison to the Persian rug on the dining room floor, which is now stained for eternity). The fourth level with which this chapter is most concerned is cultural: the blueprint for development that a group manufactures in order to maintain its socioeconomic system in a particular environmental niche. Specifically, such blueprints have a clear concept of "what an infant and child is," a temporal model of developmental sequence for the child and the related expectations of infant response to the culturally defined skill-training interaction (LeVine, 1974). As we observed in the case of Digo twins, the cultural blueprint for development, social role expections, and the availability of other caretakers are some of the ways that culture can play a contributing or hindering role in development.

Another striking example of how culture mediates child development, by prescribing training interactions and setting expectations for developmental timing, is the Digo toilet-training technique. This nurturant behavioral conditioning exchange between mother and infant begins soon after birth and involves placing the baby in particular positions when the infant shows signs of wishing to urinate and defecate. The infant soon associates the proper place and maternal sound with this position, and relatively quickly defecates and urinates only under these conditions (deVries & deVries, 1977). In the majority of cases, bowel and bladder training is achieved around the fifth month. This capacity for early training is based on the Digo idea that the child can learn from birth. The impact of the Digo values is further evident when we compare the Digo with the genetically similar Bantu group, the Kikuyu, who live north of Nairobi in the highland area of Kenya. This is a wet, often gray temperate climate where infants have greater risk of upper respiratory tract infection. The Kikuyu live in homesteads within villages. They tend to be farmers or work for wages in urban Kenya. Among Kikuyu, although they are relatively more active infant trainers than Western cultures (Leiderman, Babu, Kagia, Kraemer, & Leiderman, 1973), the concept that a child can learn from birth is less dominant than it is among the Digo. The Kikuyu view the infant as quite vulnerable at birth. For example, the child may not be carried on the back immediately as babies are in other African societies. Training is thought not immediately possible and must await a developmental growth in competence. We thus have a natural experiment; the Digo mothers are training early and their counterparts among the Kikuyu are training relatively later. Examining development milestones (see Table 13-1), we can observe the effect of training.

The timing of cultural developmental sequences may be very specific. The child may not be named for 2 to 3 months, as is the case among the Masai. The

TABLE 13-1
Differences between Digo and Kikuyu Infants in the
Accomplishment of Some Developmental Milestones

	Age at Milestone (Months)	
	Digo (N = 40)	Kikuyu (N = 40)
Sit	5–6	6–7
Stand	8–10	10–12
Walk	10–12	12–14
Vocalization	16	16
Toilet training	5	24–36
Weaning	18	6

labeling of the developmental stage transition from infant to toddler may take place at the end of the first year by the Digo, or after 3 years by the Kikuyu. The period of infancy-related vulnerability is thus prolonged among the Kikuyu and reduced among the Digo. Concepts of developmental timing and specific training techniques are culturally prescribed and have a remarkable effect on outcome, as was demonstrated in developmental milestones by the case of Fatuma's twins and by the strong tribal influence on temperament in the 3 societies in the study (deVries & Sameroff, 1984).

The model presented above focuses on the child as a process in time, in which temperament measures provide a clear operationalized description of adaptive style. The model may be clinically used to calculate risk and protection as well as help us understand in simplified form the factors that shape development in longitudinal research. Some key aspects of this model should be stressed. First of all, it is unlikely that any single component is sufficient to create problems or solutions over time—for example, the fit of "difficulty" with Masai rearing practices. Second, the multiple factors must persist over time in order to have a developmental effect. The concept of troublesomeness rather than difficulty is probably more useful then. Troublesomeness with multiple contributors such as the mother, the environment, the culture, and the individual contribution is a better way to understand the developmental outcome over time related to temperament than is the exclusive focus on the child's temperament.

The case of Bakari, given below, illustrates the situation where multiple factors influence the continuity of temperament problems over time, thereby *maintaining* and not transforming the impact of negative temperament traits. In his life, maternal and familial shortcomings as well as aspects of the physical environment exacerbated the problems created by difficult temperament.

BAKARI: THE MAINTENANCE OF RISK

I found Bakari at the age of 17, in 1991, "hanging around" the main street where he had grown up. He complained of a broken rib he had recently received while fishing for lobster to be sold to the new hotels that had developed in his lifetime along the Kenyan coast. He had been thrown by the surf against the barrier reef. Bakari's history of traumatic life events had continued to unfold. He both had a "difficult" temperament measured on the ITQ in 1974 and was considered "troublesome" by both his mother and his grandmother. Before Bakari was born, during my daily comings and goings in the village, I had noticed his mother, dressed in bright blue, sitting quietly at the fringe of activities often with her hand on her head, conspiciously immobile within the dynamic movements of Msambweni's daily routine of markets, chatter, and scurrying children: a picture of melancholia. She had not recovered from the death of her husband a year and a half previously. She now lived in the busiest part of the village in a rented room in the house of Bakari's grandmother; with her lived three of her five children, the other two being cared for by her deceased husband's family. She was not married to Bakari's biological father.

Bakari was thus born to a depressed mother under difficult economic and marital circumstances, after a pregnancy in which the mother felt "ill and weak," and during which she experienced repeated dreams that she was not going to survive. The mother expected a happy, pliable child who met the cultural ideals of an active Digo infant. Instead, fussy Bakari was born, after a painful 13-hour labor that the mother experienced as punishment. She resented this and remained angry throughout the first 2 to 3 months of Bakari's life. Depressive feelings smoldered throughout the first 2 years. Bakari was the opposite of pliable and happy; he was active, intense, and fussy. Although he soon slept through the night in his mother's bed, responded well to breast feeding, and had normal developmental milestones (except for walking somewhat late), he was a very clingy baby who could not tolerate the absence of his mother. Bakari grew up causing stress to his already stressed mother. The problem was compounded by the fact that the mother could not walk to her garden 5 miles away to cultivate her crops for both money and food. She thus became more dependent on Bakari's father for economic support, an untenable position for a traditionally independent Digo female. When Bakari was 5 months, his mother was hospitalized for abdominal surgery, which resulted in complications and left her hospitalized for more than a month. Her mother moved in to care for the three children and Bakari. Bakari was left during this crucial developmental phase. Breast feeding was terminated. He developed repeated bouts of diarrhea and was treated at the hospital several times for asthma during this period. Maternal separation, while considered psychologically significant in the West, takes on more ominous proportions in Africa in groups with subsistence economics. In the total study in Kenya of the 178 infants, maternal separation during the first 4 months of life for periods of longer than 2 weeks was significantly associated with infant illness and delayed growth and development ($r = .5$ to $r = .8$, depending on culture) (deVries & Sameroff, 1984).

The grandmother managed the often overactive and fussy Bakari by maintaining almost constant contact. When the mother returned from the hospital to recuperate, Bakari became even more clingy than before. Like her own mother, Bakari's mother now attempted to spend more time with him. This led to even greater frustration, and she occasionally beat him for his fussiness, excessive curiosity, and exploratory behavior. During this period, Bakari fell into the cooking fire twice and received minor burns. During observations of this mother-infant pair, the mother was indeed in constant contact with the child; she made no attempt to disengage herself from his grasp, but neither did she interact actively with him. They acted upon each other. The mother appeared submissive, with little involvement, eye contact, or talk. When Bakari was 4, during a subsequent pregnancy of his mother, Bakari's maternal grandmother moved in to stay.

The set of problems that marked Bakari's first year of life continued but with less intensity. At the age of 6, he was attending primary school, learning to fish, and herding his father's goats. While herding, he damaged his leg and developed a tropical ulcer, a wound that did not heal completely for 4 years, interfering with school attendance and performance. His interest in school began to ebb but improved somewhat after the wound healed. Follow-up measures of temperament in 1981, 1986, 1991, using self-report and parental report formats, demonstrated continuity of his difficult temperament with marked withdrawal. In 1991, he had quit school and was fishing for a living. He was still markedly withdrawn in social situations and had just broken his ribs chancing the reef for economic gain. Despite Bakari's complex developmental history, the contribution of his own characteristics, the impact of maternal depression, and a series of traumatic life events and illnesses that resulted in less than optimal performance socially and in school, Bakari was noticeably optimistic about the future and was hoping to enter a school for mechanics in Nairobi. This optimism was supported by his mother's brother, who gave him his formal name at the age of 14. Recently, his uncle, a more "worldly" man, had introduced Bakari to new possibilities such as trade school. As with Fatuma's twin, kin involvement and responsibility had continually saved Bakari, initially with his grandmother's help and now with the help of his mother's brother. When I left, he and his uncle were actively seeking funds for mechanics school.

SOME CONCLUSIONS

The cases of Hamadi, Enkeri, the twins, and Bakari illustrate that individual differences take on varying significances depending on diverse factors in the environment, and that these influences shift over time even for the same individual. Competence or risk at any point in early development, whether, reached through normal developmental processes or by the interventions of others, is not linearly related to the child's competence and performance at a later time. The cases make clear that in order to complete the equation of prediction one needs to add the effects of physical, social, cultural, and family environments. Development and the influence of medical and social interventions can be understood only when a larger set of environmental and personal variables are considered. The model offered in this paper provides a design for the evaluation of maternal-family, social-cultural, physical-economic, and personal-biological contributions to outcome. These afford a means of simplifying and isolating the relative contributions to development so they may be included in planning interventions.

The environmental factors, however, yield their meaning only when they are brought into relationship with individual, constitutional characteristics such as infant temperament. Temperament brings maternal activities, the cultural plan, and environmental effects into perspective. Without this focus on the individual characteristics of the infant over time, or for that matter on the person in a larger medical frame of reference, understanding the environment and developmental transactions would be impossible. Although Alex Thomas and Stella Chess originally offered the temperament concept as a reaction to environmentalism "run wild," it is now precisely the concept of temperament that allows us to illustrate and understand the complex environment-person interaction that had previously remained undetected. Professors Chess and Thomas have provided a great service by putting the individual back in the equations that evaluate developmental outcome.

REFERENCES

Bates, J. (1980). The concept of the difficult child. *Merrill-Palmer Quarterly, 26*(4), 295–319.

Bgoya, W. (1967). Child growing so big. In L. Okola (Ed.), *Drum beat* (pp. 16–17). Nairobi: East Africa Publishers.

Carey, W. B. (1970). A simplified method for measuring infant temperament. *Journal of Pediatrics, 77*, 188–194.

Carey, W. B. (1985). Temperament and increased weight gain in infants. *Journal of Developmental and Behavioral Pediatrics, 6*(3), 128–131.

Chisholm, J. S. (1983). *Navajo infancy.* New York: Aldine.

deVries, M. W. (1984). Temperament and infant mortality among the Masai of East Africa. *American Journal of Psychiatry, 141*(10), 1189–1194.

deVries, M. W. (1987a). Alternatives to mother-infant attachment in the neonatal period. In C. Super & S. Harkness (Eds.), *The role of culture in developmental disorder* (Vol. 1, pp. 119–130). New York: Academic Press.

deVries, M. W. (1987b). Cry-babies, culture and catastrophe. In N. Scheper-Hughes (Ed.), *Child survival: Anthropological perspectives on the treatment and maltreatment of children* (pp. 165–185). Dordrecht, The Netherlands: D. Reidel.

deVries, M. W. (1989). Difficult temperament, a universal and culturally embedded concept. In W. B. Carey & S.C. McDevitt, (Eds.), *Clinical and educational applications of temperament research.* Amsterdam/Lisse, The Netherlands: Swets & Zeitlinger.

deVries, M. W., & deVries, M. R. (1977). Cultural relativity of toilet training readiness. *Pediatrics, 60,* 170–179.

deVries, M. W., & Sameroff, A. J. (1984). Culture and temperament: Influences on infant temperament in three East African societies. *American Journal of Orthopsychiatry, 54*(1), 83–96.

deVries, M. W., & Super, C. M. (1978). Contextual influences on the Brazelton Neonatal Assessment Scale and implications for cross-cultural use. In A. Sameroff (Ed.), Organization and stability of newborn behavior. *Monographs of the Society for Research in Child Development, 43*(5–6, 92–101).

Konner, M. J., & Worthman, C. (1980). Nursing frequency, gonadal function and birth spacing among Kung hunter-gatherers. *Science, 207,* 788–791.

LeVine, R. (1974). Parental goals: A cross-cultural view. *Teachers College Record, 76,* 226–239.

Liederman, P., Babu, B., Kagia, J., Kraemer, C., & Leiderman, G. F. (1973). African infant precocity and some social influences during the first year of life. *Nature, 242,* 247–249.

Sameroff, A. J. (1975). Early influences on development: Fact or fantasy? *Merrill-Palmer Quarterly, 20,* 275–301.

Sameroff, A. J., & Chandler, M. (1975). Reproductive risk and the continuum of caretaking casualty. In F. Horowitz et al. (Eds.), *Review of child development research* (Vol. 4, pp. 187–244). Chicago: University of Chicago Press.

Scheper-Hughes, N. (1987). *Child survival: Anthropological perspectives on the treatment and maltreatment of children.* Dordrecht, The Netherlands: D. Reidel.

Super, C. M., & Harkness, S. (1986). Temperament, development and culture. In R. Plomin & J. Dunn (Eds.), *The study of temperament: Changes, continuities and challenges* (pp. 131–149). Hillsdale, NJ: Lawrence Erlbaum.

Thomas, A., & Chess, S. (1980). *The dynamics of psychological development.* New York: Brunner/Mazel.

Thomas, A., Chess, S., Birch, H., Hertzig, M. E., & Korn, S. (1963). *Behavioral individuality in early childhood.* New York: New York University Press.

Vogel, L. C., Muller, A. S., Odingo, R. S., Onyango, Z., & de Geus, A. (1974). *Health and disease in Kenya.* Nairobi, Africa: East African Literature Bureau.

Whiting, B., & Whiting, J. (1973). *Children of six cultures: A psychocultural analysis.* Cambridge, MA: Harvard University Press.

14

Temperament and Cultural Diversity

Edmund W. Gordon

All of us in the behavioral sciences are greatly indebted to Alexander Thomas and Stella Chess, and to the late Herbert Birch, for the important contributions they have made to our understanding of individuality in human behavioral development. Their work on temperament continues to be seminal in the shaping of our thinking and in the guidance of research studies in this area. The importance of these contributions, however, is not limited to our better understanding of temperament. Rather, their work has been a maieutic factor in the development of additional lines of thought and research concerning the processes of human development. Their struggle to define and explicate dimensions of temperament, and to account for the paradoxical relationship of change, continuity, and stability in the manifestations of this construct in the behavior of individuals, has led me to the concerns that have dominated my intellectual agenda for the past several years.

For Thomas, Chess, and Birch, temperament is a construct that is descriptive of the characteristic tempo, rhythmicity, adaptability, energy expenditure, mood, and focus of attention in the behavior of persons, independent of the content or level of any specific behavior (Thomas, 1988). It is thought to reflect patterns of neurophysiological and/or neurochemical organization, patterns that represent the characteristic modes of response of the human brain to environmental stimuli, demands, and expectations. Yet it was clear to them that this construct involves

Portions of this paper were adapted with permission from E. W. Gordon and E. Armour-Thomas (1991), Culture and cognitive development. In L. Okagaki and R. J. Sternberg (Eds.), *Directors of development: Influences on the development of children's thinking*. Hillsdale, NJ: Lawrence Erlbaum.

more than is explicit in its description. Were it not for the limitations of the human life span, I suspect the next stage of their work on this construct would have been its componential and functional analysis to reveal not simply its manifestations and some of the consequences of its presence but its subcomponents, their origins, and their meanings in human behavior. Thus, as one whose career has been significantly influenced by long association with Thomas, Chess, and Birch, I worry about the nature of temperament, its components, and origins.

The notions and works of Thomas and Chess reflect an epigeneticist and interactionist perspective. They see behavior as dynamic and dialectical, and also as the product of continuing interactions (even transactions) between organisms and their environments. In their work on temperament, they make the case for a high degree of continuity, even stability, in basic patterns of temperament. Yet they report some evidence of change and considerable variations in the consequences of particular patterns as a function of different cultural contexts. In 1977 Thomas and Chess wrote:

> As we originally began to observe clinically and impressionistically the phenomenon of temperament, we were struck by the many dramatic evidences of continuity in individuals we knew, sometimes from early childhood to adulthood. It was tempting to generalize from these instances to the concept that an adult's temperamental characteristics could be predicted from a knowledge of his behavior style in early childhood. However, such a formulation would be completely at variance with our fundamental commitment to an interactionist viewpoint, in which individual behavioral development is conceived as a constantly evolving and changing process of organism-environment interaction. (p. 156)

The problem of continuity and change in human behavior has contributed to my own concern for better understanding the intercept between culture and the origins of behavior. What is the influence of variations in cultural experiences on the developing behavior of persons? Can the tension between continuity and change in temperament and other behavioral constructs (cognitive processes, for example) be better understood as a function of differences in the cultural context in which the behavior is developed?

With respect to the componential and functional analysis of temperament, a cursory review of the several dimensions indicates that some of these categories are more likely to reflect intrinsic biological structures or states than are others. For example, one might easily conclude that rhythmicity, threshold of responsiveness, and distractibility might well reflect the status of the nervous system, while approach or withdrawal, adaptability, and quality of mood could be more responsive to differences in one's encounters with the environment. Does this possible differential response to encounters with the environment have any meaning for possible differences in the character and origin of a specific manifestation of temperament? Do the nine components as described by Thomas, Chess, and Birch refer to comparable levels of organismic organization and representation? These questions have not yet been answered, but any attempt at understanding variations in the manifestations of temperament across cultural groups pushes such questions to the forefront. Such comparative work will require that we better understand the components of the construct and their possible differential origins.

In recent years, I have become concerned with the construct disposition, the tendency to behave in certain ways or to prefer one pattern or approach over another. We think of a disposition to inquire, to explore, to suspect, to trust, to want to know. Although these appear to be tendencies that generalize to the total behavior of persons, in my own work involving self-reports (Gordon & Song, 1992), it has been clear that situations and domains mediate the influence of disposition. For example, in familiar situations the disposition to trust may be in the ascendancy; yet it sharply declines in situations of perceived threat. If this means that the directionality of disposition is a function of the situation in which it is expressed, what is the basic disposition and how do we describe or define it? Of even greater consequence is the likelihood that a behavioral phenomenon that is situationally labile is also one that has been experientially influenced if not determined. Now, several of the categories of temperament (approach or withdrawal, quality of mood, persistence) seem more like experientially produced dispositions than organismically grounded temperaments.

Chess and Thomas would no doubt lead us out of this kind of apparent contradiction by reminding us of their often-repeated notion that all behavior must be explained in the context of that which is given in the organism *and* that which is a function of environmental encounters. It is the interaction between these two forces to which we must turn for our understanding of behavior. It was in association with them that I initially advanced my own conception of the interactionist argument that all organized patterned behaviors are reflections of the interaction between living things and their environments. Encounters with environments are seen as the crucial determinants and shapers of the patterned behaviors of the individual. Specific events and circumstances are thought to be the immediate causes of behaviors or to mediate behavioral expression. This is in contrast to the view that environmental encounters cause the release of organized behavior patterns. All organized patterned behaviors are seen to exist only as the results of sensory inputs flowing from encounters between the human organism and its environment. Behavioral potentials may be said to be genetically or organismically seeded, in the sense that many physical characteristics provide the basis for certain types of behavioral responses. However, even these underlying physical characteristics may be subject to environmental influences in their development. Some biological characteristics are largely determined by genetic phenomena; however, behavioral patterns, behavioral characteristics, and the quality of behavioral function are determined by interactions between these biological characteristics and their environmental encounters. These interactions can be referred to as transactions since the processes to which the term "interactions" refers are bidirectional. Thus the nature of these interactions/transactions is crucial for the form and pattern that the behavior will take.

It is this susceptibility of behavior to environmental influences in its development that may help us to understand the problems of continuity and change in temperament as well as the fact of differential consequences for the same manifestations of the construct under conditions of cultural variance. How is it that for some subjects there appears to be a high degree of consistency in the expression of temperament from early childhood through adolescence into the adult years, while for others we see considerable discontinuity? How is it that within a Latin American subpopulation, Chess and Thomas observed that "difficult" temperament did not seem to be associated with as many behavior problems as was the case within a European-American subpopulation?

My own work on the intercept between culture and behavior may provide some insight on these questions (Gordon & Armour-Thomas, 1991). Affective and cognitive behaviors of human beings are perhaps the most complex expressions of organic matter. They are manifest expressions of the human brain, but unlike other products of mental activity, human affective and cognitive behaviors reflect transducive action by which sensory and proprioceptive information is transformed into feelings, secondary signals, schemata, and concepts, that is, symbolic representations of "real" things as well as things that are artificial, abstract, and ideational. Of possibly even greater significance and consequence for its power is the fact that human affective and cognitive behavior can be symbolic of and reactive to actual events, imaginary phenomena, and hypothetical or speculative relationships between phenomena—which have been experienced (directly or vicariously) or of which humans have simply conceived or dreamed. There are unique capacities of this organic matter that make affective and cognitive behaviors such unusual phenomena. They are the capacities of this matter (organized as brain and conditioned by culture) to manipulate symbolic representations and to achieve transformative acts whereby existing phenomena take on new characteristics, serve different purposes, or come to be or to represent other things.

Debate continues concerning the origins of organized and patterned affective and cognitive behaviors in human subjects. The nature and origin of temperament are part of this debate. The presence of certain features of human affective/cognitive behaviors that are common to the species contributes to the widely held view that they are reflections of organic matter organized in ways that are unique to human beings. The fact that there are consistencies in the patterning of behaviors that adhere to groups that share the same culture and gene pool contributes to the continuing debate over heritability of versus environmental susceptibility to development of certain characteristics of human behavior. Those of us who believe that human social experience is a powerful correlate and possible cause of human social behavior and consciousness find it difficult to dismiss the notion that, in large measure, it is human social experience, interacting with whatever is the given in human biology, to which the origins, nature, quality, and limitations of human affective and cognitive behaviors must be attributed.

If one accepts this assumption, it is to culture and to variations in cultural experience that we must turn in order to understand the nature and origins of human behavior and its differential manifestations in both individuals and groups. Temperament is not an exception. The term "culture" is usually used to refer to the cumulative and multifaceted body of symbols, beliefs, schemata, information, techniques, and values that inform the behaviors and circumstances of a group of human beings. Geertz (1973, p. 89) has provided a widely accepted definition of culture as a "historically transmitted pattern of meanings embodied in symbolic form by means of which people communicate, perpetuate, and develop their knowledge about and attitudes toward life." This conception of culture gives emphasis to language and the nonmaterial aspects of culture. In addition to shared conceptual schemata, the term "culture" refers to such structural aspects of human organization as institutions, social divisions, ways of doing things, and the technologies of a social group. Thus culture includes humanmade objects; art forms and objects; belief systems; and patterns of economic, political, and social intercourse.

There are also functions that are served by culture that elude efforts at definition. Culture is not only a product of human action but also a cause of human action. Organized, patterned human behavior is a cultural product. We assert that without culture what we think of as the species-typical behaviors of humans would not emerge. Humans are essentially social beings. We require social interactions, initially, simply to survive. Human beings experience longer periods of infancy and childhood than do any other animals. Beyond the first years of life, it is thought that this extended social dependency is more of social developmental than biological developmental necessity. Some cognitive developmentalists—Piaget, for example—argue that cognitive development is a natural consequence of being a human animal "intentionally rational and scientific . . . striving to adapt or accommodate intelligence to the demands of common reality" (Piaget, as cited by Shweder & LeVine, 1984, p. 49). Other cognitive scientists see the genesis of human thought in the social interactions/transactions between the developing human organism and the culture that forms the context for development. In contrast to Piaget's implied self-constructed knowledge, D'Andrade (1980, p. 186) attributes human affective and cognitive functions to "other-dependent learning," in which, through informally guided discovery, we learn from social interactions with others. Whether we refer to cognitive behavior or to nonreflexive but otherwise organized human behavior, they are the context and content provided by one's culture that shape such human behaviors.

If the roots of organized and patterned human behavior are in cultural experience, what are the mechanisms by which experience becomes transformed into human characteristics and behavior tendencies such as dispositions and temperament? Several possibilities must be entertained. Among these are (1) neural cell differentiation, (2) synaptogenesis, and (3) model replication and social learning.

According to Hebb (1949), it is the function of experience, in human behavioral development, to enable the differentiation of neural cells to produce what he called cell assemblies. As a result of one's experiences, brain cells become organized into multiple assemblies and, once so associated, return to a specific assembly in the presence of specific patterns of stimulation. By this line of reasoning, it is culture that provides the stimuli, the models, and the contexts by which experience comes to be reflected in differential potentials for neural cells to be so organized; and it is social experience that provides instances for such potential to be expressed.

Synaptogenesis occurs in late prenatal and early postnatal development and involves the overproduction and later pruning of synaptic connections. Greenough, Black, and Wallace (1987) assert that while overproduction is maturationally regulated, the process of selective pruning seems to be a function of experience. In agreement with Hebb, they argue that experience triggers neural activity that commits a set of synapses to a particular pattern. Synapses not needed for that patterning are pruned. The residual synapses are manifested in subsequent relevant neural activity. Again, culture is the source of the necessary stimulation, the models that inform the patterning of these synapses, and the stimulus situations that subsequently call them into play.

Model replication and social learning are the concepts used to explain much of organized human behavior. Other human beings provide the models, and the ubiquitous press of social interdependency is the driving force. It is to Vygotsky (1978) that we turn for theoretical explication. His cultural-historical theory advances four processes that are foundational to the argument that culture shapes affective/cognitive development. Those concepts are (1) transmission of knowledge, (2) transmission of skills, (3) cultivation of nascent abilities, and (4) encouragement of abilities. He argues that knowledge of one's culture is socially transmitted by adults and capable peers; that social participation in a range of activities, determined by the culture, allows for skills to be demonstrated and practiced; that new abilities are cultivated through the sharing of initiative and responsibility with the child for culturally important tasks that have been modeled by the adult; and that abilities are encouraged and reinforced through apprentice-type encounters between older and younger members of the culture. Working with children in their "zone of proximal development," (Vygotsky as cited by Gordon & Armour-Thomas, p. 93, 1991), the adult models the task-appropriate behaviors, directs the children's attention to alternative procedures and approaches to the task, and encourages the children to try out and practice their embryonic skills.

Although this line of reasoning clearly holds for socially acquired behaviors, in the case of temperament there is some ambiguity. Are the patterns of neurophysiological and/or neurochemical organization which represent modes of response of the human brain intrinsic to the organism? Or are they the results of adaptations (neural cell differentiations) in response to environmental encounters? The best evidence we have comes from a consideration of the ages at which manifestations of temperament have been first identified. The initial subjects included in the Thomas, Chess, Birch, Hertzig, and Korn studies (1963) were infants less than 6 months of age. The nine categories by which temperament is classified by them were developed from these data. We must conclude that the basic patterns were and are discernible at a very early age, before the infants had extensive opportunities for socialization or even acculturation. In addition, in my own neonatal work, Turkewitz, Birch, and Gordon (1964) observed what may at least be precursors of these patterns of temperament in neonates less than 72 hours old. If these patterns are intrinsic to the organism, our cultural explanations speak to their continuity and change and are less useful in addressing their origins.

Unfortunately, there appear to be available no systematically collected cross-cultural data concerning manifestations of temperament in different population subgroups. Chess and Thomas did conduct a series of studies with a Puerto Rican population that did not result in new categories of temperament or patterns of its expression; however, they did note differential life adjustment consequences associated with culture-related parental child-rearing practices. As far as the basic categories are concerned, it appears that we have no evidence that indicates variations in the basic patterns as a result of differences in cultural experience. The impact of culture or environmental input generally appears to be reflected in the ways in which manifestations of temperament get played out in the lives of persons.

Thomas and Chess (1977) remind us:

> Temperament is a phenomenologic term in which the categorization of any individual is derived from the constellation of behaviors exhibited at any one age period. These behaviors are the result of all the influences, past and present, which shape and modify these behaviors in a constantly evolving interactive process. Consistency of a temper-

amental trait or constellation in an individual over time, therefore, may require stability in these interactional forces, such as environmental influences, motivations and abilities. (pp. 171–172)

What is being argued here is that temperament is a dynamic phenomenon that can appear to be stable if the environmental input is stable. Whether the source of input is culture or something else, if its pattern is constant, its product is likely to maintain a consistent course. Also implied is the likelihood that, as a dynamic developmental phenomenon, the manifestations of temperament in the life course of the person are dependent upon the pattern of environmental encounters to which the person is exposed. Thus we see in the development of a group of children whose socialization experiences are less structured and demanding of conformity less deleterious consequences for the "difficult child" or the "slow-to-warm-up child."

Future research focused on the construct temperament will need to be directed at the systematic examination of the relationship of specific patterns of cultural experience to the manner in which patterns of temperament are maintained and changed, and to the consequences for behavioral adaptation of specific patterns of temperament in interaction with specific variations in cultural experience. Such cross-cultural work conducted in the longitudinal tradition that has been characteristic of the Thomas and Chess work is likely to lead to a fuller understanding of the construct itself, as well as of the problems associated with continuity and change in the manifestations of temperament.

REFERENCES

D'Andrade, R. (1980). The cultural part of cognition. *Cognitive Science, 5*, 179–196.

Geertz, C. (1973). *Interpretation of cultures.* New York: Basic Books.

Gordon, E. W., & Song, L. D. (1992). *Variations in the experience of resilience.* Proceedings of the Temple University Invitational Conference on Resilience, Philadelphia.

Gordon, E.W., & Armour-Thomas, E. (1991). Culture and cognitive development. In L. Okagaki & R. J. Sternberg (Eds.), *Directors of development.* Hillsdale, N.J.: Lawrence Erlbaum.

Greenough, W. T., Black, J. E., & Wallace, C. S. (1987). Experience and brain development. *Child Development, 58*, 539–559.

Hebb, D. O. (1949). *The organization of behavior: A neuropsychological theory.* New York: John Wiley.

Shweder, R. A., & LeVine, R. A. (1984). *Culture theory: Essays on mind, self, and emotion.* New York: Cambridge University Press.

Thomas, A. (1988). Affective response tendency. In E. W. Gordon et al. (Eds.), *Human*

Prevention and Early Intervention

diversity and pedagogy. New Haven, CT: Center in Research on Education, Yale University.

Thomas, A., & Chess, S., (1977). *Temperament and development.* New York: Brunner/Mazel.

Thomas, A., Chess, S., Birch, H., Hertzig, M., & Korn, S. (1963). *Behavioral individuality in early childhood.* New York: New York University Press.

Turkewitz, G., with Birch, H., & Gordon, E. W. (1962, November). Head movement in human neonates. *American Zoologist, 2* (4).

Vygotsky, L. S. (1978). *Mind in society.* Cambridge, MA: Harvard University Press.

15

Variations in Cultural Influences in Hawaii

Anita L. Gerhard,
John F. McDermott, Jr., and
Naleen N. Andrade

Our understanding of the effects of culture on temperament is in its infancy compared to the rest of the knowledge base on temperament. Of necessity, the original New York Longitudinal Study (NYLS) attempted to control for environmental factors and thus examined a relatively homogeneous cultural group in order to ferret out individual characteristics. Later, however, Chess and Thomas laid the foundation for further research on culture and temperament in the NYLS Puerto Rican study. Super and Harkness and other authors (this volume) have elaborated on this issue, making significant contributions to the field.

Even though the body of knowledge on culture is small, preliminary findings have contributed to such important concepts as "goodness of fit" and have led many to agree with Chess and Thomas (1991) that "cross-cultural studies promise to . . . provide opportunities for refinement and application of the concept of goodness of fit" (p. 157).

In this chapter we will speculate about this developing picture of culture and temperament from our own cross-cultural vantage point in Hawaii's multiethnic society. While some of what we say may appear as flights of fancy, we share the findings from our current research and clinical experience in order to honor Chess and Thomas on this occasion, being inspired by their work as are other authors in this volume.

Our presentation is based on three fundamental observations: (1) that temperament is not fixed but is influenced by culture, (2) that the relationship of culture and temperament may change with time, and (3) that goodness of fit may vary developmentally in a given culture. A review of the general literature on culture and temperament and our own specific cross-cultural family studies will lead to further consideration of these basic principles.

BACKGROUND

The original conceptions of temperament assumed a set of innate biological characteristics that would remain constant over time. Soon, however, this thinking evolved to an interactionist viewpoint. Of their own seminal study, Chess and Thomas (1991) themselves observed: "As our young children became older, we have found that such continuities have not always been the case. And, in reflection, how could it be so? All other psychological phenomena can and do change over time. How could it be otherwise for temperament?" (p. 151). Indeed, they reflected that cultural evolution is in some ways like Lamarkian evolution, in which social experience is transmitted rapidly through social institutions (Thomas & Chess, 1980, p. 18).

Nevertheless, the range of factors that influence continuities and discontinuities in temperament is beyond the scope of this chapter. Our focus will be on an examination of the spectrum of cultural influences on these continuities and discontinuities. Part of this spectrum has yet to be elucidated.

Some researchers have focused on differences in temperament found among different cultural groups (Hsu, Soong, Stigler, Hong, & Liang, 1981; Weissbluth, 1982). Others (e.g., Freedman, 1974; Freedman & Freedman, 1969) have considered these differences as reflections of different gene pools between cultures, for example, Asian and European. One study on how culture may affect biological outcome has even considered the effect of the mother's emotional state on prenatal physiology (Chisholm & Heath, 1987). In one classic study, cultural influences on infant temperament in three East African societies were described (deVries & Sameroff, 1984). Methodological and conceptual problems that complicate comparative studies of temperament have also been considered in some detail (Super & Harkness, 1986). One study of temperament in Malay children (Banks, 1989) interpreted as cultural differences what may have been artifacts due to translation and elimination of items.

The study of temperament and infant mortality among the Masai of East Africa (deVries, 1984; also see Chapter 13 of this volume) is the most often quoted regarding the goodness of fit between culture and temperament because the findings were both unexpected and dramatic. Under conditions of drought and famine, infants with difficult temperament had the best goodness of fit, while infants of easy temperament had a much higher mortality rate. The investigators concluded that in desperate times difficult temperament may lead to better adaptation than an easy temperament because the infant with difficult temperament cries and fusses and thus is fed more.

Less dramatic, but conceptually as important, is the comparison of children from the Puerto Rican NYLS group with the original NYLS group (Korn & Gannon, 1983). The significance of that study was that the "difficult" cluster did not lead to behavior problems in the first 5 years because of the greater flexibility of the home environment but that after that problems arose when the children mingled in the dominant culture with its stricter requirements.

The research reports reviewed so far suggest that culture is an essential determinant of the goodness of fit between a child and the environment. The next logical question is whether culture acts as a constant determining factor over development, or whether the relationship between culture and temperament changes with time. As we have seen, most studies have focused on the relationship between temperament and culture in infancy and early childhood. What happens during adolescence, a later stage of rapid biological and emotional growth? Two family studies, one of Japanese and Caucasian families in Hawaii, and the other of Vietnamese adolescents and their parents in Oklahoma, may shed some light on this extension of the developmental question.

CULTURAL VARIATIONS AMONG ADOLESCENTS AND FAMILY VIEWS OF THEIR BEHAVIOR

In these studies, temperament was not measured. However, a particular aspect of the nature-nurture interaction *was* investigated—what individuals bring to their own development, including gender, and how it seemed to be influenced by the cultural environment as defined by family values.

An interdisciplinary team of investigators at the University of Hawaii School of Medicine conducted studies of family functioning around adolescent development using a cross section from the community representing several major ethnic groups, Caucasian, Chinese, Japanese, and Hawaiian. This work has been described in detail elsewhere (McDermott et al., 1983a,b), so only the findings pertinent to this issue will be discussed here. A subgroup of the sample, 158 Japanese-American and Caucasian families with two or more adolescent offspring, was surveyed for family attitudes and values. Statistically significant ethnic differences appeared in two major areas—cognitive versus emotional expression and group versus individual orientation. Japanese families were oriented toward collective action and cognitive approaches toward tasks. Caucasian parents, on the other hand, favored individual initiative and shared affective expression. However, the most interesting findings for the purpose of this chapter were in the specific areas in which *differences* between the generations on questions of authority and responsibility were examined. The influence of ethnicity gave way to gender differences between adolescent boys and girls. Girls valued family affiliation, closeness, and emotional expression significantly more highly than did the boys, who valued autonomy and independence.

One could argue that these findings simply represent blurring of ethnic distinctions through acculturation in the younger generation. However, follow-up findings on the youngsters 3 years later suggest that ethnic differences may reappear more strongly as they reach young adulthood. In any case, these findings challenge the notion that adolescent boys and girls have the same family experience. Gender is a powerful influence on adolescent development. Perhaps adolescents, or at least middle-class adolescents regardless of cultural background, have a common experience in adolescence that binds them more closely than their culture does. The interaction between biology, in this case represented by gender, and culture, in this case mediated through the family, may be a shifting and changing one throughout development, biology being a more powerful influence at one point, culturally learned values at another.

In another study (Nguyen & Williams, 1989) of Vietnamese refugee parents and their adolescent children in Oklahoma City, further evidence can be found for this changing interactional hypothesis. The investigators used a questionnaire for family values largely based on that used in the Hawaii Family Study (McDermott et al., 1983a,b), so that direct comparisons are possible. Quoting directly from their conclusions:

> Overall, the data on generation differences and gender differences are similar to those of McDermott et al. (1983a,b). This replication is rather remarkable when one considers the notable differences between the Hawaii and Oklahoma samples in terms of ethnic background, stage of acculturation of the Asian respondents to American society, and the very different environments of the two communities. (Nguyen & Williams, 1989, p. 514)

The Oklahoma researchers concluded that such concordance implies a degree of construct validity for the method. Comparing traditional Vietnamese family values with the degree of adolescent independence, they found considerable Vietnamese parental ambivalence toward the independence of their adolescent children. They speculated that this generational discrepancy would place considerable strain on the teenagers as mixed messages from their parents when they faced the cultural realities of American society.

IMPLICATIONS FOR UNDERSTANDING TEMPERAMENT

What does all this have to do with temperament? Family values and expectations are clearly part of the cultural environment surrounding any given child. Although they are only part of what the given culture contributes to a "developmental niche," they are not an insignificant part. How they might influence goodness or poorness of fit for youngsters with a given temperament is a critical question. Yet in the two family studies just reviewed, culture does not appear to be nearly as important as gender, at least temporarily during adolescence, nor is it as important as adolescence itself. What these teenagers brought to their own development appeared more influential than the culture in which it evolved. Temperament is an important component of what youngsters bring to their own development. And while temperament was not specifically measured in these two studies, they suggest that culture has less influence in determining goodness of fit in adolescents than it does in preschool or school-age children because adolescents appear to renounce its influence, at least temporarily.

A second question is raised by these studies—does culture derived from ethnicity have as much influence on goodness of fit as peer culture during this adolescent phase of development? Another related question is whether critical periods exist in which culture exerts a major influence on temperament and development. In the case of the Masai infants of East Africa during the drought and famine of 1974, the central issue was life or death (deVries, 1984). What did those of easy temperament who survived look like later as adolescents? More at risk during infancy, were they more or less at risk in adolescence? For example, were they better able to fit the cultural ideal of assertiveness and boldness because of their greater tendency for adaptability to change? How was gender important? (See the chapter by deVries, this volume.) In any case, we must now consider the concept of a constantly changing *interaction* between temperament and culture as part of the central interactional concept of temperament advanced by Chess and Thomas (1977, 1980, 1991).

Suppose temperament had been measured in the family studies we have presented above. In the Vietnamese study, one might wonder whether those teenagers with difficult temperament would be more vulnerable to reacting unfavorably to the mixed parental messages, and more prone to behavioral disturbances. Yet as infants, just like the Masai, these refugees' offspring might have had a better goodness of fit with their environment if they had been of *difficult* temperament, because of the rigors and dangers of life on the move. Or, would their greater inflexibility and complaining make it more likely that they would be abused or abandoned? Either way, culture, interacting with the environment, produces a changing medium for the evolution of temperament.

Many indigenous peoples as well as immigrant groups in our society face the problems of high infant and childhood mortality, as well as high rates of teenage delinquency, alcoholism, and gang membership. Is the child with difficult temperament *always* at highest risk throughout the life span? Or does the risk vary with the conditions he or she encounters? One might wonder whether conditions in which one culture colonizes another create developmental niches in which infants of difficult temperament have better survival in infancy only to experience greater trouble in adolescence. Could this relationship between culture, temperament, and goodness of fit offer a mechanism to explain what happens in societies in which minority groups are victims of cultural oppression? Does, for example, the intensity of difficult temperament produce the nationalistic leaders who so often emerge out of such adversity? We do not know! But think of our indigenous peoples living on reservations in this country, many of them under conditions close to starvation. Is it possible that a process of natural selection occurs by which children of difficult temperament have preferential survival, only to be more vulnerable to teenage alcoholism and delinquency? Not as farfetched as we might think. Although there are few studies on temperament in adolescence, some have shown a clear association between difficult temperament and substance abuse (Windle, 1991). Prevention and early intervention models based on temperament research have been extensively described for infancy and middle childhood (see this volume) but hardly at all for preadolescence or adolescence. While there are many complex factors contributing to depression and associated problems such as substance abuse in the youngsters of disadvantaged groups, perhaps those with difficult temperament in some cultural settings should receive the highest priority for intervention by clinicians. On the basis of experience from our family studies, we wonder whether the adolescents at highest risk aren't those with poorest "goodness of fit" in a setting with rapid cultural change or culture clash in which mixed messages on family values predominate. Closer attention to "developmental niche" may help clinical interventions.

Large-scale interventions with adolescents in the hope of preventing substance abuse have been made with little demonstrated success, while the single most effective drug prevention effects have come from the one-page ad showing an egg frying in a skillet. The caption simply states: "This is your brain on drugs. Any questions?" (Kleber, 1991). Perhaps there is a better developmental niche, for example, with 9-, 10-, or 11-year-olds in a given culture in which smaller interventions are more helpful.

The Hawaii and Oklahoma studies suggest that the influence of gender, as well as culture, needs to be reexamined. In the original NYLS study, sex differences in temperament in young children were not found significant (Chess & Thomas, 1984). Other work has shown divergence of temperament in middle childhood between boys and girls (Clarke-Stewart, 1988; Korn, 1984). Do critical periods exist in which gender is more relevant than at other times? The parallels we have discussed between the family studies lead us to wonder whether this relationship may be different in different cultures. How does our temperament knowledge base fit with the newly emerging data about differences in male and female adolescent development? How do the current concepts of male emphasis on individual autonomy and female orientation to relationships and interdependence interact with temperament to produce goodness or poorness of fit? In a recent study of sex differences in the interaction between temperament and parenting (Bezirganian & Cohen, 1992), gender-specific effects on the evolution of difficult temperament were in fact found. Although the role of culture was not explicitly examined, parenting styles are clearly very heavily influenced by culture. This study may serve as a model for launching an investigation into the complex interactions between gender, temperament, and culture.

The surprises found in the family studies of adolescents raise other theoretical questions as well. For example, the three classic temperament categories (easy, difficult, and slow to warm up) were formulated after qualitative analysis and factor analyses from a set of nine categories (activity level, rhythmicity, approach or withdrawal, adaptability, threshold of responsiveness, intensity of reaction, quality of mood, distractibility, and attention span/persistence). A study on the structure of temperament among young Japanese adults (Iwawaki, 1985) found large cultural differences in the adaptability/approach-withdrawal dimensions. Perhaps newer constructs are needed in examining the *changing* goodness-of-fit relationship between culture and development that we hypothesize.

CONCLUSION

In summary, we have considered the research on culture and temperament. From it, and our own experience, we hypothesize that (1) the relationship between culture and temperament may constitute a dynamic fusion that changes with time (developmental stages) in a nonlinear, but not random way, and (2) "goodness of fit" varies with developmental stage and may have its own critical time periods. We do not suggest a concept of rigid critical periods associated with fixation and irreversibility that led to such disenchantment with critical period theory in the 1980s, but a new concept in which temperament may be significantly influenced depending on the timing and force of outside influences. A new method of thinking may be needed to incorporate these complex, constantly interacting systems. For example, we are struck by the similarities in our struggle to understand the relationship between culture, temperament, and development and those encountered by nonlinear mathematicians in their attempt to look at other complex systems (Cotton, 1991). We can well remind ourselves of the early wisdom of Chess and Thomas when they proposed that temperament has stability, yet is not fixed, but influenced by culture. We hope that cross-cultural research currently in progress, including our own, will in the future add further to our understanding of this dynamic interaction.

REFERENCES

Banks, E. (1989). Temperament and individuality: A study of Malay children. *American Journal of Orthopsychiatry, 59*(3), 390–397.
Bezirganian, S., & Cohen, P. (1992). Sex differences in the interaction between temperament and parenting. *Journal of the American Academy of Child and Adolescent Psychiatry, 31*, 790–801.
Chess, S., & Thomas, A. (1984). *Origins and evolution of behavior disorders.* New York: Brunner/Mazel.
Chess, S., & Thomas, A. (1991). Temperament. In M. Lewis (Ed.), *Child and adolescent psychiatry: A comprehensive textbook.* Baltimore: Williams & Wilkins.
Chisholm, J. S., & Heath, G. (1987). Evolution and pregnancy: A biosocial view of prenatal influences. In C. M. Super & S. Harkness (Eds.), *The role of culture in developmental disorder.* New York: Academic Press.
Clarke-Stewart, K-A. (1988). Parents' effects on children's development: A decade of progress. *Journal of Applied Developmental Psychology, 9*, 41–84.
Cotton, P. (1991). Chaos, other nonlinear dynamics research may have answers, applications for clinical medicine. *Journal of the American Medical Association, 266*(1), 12–18.
deVries, M. W. (1984). Temperament and infant mortality among the Masai of East Africa. *American Journal of Psychiatry, 141*, 1189–1194.
deVries, M. W., & Sameroff, A. J. (1984). Culture and temperament: Influences on infant temperament in three East African societies. *American Journal of Orthopsychiatry, 54*(1), 83–96.
Freedman, D. G. (1974). *Human infancy: An evolutionary perspective.* Hillsdale, NJ: Lawrence Erlbaum.
Freedman, D. G., & Freedman, N. C. (1969). Behavioral differences between Chinese-American and European-American newborns. *Nature* (London), *224*, 1227.
Hsu, C. C., Soong, W. T., Stigler, J. W., Hong, C. C., & Liang, C. C. (1981). The temperamental characteristics of Chinese babies. *Child Development, 52*, 1337–1340.
Iwawaki, S., Hertzog, C., Hooker, K., & Lerner, R. M. (1985). The structure of temperament among Japanese and American young adults. *International Journal of Behavioral Development, 8*, 217–237.
Kleber, H. (1991). *Drug abuse, psychiatry and public policy.* Paper presented at the American College of Psychiatrists annual meeting, Fort Lauderdale, FL.
Korn, S. (1984). Continuities and discontinuities in difficult/easy temperament: Infancy to young adulthood. *Merrill-Palmer Quarterly, 30*(2), 189–199.
Korn, S. J., & Gannon, S. (1983). Temperament, cultural variations, and behavior disorder in preschool children. *Child Psychiatry and Human Development, 13*(4), 203–212.
McDermott, J. F., Char, W. F., Robillard, A. B., Hsu, J., Tseng, W. S., & Ashton, G. C.

(1983a). Cultural variations in family attitudes and their implications for therapy. *Journal of the American Academy of Child Psychiatry, 22*(5), 454–458.

McDermott, J. F., Robillard, A. B., Char, W. F., Hsu, J., Tseng, W. S., & Ashton, G. C. (1983b). Reexamining the concept of adolescence: Differences between adolescent boys and girls in the context of their families. *American Journal of Psychiatry, 140*, 1318–1322.

Nguyen, N. A., & Williams, H. L. (1989). Transition from east to west: Vietnamese adolescents and their parents. *Journal of the American Academy of Child and Adolescent Psychiatry, 28*(4), 505–515.

Super, C. M., & Harkness, S. (1981). Figure, ground and gestalt: The cultural context of the active individual. In R. M. Lerner & N. A. Busch-Rossnagel (Eds.), *Individuals as producers of their development.* New York: Academic Press.

Super, C. M., & Harkness, S. (1986). Temperament, development, and culture. In R. Plomin & J. Dunn (Eds.), *The study of temperament: Changes, continuities and challenges.* Hillsdale, NJ: Lawrence Erlbaum.

Thomas, A., & Chess, S. (1977). *Temperament and development.* New York: Brunner/Mazel.

Thomas, A., & Chess, S. (1980). *The dynamics of psychological development.* New York: Brunner/Mazel.

Weissbluth, M. (1982). Chinese-American infant temperament and sleep duration: An ethnic comparison. *Journal of Developmental and Behavioral Pediatrics, 3*(2), 99–102.

Windle, M. (1991). The difficult temperament in adolescence: Associations with substance use, family support, and problem behaviors. *Journal of Clinical Psychology, 47*(2), 310–315.

PART V

GOODNESS OF FIT:
THEORETICAL ISSUES

16

Explorations of the Goodness-of-Fit Model in Early Adolescence

Jacqueline V. Lerner and Richard M. Lerner

The theory and research of Alexander Thomas and Stella Chess (e.g., Chess & Thomas, 1984; Thomas & Chess, 1977, 1981; Thomas, Chess, & Birch, 1968; Thomas, Chess, Birch, Hertzig, & Korn, 1963) have changed the field of human development. They have made at least four pioneering contributions. First, and superordinately, their productive and high-quality research careers have exemplified the fact that theoretically important and methodologically creative research can have profound clinical significance.

Second, their theoretical conception of human development has championed the view that, across the entire span of life, development involves dynamic, that is, bidirectional, relations between the person and his or her context (e.g., Thomas & Chess, 1977, 1981). This perspective has been labeled "developmental contextualism" (Lerner, 1986, 1991; Lerner & Kauffman, 1985). Third, Thomas and Chess have promoted a methodological approach to appraising these changing person-context relations—that is, a multicohort, multivariate longitudinal one; this approach helped foster a zeitgeist in contemporary social and behavioral science for the primacy of such design strategies in the appraisal of human development (cf. Baltes, Reese, & Nesselroade, 1977).

Fourth, the substantive focus of their work—temperament—has revolutionized

The preparation of this manuscript was supported in part by grants to Richard M. Lerner and Jacqueline V. Lerner from the W. T. Grant Foundation and by the NICHD (HD23229-03).

the way in which the functional significance of human individuality is conceptualized in contemporary social science. Indeed, today, most approaches to the study of temperament view this aspect of personality as pertaining to the stylistic component of an individual's mental or behavioral repertoire (Buss & Plomin, 1984; Windle, 1988). That is, following Thomas and Chess, most scientists conceptualize temperament as *how* the person does whatever is done. Thus, from this perspective neither the content of, nor the motivation underlying, behavior is of primary concern in the study of temperament. Instead, individual differences in the style in which a person manifests otherwise identical behaviors are of prime interest.

For example, all children eat and sleep; as such, focus on these contents of the behavioral repertoire would not readily differentiate among children. However, children may differ in the rhythmicity of their eating or sleeping behaviors and/or in the vigor, activity level, or mood associated with these behaviors; such characteristics of individuality are temperamental attributes by the Thomas and Chess (1977; Thomas et al., 1963) definition.

Through the influence of Thomas and Chess, a significant growth has occurred in the study of temperament over the past two decades, especially during infancy and childhood (Lerner & Lerner, 1986). One reason for this growth in scientific attention is the theoretical role that Thomas and Chess have specified for the functional significance of individual differences in temperament, especially for person-context social relations (Chess & Thomas, 1984; Lerner & Lerner, 1983, 1986; Thomas & Chess, 1977). This theoretical conceptualization, which involves what we term a developmental contextual view of human development, helps account for the ways in which interindividual differences in temperament are related to an individual's success at coping with the stressors or demands encountered in the key settings of life (e.g., the family, the school, or the peer group).

Reflecting the emphases in the contemporary human development literature, our interest in the study of temperamental individuality derives from a concern with testing ideas associated with developmental contextualism. As noted above, this perspective involves the idea that development occurs through reciprocal relations, or "dynamic interactions" (Lerner, 1978), between people and their contexts. A notion of integrated, or "fused," levels of organization is used to account for these dynamic interactions (Novikoff, 1945a,b; Schneirla, 1957; Tobach, 1981). Variables from levels of analysis ranging from the inner-biological through the psychological to the sociocultural all change interdependently across time (history); as such, variables from one level are both products and producers of variables from the other integrated levels (Lerner, 1982; Lerner & Busch-Rossnagel, 1981). Accordingly, models where one represents the *relations* among levels, and not any level in isolation, are needed to study these dynamic interactions and their functional significance.

THE GOODNESS-OF-FIT MODEL

One such model is found in the goodness-of-fit concept detailed by Thomas and Chess (1977; Thomas, Chess, & Korn, 1982) and tested in the research in our laboratory (e.g., Lerner & Lerner, 1986, 1987, 1989). The goodness-of-fit concept derives from the view that the person-context interactions depicted within developmental contextualism involve "circular functions" (Schneirla, 1957), that is, person-context relations predicated on others' reactions to a person's characteristics of individuality: As a consequence of their characteristics of physical and behavioral individuality, people evoke differential reactions in the other people in their context; these reactions constitute feedback to people and influence their further interactions (and thus their ensuing development).

The goodness-of-fit concept, introduced in the temperament literature by Thomas and Chess, allows the valence of the feedback involved in these circular functions to be understood (Chess & Thomas, 1984; Lerner & Lerner, 1986, 1987, 1989; Thomas & Chess, 1977; Thomas et al., 1963). That is, the goodness-of-fit concept emphasizes the need to consider both the characteristics of individuality of the person and the demands of the social environment, as indexed for instance by expectations or attitudes of key people with whom the person interacts (e.g., parents, peers, or teachers). If a person's characteristics of individuality match, or fit, the demands of a particular social context, then positive interactions and adjustment are expected. In contrast, negative adjustment is expected to occur when there is a poor fit between the demands of a particular social context and the person's characteristics of individuality.

To illustrate, if a particular characteristic of temperament (e.g., regular sleeping habits) is expected within a given social context (e.g., the family) by a significant caretaker (e.g., the mother), then a child who possesses or develops that behavior will have a good fit with his or her environment. In such cases these children are expected to show positive behavioral interactions in regard to this characteristic, and ensuing developments are predicted to be favorable. If a child does not possess or develop behavior that matches or fits the demands of the context, then negative interactions and unfavorable outcomes are predicted.

In essence, then, within the framework of a developmental contextual perspective, we see temperament as a key instance of behavioral individuality. Through testing the goodness-of-fit concept, we seek to determine whether the functional significance of temperamental individuality for concurrent person-context relations and for subsequent development lies in the nature of the fit between (1) the person's characteristics of temperamental individuality (i.e., temperamental style); and (2) the demands (e.g., the expectations or attitudes) regarding temperamental style that are maintained by the significant others in the person's key contexts (e.g., the home, the peer group, the school).

TESTING THE GOODNESS-OF-FIT MODEL DURING EARLY ADOLESCENCE

Our laboratory has been engaged over the course of about a decade with research testing this developmental contextual model of the functional significance of temperamental individuality for adaptive development. Much of this work has been reviewed elsewhere (e.g., J. Lerner, 1984; Lerner, Nitz, Talwar, & Lerner, 1989; Lerner & Lerner, 1983, 1987, 1989; Talwar, Nitz, Lerner, & Lerner, 1991). Here, then, it may be of most use to present some of our more recent findings devoted to appraising the functional significance of individual temperament-context relations.

This research may be divided into several areas (Lerner et al., 1989; Talwar et al., 1991). However, because of its explicit relevance to the theory and research tradition pioneered by Alexander Thomas and Stella Chess, we focus here on our work pertinent to two short-term longitudinal studies of early adolescence, the Pennsylvania Early Adolescent Transitions Study (PEATS), and the Replication and Extension of the Pennsylvania Early Adolescent Transitions Study (REPEATS). In both investigations temperament-context fit has been related to psychosocial adjustment during the transition from elementary school to junior high school or to middle school.

We should note that Chess and Thomas (1984) have reported that in their analysis of the New York Longitudinal Study (NYLS) goodness of fit was relevant for the onset of new behavior problems up until about age 10. Our investigations of goodness of fit and adjustment in children have involved older samples for a number of reasons. First, we are interested not only in how goodness of fit is implicated in the onset and development of behavior problems. Our research has involved, in general, an attempt at delineating the role of temperamental individuality in children's functioning in the family, the school, and the peer context. The goodness-of-fit concept been an important one for us in our attempts at looking at early adolescent development with a broader developmental contextualism framework.

The PEATS And The REPEATS

Many of our tests of the goodness-of-fit concept have occurred within our conducting of the PEATS, a short-term longitudinal study of approximately 150 northwestern Pennsylvania young adolescents from the beginning of sixth grade across the transition to junior high school and to the end of the seventh grade, and the REPEATS, a cohort-comparative longitudinal study of two successive groups of central Pennsylvania youth from the beginning of sixth grade (or the start of middle school) to the end of eighth grade (or the completion of eighth grade).

Temperament has been assessed in these studies through the use of the Dimensions of Temperament Survey (DOTS; Lerner, Palermo, Spiro, & Nesselroade, 1982) and the DOTS-Revised (Windle & Lerner, 1986). These questionnaires are based on the nine original temperamental dimensions found in the NYLS. To assess demands, parents and peers respond to questionnaires designed to assess their expectations for the behavioral style characteristics. A child's "fit" is then determined by comparing his or her actual rated temperamental characteristics with the demands for those characteristics as reported by parents or peers.

To illustrate our work here, we may note that East and colleagues (1992) determined the relationships between the temperamental fit of the PEATS adolescents' and the contextual demands of their peers, their peer relations, and their psychosocial competence. Analyses of autocorrelations indicated that all variables (fit, peer relations, and competence) were highly stable across all times of testing. Results from within time-across domain correlations revealed that for each time of testing early-adolescent peer group fit for adaptability was positively related to favorable peer relations; early-adolescent peer group fit for adaptability and task rhythmicity was positively related to both self- and teacher-rated competence; and peer relations were highly correlated with both self- and teacher-rated competence. Additional analyses revealed many across time-across domain patterns of covariation.

Nitz, Lerner, Lerner, and Talwar (1988) found similar results regarding temperamental fit with parental demands and adolescent adjustment among the PEATS participants. At the beginning of sixth grade, temperamental fit of the adolescents with their parents' demands was not related to adjustment in significantly more ways than was simply the temperament of the adolescent. However, over time, at both the middle and the end of sixth grade, adolescent temperament-parental demand fit was related more frequently to adolescent adjustment than was adolescent temperament alone. Moreover, and underscoring the interconnections among the child-family relation and the other key contexts comprising the ecology of human development, such as the school context, Nitz and colleagues (1988) found almost interchangeable results when fit scores with the peer demands were considered.

In a related study of the PEATS data set, Talwar, Nitz, and Lerner (1990) found that at the end of sixth grade poor fit with parental demands (especially in regard to the attributes of Mood and Approach-Withdrawal) was associated in seventh grade with low teacher-related academic and social competence and with negative peer relations. Corresponding relations were found in regard to fit with peer demands. Moreover, and again underscoring the importance of considering the context within which organismic characteristics are expressed, goodness-of-fit scores (between temperament and demands) were more often associated with adjustment than were temperament scores alone; this was true in regard to both peer and parent contexts at the end of sixth grade, and for the peer context after the transition to junior high school (at the beginning of seventh grade). Finally, Talwar and colleagues grouped the PEATS subjects into high versus low overall fit groups (by summing fit scores across all temperament dimensions). Adolescents in the low-fit group in regard to peer demands received lower teacher ratings of scholastic competence, and more parent ratings for conduct and school problems, than did the adolescents in the high-fit group in regard to peer demands. Comparable findings were found in regard to low versus high fit in regard to parent demands.

Using the REPEATS data set, Schwab and Lerner (1991) examined the relation between temperament, adjustment, and social context by assessing the links between temperament and measures of coping and of parent and peer social support. On the basis of past research, it was expected that parental support and peer support (constructs construed to reflect good fit with parents and with peers, respectively) would moderate the link between temperament and coping. Results indicted that, as expected, there were few significant relations between temperament and coping (e.g., mood was not related to the adolescent's expression of negative feelings during coping). However, in support of the hypothesis that parental and peer support would moderate the link between temperament and coping, path models involving temperament *and* support in relation to coping responses were significant. For example, adolescent mood *and* peer support together contributed significantly to the expression of negative feelings during the coping response.

CONCLUSIONS AND FUTURE DIRECTIONS

Together, the concepts of organismic individuality, of context, and of the relations between the two, found in a developmental contextual perspective, are quite complex. The simultaneous consideration of these concepts imposes formidable challenges on those who seek to derive feasible research from this perspective. The careers of Thomas and Chess stand as an exemplar of the fact that such research can be accomplished with scientific rigor and applied (e.g., clinical) significance. Moreover, as stressed by Thomas and Chess, this developmental contextual perspective leads to an integrated, multilevel concept of development, one in which the focus of inquiry is the person-environment dynamic interaction. Furthermore, such an orientation places an emphasis on the potential for intraindividual change in structure and function—for plasticity—across the life span (R. Lerner, 1984).

One reasonably successful path we have taken for exploring the usefulness of a developmental contextual perspective involves the testing of the Thomas and Chess (1977; Thomas et al., 1963) goodness-of-fit model of person-context relations. Nevertheless, the goodness-of-fit model is not the only conception of person-context relations that can be derived from a developmental contextual orientation. There are perhaps an infinity of possible interlevel relations that may occur, and a potentially similarly large array of ways to model them. In the future, those testing these perspectives should consider incorporation of multiple measures within each of the levels modeled. Indeed, since current tests of other models derived from a developmental contextual or life-span perspective also have found considerable empirical support (e.g., Baltes, 1987), we can expect that such extensions will be important additions to an already significant foundation. As such, the seminal scientific and clinical contributions of Alexander Thomas and Stella Chess will continue to expand for generations to come.

REFERENCES

Baltes, P. B. (1987). Theoretical propositions of life-span developmental psychology: On the dynamics between growth and decline. *Developmental Psychology, 23*, 611–626.

Baltes, P. B., Reese, H. W., & Nesselroade, J. R. (1977). *Life-span developmental psychology: Introduction to research methods.* Monterery, CA: Brooks/Cole.

Buss, A. H., & Plomin, R. (1984). *Temperament: Early developing personality traits.* Hillsdale, NJ: Lawrence Erlbaum.

Chess, S., & Thomas, A. (1984). *The origins and evolution of behavior disorders: Infancy to early adult life.* New York: Brunner/Mazel.

East, P. L., Lerner, R. M., Lerner, J. V., Soni, R., Ohannessian, C., & Jacobson, L. P. (1992). Early adolescent peer-group fit, peer relations, and psychosocial competence: A short-term longitudinal study. *Journal of Early Adolescence, 12*, 132–152.

Lerner, J. V. (1984). The import of temperament for psychosocial functioning: Tests of a "goodness of fit" model. *Merrill-Palmer Quarterly, 30*, 177–188.

Lerner, J. V., & Lerner, R. M. (1983). Temperament and adaptation across life: Theoretical and empirical issues. In P. B. Baltes & O. G. Brim, Jr. (Eds.), *Life-span development and behavior* (Vol. 5, pp. 197–231). New York: Academic Press.

Lerner, J. V., & Lerner, R. M. (Eds.). (1986). Temperament and social interaction in infants and children. *In New directions for child development.* San Francisco: Jossey-Bass.

Lerner, J. V., Nitz, K., Talwar, R., & Lerner, R. M. (1989). On the functional significance of temperamental individuality: A developmental contextual view of the concept of goodness of fit. In G. A. Kohnstamm, J. E. Bates, & M. K. Rothbart (Eds.), *Temperament in childhood* (pp. 509–522). Chichester, England: John Wiley.

Lerner, R. M. (1978). Nature, nurture and dynamic interactionism. *Human Development, 21*, 1–20.

Lerner, R. M. (1982). Children and adolescents as producers of their own development. *Developmental Review, 2*, 342–370.

Lerner, R. M. (1984). *On the nature of human plasticity.* New York: Cambridge University Press.

Lerner, R. M. (1986). *Concepts and theories of human development* (2nd ed.). New York: Random House.

Lerner, R. M. (1991). Changing organism-context relations as the basic process of development: A developmental contextual perspective. *Developmental Psychology, 27*, 27–32.

Lerner, R. M., & Busch-Rossnagel, N. (1981). Individuals as producers of their development: Conceptual and empirical bases. In R. M. Lerner & N. A. Busch-Rossnagel (Eds.), *Individuals as producers of their development: A life-span perspective.* New York: Academic Press.

Lerner, R. M., & Kauffman, M. B. (1985). The concept of development in contextualism. *Developmental Review, 5*, 309–333.

Lerner, R. M., & Lerner, J. V. (1987). Children in their contexts: A goodness of fit model. In J. B. Lancaster, J. Altmann, A. S. Rossi, & L. R. Sherrod (Eds.), *Parenting across the life span: Biosocial dimensions.* Chicago: Aldine.

Lerner, R. M., & Lerner, J. V. (1989). Organismic and social contextual bases of development: The sample case of adolescence. In W. Damon (Ed.), *Child development today and tomorrow.* San Francisco: Jossey-Bass.

Lerner, R. M., Palermo, M., Spiro, A., III, & Nesselroade, J. R. (1982). Assessing the dimensions of temperamental individuality across the life-span: The Dimensions of Temperament Survey (DOTS). *Child Development, 53*, 149–159.

Nitz, K., Lerner, R. M., Lerner, J. V., & Talwar, R. (1988). Parental and peer demands, temperament, and early adolescent adjustment. *Journal of Early Adolescence, 8*, 243–263.

Novikoff, A. B. (1945a). The concept of integrative levels of biology. *Science, 101*, 405–406.

Novikoff, A. B. (1945b). Continuity and discontinuity in evolution. *Science, 101*, 405–406.

Schneirla, T. C. (1957). The concept of development in comparative psychology. In D. B. Harris (Ed.), *The concept of development.* Minneapolis: University of Minnesota Press.

Schwab, J., & Lerner, J. V. (1991, April). Temperament, coping, and social support in early adolescents. Poster presented at the Biennial Meeting of the Society for Research in Child Development, Seattle.

Talwar, R., Nitz, K., & Lerner, R. M. (1990). Relations among early adolescent temperament, parent and peer demands, and adjustment: A test of the goodness of fit model. *Journal of Adolescence, 13*, 279–298.

Talwar, R., Nitz, K., Lerner, J. V., & Lerner, R. M. (1991). The functional significance of organismic individuality: The sample case of temperament. In J. Strelau & A. Angleitner (Eds.), *Explorations in temperament: Contemporary conceptualizations, measurement, and methodological issues* (pp. 29–42). New York: Plenum Press.

Thomas, A., & Chess, S. (1977). *Temperament and development.* New York: Brunner/Mazel.

Thomas, A., & Chess, S. (1981). The role of temperament in the contributions of individuals to their development. In R. M. Lerner & N. A. Busch-Rossnagel (Eds.), *Individuals as producers of their development: A life-span perspective* (pp. 231–255). New York: Academic Press.

Thomas, A., Chess, S., & Birch, H. (1968). *Temperament and behavioral disorders in childhood.* New York: New York University Press.

Thomas, A., Chess, S., Birch, H. G., Hertzig, M. E., & Korn, S. (1963). *Behavioral individuality in early childhood.* New York: New York University Press.

Thomas, A., Chess, S., & Korn, S. J. (1982). The reality of difficult temperament. *Merrill-Palmer Quarterly, 28,* 1–20.

Tobach, E. (1981). Evolutionary aspects of the activity of the organism and its development. In R. M. Lerner & N. A. Busch-Rossnagel (Eds.), *Individuals as producers of their development: A life-span perspective.* New York: Academic Press.

Windle, M. (1988). Psychometric strategies of measures of temperament: A methodological critique. *International Journal of Behavioral Development, 11,* 171–201.

Windle, M., & Lerner, R. M. (1986). Reassessing the dimensions of temperamental individuality across the life span: The Revised Dimensions of Temperament Survey (DOTS-R). *Journal of Adolescent Research, 1,* 213–230.

17

Genetics and Individual Differences: How Chess and Thomas Shaped Developmental Thought

Sandra Scarr

In our analysis of the dynamics of the origins and evolution of behavior disorders, we have found the concept "goodness of fit" and the related ideas of consonance and dissonance to be very useful. . . .

When the organism's capacities, motivations and style of behaving and the demands and expectations of the environment are in accord, then goodness of fit results. Such consonance between organism and environment potentiates optimal positive development. Should there be dissonance between the capacities and characteristics of the organism on the one hand and the environmental opportunities and demands on the other hand, there is poorness of fit, which leads to maladaptive functioning and distorted development. (Chess & Thomas, 1984)

The theoretical clarity and elegance of expression that characterize Stella Chess and Alexander Thomas's thinking about development make their work particularly appealing. Ever since I read their 1968 book (Chess, Thomas, & Birch, 1968),

I knew I had found kindred spirits. It is not so much their research—interesting and unique as it is—as their insights that make their contributions outstanding. It is with great pleasure that I write about their influence on my thinking about development.

GOODNESS OF FIT

Their concept of goodness of fit incorporates organism and environment in a system that promotes development or impedes it. In an era of rabid environmentalism, Chess and Thomas stood up for the organism's role in its own development. Children were not pawns of their environments; they were active players in their adult destinies. Yet, children were also vulnerable to the vicissitudes of their rearing environments: A poor fit between a child's temperament and parental demands could create disturbance in the child's adjustment.

Beginning in 1957, Thomas and Chess (1957) promoted interactionism of the sort advocated by Jean Piaget (Piaget, 1954). In this view development depends on the interplay between organism and environment, not on the characteristics of either alone. Notice that there is no requirement to assign virtue or priority to either organism or environment; both are required and both contribute to normal human development. My own conclusions are that genes drive experience and that interaction results primarily from the biological individuality of the child.

Piaget concerned himself only with species-typical development, in a stage theory of intellectual change. He was not at all interested in individual differences in development—their course or their etiology. Piaget attempted to describe the course of normal human development in contexts that promoted normal development, and he did not concern himself with variations in the fit between child and environment.

Chess and Thomas's version of interactionism takes individual differences into account in ways that the more traditional developmentalists do not. It is this concern with individual adjustment that gives these authors their distinction. They promoted the idea and conducted their research on individual differences in adjustment resulting from good to poor fits between children and their environments.

ORGANISMS AND ENVIRONMENTS

For all children, an environment within the range that is normal for the species is crucial. Chess and Thomas focus more on variations within those normal limits. Within the ranges of normal organisms and normal or "average expectable" environments (Hartmann, 1958), what is important for the child's development is the "match" (Piaget, 1954) between the two. An "easy" child, one who is adaptable, predictable, and low in intensity of reaction, is more likely to have good behavioral outcomes because of the ease with which parents can deal with the child and because of the ease with which the child can negotiate new and stressful situations. Even nervous and demanding parents have a better chance of providing acceptable parenting to an undemanding, calm, and easy child than to a highly reactive, intense, difficult child. The latter kind of child requires specially calm, undemanding, and accepting parents to achieve good outcomes (Chess et al., 1968; Thomas, & Chess, 1980; Chess & Thomas, 1984). The goodness of fit between parental style and child temperament is crucial for all children, because some "easy" children can be come maladjusted with family maladjustments, parental death, conflicts, and the like (Thomas & Chess, 1980). But children at risk for maladjustment in adolescent and young adult years are more likely to be those with difficult child temperaments.

CHILDREN AFFECT PARENTING

Although Chess and Thomas certainly recognized the importance of a genetically/biologically normal organism (e.g., Chess & Thomas, 1984, Chapter 15), reactions of parents to vulnerable children, who do not always meet parental expectations, provide some of their most tender case histories. Even in the case of brain damage, they stress the importance of a good match between the child's characteristics—temperamental and intellectual—and the parents' expectations and demands. Parental level of demandingness can significantly ease or exacerbate a child's hyperactivity.

Having read the Chess and Thomas books, I was forewarned about the overdiagnosis of hyperactivity when I began a large research project in Bermuda in 1978. The first phase of the project included 125 families with 2-year-olds. Later phases of the project involved nearly a thousand families. The families varied from poorly to well educated, from low to high income. Mothers rated their children on activity levels and other temperamental characteristics, as did observers of the children over the course of several hours of interaction. Too many parents scored their children in the ranges of hyperactivity on our measures. And our graduate student observers thought about 10% of the children were hyperactive.

To evaluate the 2-year-olds, we subjected them to an experimental teaching task with their mothers, to several other observations and tasks, and to an IQ assessment with mothers present. Now, 24-month-olds are among the most difficult creatures to test with the Bayley Mental Development Scales or the Stanford-Binet Intelligence Test; they are age-appropriately impatient with the tests' demands.

Thus, we had ample opportunity to observe the ways in which mothers handled their children in stressful situations.

About 10% of the 2-year-olds were scored as "hyperactive" by mothers and observers, but I saw only one child of the first 125 I could classify as hyperactive— Chris, a bright boy of 24 months. His speech and language were superior, but he was a disaster to test. Although he scored 115 on the Bayley at 24 months, one knew he could have done better if he had been able to pay closer attention to the tasks. His mother was patient and caring with him. She held him on her lap throughout testing, said encouraging things, even promised him a candy reward if he could finish the test. Without being punitive, she persistently tried to get him to focus on the task demands. Here was a bright, overly active child with a patient, skillful parent.

I tested him again at 42 months. At that time, he was still hyperactive, and his mother was both more cognizant and more accepting of his difficulties. His mother helped him to control himself by patient interventions and encouragement to attend to the tasks and to take frequent, defined breaks (which I agreed to, at her suggestion) during the testing. She recognized his extreme problems with attention and control of activity, and she remained calm, supportive, and appropriately helpful to him. She sat him in her lap until he wriggled free ("Mommy, I *have* to get down"). By this age, Chris had learned some methods of self-control, however external. He used speech to try to control himself with self-instructions to sit still, to stop fidgeting, to do the tasks. Yet he climbed on my desk repeatedly, vaulted off the desk onto a sofa, climbed over the back of the sofa onto a chair, wandered around the room endlessly—all while being tested. At home, his mother reported that he had several times walked or run through the patio screen door.

His mother and I kept him from harm but conducted the assessments in accord with his limitations. This boy virtually climbed the walls during our testing session, all the while trying hard not to do so ("Oh, Mommy, I wish I could sit down" and "I'm going to do it"). It was clear that patience in dealing with his attentional and activity problems paid off in a superior performance on the intellectual assessments (IQ: 135), but he was an exhausting experience for even a few hours. It is unlikely that school personnel will look kindly upon this child's hyperactivity and distractibility.

The other children I saw at 24 and 42 months who were called "hyperactive" by their mothers and by our observers had more problems from poor parental management than from intrinsic behavior problems. Yes, they presented challenges to parenting that calmer, less active children did not present. These children would not win any prizes for easy-child-of-the-month. But they could be managed with the same kind of patient, calm, and undemanding parenting behaviors that Chris's mother showed in abundance, but with so little success in Chris's outcomes.

Most often, mothers of overly active–naughty children exhibited what I called the "limp-wrist syndrome": The mother had given up trying to manage the child. She sat in a chair watching the child's misbehaviors, arms dangling at her side, while verbally complaining at the child, but not enforcing any controls. Children of tired, limp-wrist mothers got away with overly active misbehaviors while receiving the message that they were bad, irritating children. This reinforcement pattern undoubtedly increased these children's acting out and did nothing to reduce those behaviors that schools (and testers) find so unacceptable.

I learned from reading Chess and Thomas that interactions between children and parents are crucial in predicting children's behavioral outcomes, both because some children require unusual adaptations from parents, and because some parents are unable to handle the challenges that even normal children present. No child is destined by genes to be a behavior problem, but some children are more likely to develop in problematic directions with ordinary parents unless there is intervention in their developmental course.

CHILDREN AND THEIR OWN DEVELOPMENT

It is commonly observed that children in the same family resemble each other to some extent. Identical twins are very similar on all behavioral measures. Plomin (this volume) notes the common observation that degree of behavioral similarity follows genetic relatedness, not environmental relatedness, because identical twins reared in different homes are very similar whereas adopted children reared in the same home hardly resemble each other at all (see Scarr, 1992).

I argue that the role of the child in the kind of parenting the child evokes and reinforces has been underestimated (Scarr, 1992; Scarr & McCartney, 1983). The idea that people make their own environments runs counter to the mainstream of developmental psychology. A large base of literature examining the relationships between familial, parental, and child characteristics has found that these characteristics are, indeed, related to each other. Developmentalists most often interpret these findings as evidence that the rearing conditions that parents provide for their children make differences in the children's life chances and eventual adult statuses—both socioeconomic achievements and mental health. Thus, although some developmentalists have suggested that children may affect their environments as well as vice versa (Chess et al., 1968; Thomas & Chess, 1980; Chess & Thomas, 1984; Bell, 1968), the theory that children actually construct their own environments challenges the basic tenets of much of mainstream developmental psychology.

GENERAL THEORY

In the theory of how people make their own environments, there are three ways by which genotypes and environments become correlated. First, one must take into account the fact that most biological parents provide their children with both genes and home environments. The fact that parents provide both genes and environments means that the child's genes and environment will necessarily be positively correlated. For example, parents who read well and who like to read will be likely to subscribe to magazines and papers, buy and borrow books, take books from the local library, and read to the child. Parents who have reading problems are less likely to expose themselves to this world of literacy, so that their children are likely to be reared in a less literate environment. Those same children are also more likely to have reading problems themselves and to prefer nonreading activities. Thus, the reading abilities of parents are likely to be correlated with the reading abilities of their children and with the environments parents provide for their children—a positive genotype–environments effect. Of course, parents can provide interventions, such as tutoring for reading disabilities, that will result in a negative genotype–environment correlation for the duration of the treatment. It is unlikely, however, that such interventions will last long enough or have sufficient effects to alter the generally positive $g \rightarrow e$ effect for most children, most of the time. Without professional intervention, most difficult children are likely to receive irritable parenting most of the time.

Second, each person at each developmental stage *evokes* from others responses that reinforce positively or negatively that person's behaviors. Evocative effects have profound effects on a person's self-image and self-esteem throughout the life span. Smiling, cheerful infants who evoke positive social interactions from parents and other adults (Wachs & Gruen, 1982) seem likely to form positive impressions of the social world and its attractions. Infants who are fussy and irritable and who have negative or neutral interactions with their care givers and others would seem less likely to form the impression that social interactions are a wonderful source of reinforcement. Young children who exceed their parents' patience for hyperactive behaviors can evoke environments that are punitive or that reward misbehaviors. Few hyperactive children have tolerant parents as Chris did; most are rejected as intolerable annoyances. School-age children from disadvantaged families who are more intelligent and more "spunky" (Scarr, 1985) are more likely to be given positive attention and encouragement by teachers than less intelligent or less "spunky" children from the same type of environment. Thus, a person's own characteristics evoke from others responses that are correlated with that person's developmental status and individual differences—for better and for worse.

Third, each person makes choices about what environments to experience. Past infancy, people who are in a varied environment choose what to attend to and what to ignore.[1] Depending on their personal interests, talents, and personality, people choose pursuits, whether educational, occupational, or leisure activities. Children who are athletic hang out on playing fields and usually read less than children who are less athletic or more skillful readers. Musical children are attracted to opportunities to play instruments and participate in musical activities. There are no surprises here, only common observations that this theory makes explicit.

FAMILIES AS ENVIRONMENTS

Attention has been focused on differences among families in the opportunities they provide for their children. Beginning with family differences in social class, it has been assumed that observations of ubiquitous correlations between family education, occupational status, and income and children's intellectual and other outcomes were caused by differences among families' *environments* (Scarr, 1985). Clearly, there are family differences; it is not clear that most of those differences are environmental. In fact, among families in the mainstream of Western European and North American societies, differences in family environments seem to have little effect on intellectual and personality outcomes of their children. This point is worth pondering. How can it be that parents have little effect on the intellectual or personality development of their children? To parents who care, it seems impossible that this could be the case. This is not to say that parents may not have effects on children's self-esteem, motivation, ambitiousness, and other important characteristics. It is to say that parental *differences* in rearing styles, social class, and income have a small effect on the measurable *differences* in intelligence, interests, and personality among their children.

Family differences have been assumed to be environmental differences. However, research on adoptive families and on twins suggests that a large proportion of differences between children from different families is related to genetic differences among parents, which genetic variability is transmitted to their children. Thus, their children have different assortments of interests, talents, and personalities. Those differences among the children cause them to evoke different types of parenting and to take advantage of different opportunities inside and outside of the family.

In fact, the same body of behavioral genetic literature that illustrates the impor-

---

[1]The entire theory depends on people having a varied environment from which to choose and construct experiences. The theory does not apply, therefore, to people with few choices or few opportunities for experiences that match their genotypes. This caveat applies particularly to children reared in very disadvantaged circumstances and to adults with little or no choice about occupations and leisure activities.

tance of genetic variation also highlights the importance of environmental variation. One of the most striking findings of the behavior genetic literature is that, for a variety of traits, most of the environmental variance is contributed by nonshared environmental influences. Nonshared environmental influences are those that are not shared by members of a family; that is, they act to make members of a family different from one another. As Plomin and Thompson (1987) highlight, the above finding "implies that the unit of environmental transmission is not the family, but rather micro-environments within families" (p. 20).

GOOD-ENOUGH PARENTS

Good-enough, ordinary parents probably have the same effects on their children's development as culturally defined super-parents. This supposition gives parents a lot more freedom to care for their children in ways they find comfortable for them, and it gives them more freedom from guilt when they deviate (within the normal range) from culturally prescribed norms about parenting. There are children whose outcomes will not be wonderful, regardless of the efforts of patient, nondemanding parents. There are children whose outcomes could be better if they had patient, supportive, nondemanding parents. But most of the variations among children seem to be due to their genetic differences and to the environments they evoke and select.

Venturing advice to parents, I would say that the research supports the idea that parents need to provide *opportunities, not prescriptions* for their children. A rich and varied environment of opportunities afforded by the family will provide children the possibility of becoming the best they can be. For some parents with fixed ideas about their offsprings' outcomes, this will be anxiety-provoking advice, but given that nearly all parents want their children to grow up to be well-functioning and happy adults, this is good advice, based on behavior genetic research.

SUMMARY

Following and elaborating on Chess and Thomas's views, I have proposed additional points regarding observed relationships between parental and child characteristics. First, the traditional widely held belief that such observed relationships are necessarily indicative of parental effects on their children's development is questionable. It is now quite evident that children can and do influence their own environments. Second, the field of behavior genetics has provided data that illustrate that for many traits, there is more variation within families than between families. Thus, the assumption that differences between families cause differences between children is called into question. Unless children have a seriously deprived and unsupportive environment, differences in their outcomes are caused more by their characteristics than by differences in opportunities in their environments. Third, given objectively "similar" environments, not all individuals respond in the same ways. Such responses often vary on the basis of characteristics that the child brings to the situation.

Finally, I do not claim that differences in environments cannot influence differences among individuals, especially in deficient and unsupportive situations, but that the effective "environment" for development is not indexed by traditional family measures. Rather, children have profound effects on their own environments, and the match between child characteristics and rearing environment is what matters. Perhaps, Chess and Thomas will think I have gone too far. Regardless, they have profoundly influenced my thinking, and I am very grateful to them for it.

REFERENCES

Bell, R. Q. (1968). A reinterpretation of the direction of effects in studies of socialization. *Psychological Review, 75*, 81–95.

Chess, S., & Thomas, A. (1984). *Origins and evolution of behavior disorders for infancy to early adult life.* New York: Brunner/Mazel.

Chess, S., Thomas, A., & Birch, H. G. (1968). *Temperament and behavior disorders in children.* New York: New York University Press.

Garmezy, N., Masten, A., & Tellegen, A. (1984). The study of stress and competence in children: A building block for developmental psychopathology. *Child Development, 55*, 97–111.

Hartmann, H. (1958). *Ego psychology and the problem of adaptation.* New York: International Universities Press.

Hunt, J. McV. (1961). *Intelligence and experience.* New York: Ronald Press.

Piaget, J. (1954). *The construction of reality in the child.* New York: Basic Books.

Plomin, R., & Thompson, R. (1987). Life-span developmental behavioral genetics. In P. B. Baltes, D. L. Featherman, & R. M. Lerner (Eds.), *Life-span development and behavior* (Vol. 8). Hillsdale, NJ: Lawrence Erlbaum.

Scarr, S. (1985). Constructing psychology: Making facts and fables for our times. *American Psychologist, 40*, 499–512.

Scarr, S. (1992). Developmental theories for the 1990s: Development and individual differences. *Child Development, 63*, 1–19.

Scarr, S., & McCartney, K. (1983). How people make their own environments: A theory of genotype —> environment effects. *Child Development, 54*, 424–435.

Thomas, A., & Chess, S. (1957). An approach to the study of sources of individual differences in child behavior. *Journal of Clinical and Experimental Psychopathology and Quarterly Review of Psychiatry and Neurology, 18*, 347–357.

Thomas, A., & Chess, S. (1980). *The dynamics of psychological development.* New York: Brunner/Mazel.

Wachs, T. D., & Gruen, G. (1982). *Early experience and human development.* New York: Plenum Press.

18

Interface of Nature and Nurture in the Family

Robert Plomin

I first became acquainted with the temperament research of Alexander Thomas and Stella Chess with their 1970 *Scientific American* article, "The Origin of Personality." I went on to read their 1963 book, *Behavioral Individuality in Early Childhood* (Thomas, Chess, Birch, Hertzig, & Korn) and their 1968 book, *Temperament and Behavior Disorders in Children* (Thomas, Chess, & Birch), and have kept on reading their books with pleasure (Chess & Thomas, 1984; Thomas & Chess, 1977, 1980). In the early 1970s, I was interested in genetic influences in personality development, at a time, just 20 years ago, when it was literally dangerous to consider genetic influence in human development. Although times were changing, environmentalism continued to have a stranglehold on psychological, especially developmental, research. For this reason, it was comforting for me to hear Thomas and Chess, speaking as much from their vast experience as clinicians as from their research, boldly shout that the emperor of environmentalism has no clothes, or at the least is quite skimpily clad. They spoke out against what they called the *mal de mère* syndrome, in which all maladjustment was laid at the doorstep of the mother. They argued that parents reflect as much as they affect temperamental dispositions of their children in a dynamic process of interaction. In 1956, they had launched their New York Longitudinal Study, which, a decade later, provided strong support for their view that children are temperamentally dif-

Preparation of this chapter was supported in part by grants for the Colorado Adoption Project from the National Science Foundation (BNS-91-08744) and the National Institute of Child Health and Human Development (HD-10333 and HD-18426) and for the Nonshared Environment in Adolescent Development Project from the National Institute of Mental Health (MH-43373).

ferent early in life and that these temperamental dimensions show increasing stability throughout the life course and increasing ability to predict later behavioral problems.

In this way, the work of Thomas and Chess helped to legitimize the study of genetic influence in personality, even though their theory of temperament did not demand the demonstration of genetic influence. Research on this topic blossomed during the past two decades (e.g., Eaves, Eysenck, & Martin, 1989; Loehlin, 1992; Plomin, Chipuer, & Neiderhiser, 1990). It was at first important merely to document that genetic factors could affect developmental phenomena as complex as personality. That has been accomplished. Significant genetic influence appears to be nearly ubiquitous in the domain of personality, although there is some evidence that the EAS temperaments of emotionality (neuroticism in adulthood), activity, and sociability/shyness (extraversion/introversion in adulthood) are among the most heritable (Buss & Plomin, 1984).

A chapter by Sandra Scarr in this volume focuses on genetic research. The present chapter discusses two findings that lie at the hyphen in the phrase nature–nurture, at the interface of nature and nurture. The first involves the possibility of genetic involvement in measures of the family environment. The second finding is that environmental influences that affect personality do not make children in the same family similar to one another. These findings may have even greater relevance to clinicians than the basic finding of ubiquitous genetic influence on temperament. For example, a finding of a genetic contribution on measures of parenting suggests either that parents are responding to genetically influenced characteristics of their children or that genetically influenced characteristics of the parents themselves are involved in their parenting. This adds a new dimension to thinking about the dynamics of the family system. The most obvious implication of the second finding, called nonshared environment, is that the clinician cannot assume that the family environment is the same for different children in the same family. Implications of such genetic research for clinicians are discussed elsewhere (Baker & Clark, 1990).

Before I launch a discussion of these two topics, two prefatory remarks are in order concerning genotype–environment interaction and correlation and concerning the magnitude of genetic influence for mental health. On the first topic, it may surprise the reader familiar with the work of Thomas and Chess that this discussion of the interface between nature and nurture does not include the topic of genotype–environment interaction. Thomas and Chess have from early on emphasized the importance of interaction in development—for example, "the dynamics of development as a continuous dialectical unity of opposites—heredity and environment, biological and cultural, continuity and change" (Thomas & Chess, 1980, p. 250). Even though the process by which genes work out their influence during development involves interactions with the environment, the quantitative genetic construct of genotype–environment interaction is much more limited. In quantitative genetics, the phrase "genotype–environment interaction" uses the word "interaction" in the statistical sense of joint effects of two variables (i.e., genes and environment) that affect the dependent variable beyond the main effects of either of the variables. It is a conditional relationship in which the effect of one variable depends on the other. Specifically, genotype–environment interaction refers to environmental effects that depend on genotype (or, vice versa, genetic effects that depend on environment). Thomas and Chess (e.g., 1980) distinguish this sort of model, which they call *interactive*, from their more dynamic model for which they have used the contrasting term *interactionalist*. There are many other ways to construe the coaction of predictor variables as they relate to an outcome variable, only some of which can be detected as statistical interactions (Rutter & Pickles, 1991). Although the quantitative genetic approach to genotype–environment interaction is limited, it is at least testable. The problem is that even this limited focus has not made it easy to find genotype–environment interaction. Part of the problem is that environmental measures have not often been incorporated in genetic studies, and without environmental measures genotype–environment interaction cannot be examined (Plomin, DeFries, & Loehlin, 1977; Eaves et al., 1989). Nonetheless, in the few studies that have included measures of the environment, it has been difficult to identify specific interactions between genotypes and environments (Plomin & Hershberger, 1991).

More progress has been made conceptually and empirically in understanding genotype–environment correlation than genotype–environment interaction (Plomin, 1986). Genotype–environment correlation refers to the covariance rather than interaction between genetic and environmental deviations. It occurs when individuals are exposed to or construct environments on the basis of their genetic propensities (Scarr, 1992). For example, musically gifted children might be selected as gifted and given special opportunities that foster their talent. In contrast, genotype–environment interaction occurs when the effects of environment depend on genetic differences among individuals. For example, the effect of musical training might be greater for musically gifted children. It is interesting that the Lerners, who have provided much of the empirical work for the Thomas/Chess interaction construct of goodness of fit (e.g., Lerner et al., 1986), have also begun to consider goodness of fit in terms of person–context correlation rather than person–context interaction (Windle & Lerner, 1986). Although the present chapter will not focus on genotype–environment correlation (see the chapter by Scarr in this volume), its first major topic, genetic influence on environmental measures, can be best construed as genotype–environment correlation.

The second prefatory point involves the magnitude of genetic influence. The disavowal of extreme environmentalism has been so extreme that the pendulum may be beginning to swing too far in the other direction, toward extreme biological determinism. For this reason, it should be emphasized that behavioral genetic evidence for significant and substantial genetic influence by no means implies that temperament is entirely genetic in origin. To the contrary, these same behavioral genetic data provide the best available evidence for the importance of nongenetic factors. Rarely does heritability, the proportion of phenotypic variance due to genetic variance, exceed 50%. Accounting for 50% of the variance in the behavioral sciences is a major achievement because rarely do findings explain even 5% of the variance. However, the message today is that this is just half of the story—the rest of the variance is nongenetic. The most concrete exemplar of this general finding is that identical twin correlations for personality rarely exceed .50, even though these individuals are genetically identical. No genetic explanation can account for this finding. As discussed later in relation to the second nature–nurture topic, these findings imply that environmental influences affect personality development in a dramatically unorthodox manner.

THE NATURE OF NURTURE

If, as Thomas and Chess have emphasized for the past 30 years, parents respond to temperamental dispositions of their children, and if temperamental dispositions are influenced by genetic factors, then parental interactions with their children should show genetic influence.

This syllogism reflects a hypothesis that temperament contributes to a finding consistently emerging from a new research literature: Widely used measures of the environment, especially measures of the family environment, show significant genetic influence. The implications of this finding for research on prevention and early intervention are profound. At the most general level, this finding supports an active view of the developmental transaction between children and their environments, a view in which children construct their own environments based on genetic propensities including temperament (Scarr, 1992).

More specific implications for intervention and prevention emerge from the recognition that labeling a measure "environmental" does not make it an environmental measure. If environmental measures as well as outcome measures show genetic influence, then associations between environmental measures and outcome measures can be mediated by genetic rather than environmental mechanisms. Interventions planned on the basis of an association between an environmental measure and an outcome measure usually make the unwarranted assumption that the association is mediated environmentally. Such interventions are unlikely to succeed if the association is due to genetic rather than environmental factors. Intervention and especially prevention research can profit from considering the family as a genetic as well as an environmental system in which links between parental behavior and child outcomes may be mediated genetically.

How is it possible that environmental measures show genetic influence? Although environments have no DNA, measures of the environment, especially measures of the family environment, may be perfused with genetically influenced characteristics of individuals such as temperament. To the extent that this is the case, measures of the environment can show genetic influence, and this is what the first studies in this area consistently show. For example, in four twin studies, children's perceptions of their parents' behavior toward them yielded significant genetic influence (Bouchard & McGue, 1990; Rowe, 1981, 1983a; Plomin, McClearn, Pedersen, Nesselroade, & Bergeman, 1988). Even reports of life events appear to be influenced genetically, especially reports of controllable life events (Plomin, Lichtenstein, Pedersen, McClearn, & Nesselroade, 1990). Evidence for genetic influence has also been found in comparisons between nonadoptive and adoptive siblings for videotaped observations of maternal behavior (Dunn & Plomin, 1986) and for a widely used observation/interview measure of the home environment (Braungart, Plomin, Fulker, & DeFries, 1992). Measures of the environment often show as much genetic influence as do measures of personality.

These findings are surprising only if we forget that in families, with the exception of adoptive families, parents and children are genetically related. Thus, their behavior toward one another (which is what measures of the family environment assess) could reflect genetic influence, especially when we consider how widespread genetic influence on behavior appears to be.

The importance of genetic influence on widely used measures of the environment has recently been reviewed in a *Behavioral and Brain Sciences* target article (Plomin & Bergeman, 1991a), which was published with 30 commentaries and a response to the commentaries (Plomin & Bergeman, 1991b). Subsequently, results have become available from a behavioral genetic study that focuses on environmental measures. The Nonshared Environment in Adolescent Development Project is a study of 720 pairs of adolescent siblings from 10 to 18 years of age in a novel design that includes identical and fraternal twins; full siblings in intact families; and full siblings, half siblings, and unrelated siblings in step families (Reiss et al., in press). For 88 measures of the familial and extrafamilial environment, significant genetic influence was found for 68 measures, and the average heritability for the 88 measures was .27, suggesting that over a quarter of the variance of these environmental measures can be accounted for by genetic differences among children (Plomin, Reiss, Hetherington, & Howe, 1992). Genetic influence was greatest for measures of peers, intermediate for measures related to parental behavior, and least for measures involving relationships with siblings and friends.

As mentioned earlier, a major implication of these findings is that correlations between environmental measures and developmental outcomes cannot be assumed to be environmental in origin. For example, parental "warmth" (cohesiveness and expressiveness) is related to infant "easiness" (low emotionality and difficultness, and high sociability and soothability). One approach to disentangling genetic and environmental components of covariance between environmental measures and personality is to compare environment–development associations in nonadoptive families and adoptive families (Plomin, Loehlin, & DeFries, 1985). Genetic mediation of environment–outcome associations is suggested when environment–outcome correlations are lower in adoptive families, in which parents and children are unrelated genetically, than in nonadoptive families. Analyses of this type suggest that fully half of environment–development associations in infancy and early childhood appears to be mediated genetically (Plomin, DeFries, & Fulker, 1988). In the specific example of parental warmth and infant easiness, correlations in nonadoptive families are significantly greater than correlations in adoptive families at both ages where data were available, when the children were 1 and 3 years of age. Model-fitting analyses suggest that nearly all of the phenotypic correlation between parental warmth and child easiness is mediated genetically. Multivariate quantitative genetic models can also be used with twin data to investigate the extent to which associations between ostensible environmental measures and developmental outcomes are mediated genetically. The first analysis of this type used data from a study of twins reared apart and matched twins reared together (Chipuer et al., 1992). Multivariate model-fitting analyses suggested that genetic influence on perceptions of family environment can be explained somewhat by genetic influence on extraversion and neuroticism, but most genetic influence on these environmental measures is independent of these two major dimensions of personality.

A major direction for research on the nature of nurture is to investigate genetically influenced characteristics of children and their parents that are responsible for genetic influence on measures of the environment. Temperament is perhaps the best candidate, as implied in the writings of Thomas and Chess over the past 25 years.

NONSHARED ENVIRONMENT

The second finding at the nature–nurture interface does not appear to have been anticipated by Thomas and Chess. This is understandable because Thomas and Chess, and nearly all other developmental researchers, primarily studied one child per family. When you study more than one child per family, you cannot help but be struck by how different siblings are even though they are growing up in the same family. Why are siblings in the same family so different? Genetics is part of the answer, because the first law of genetics is that like begets like and the second law is that like does not beget like. That is, first-degree relatives share half of their segregating genes, but this also means that they do not share half of their segregating genes. But the more surprising part of the story concerns nurture rather than nature.

One of the most important findings that has emerged from human behavioral genetics research is that environmental influences on development, especially personality and psychopathology, largely operate to make children growing up in the same family different from one another, not similar to one another as most theories of socialization would implicitly predict. This class of environmental influence has been called nonshared in the sense that these environmental influences are not shared by children growing up in the same family. Siblings resemble each other, for example in personality, but mostly because of shared heredity, not shared experience. Implications of this finding for clinicians are the topic of a recent paper (Dunn & Plomin, in press).

The importance of nonshared environment for personality was first emphasized in a 1976 study of high school twins (Loehlin & Nichols, 1976), and data from family, twin, and adoption research have consistently converged on this conclusion. Evidence for this conclusion was summarized in another *Behavioral and Brain Science* target article (Plomin & Daniels, 1987a), published with 32 commentaries and a response to the commentaries (Plomin & Daniels, 1987b). An update and greater detail concerning this evidence are available (Plomin et al., in press). One of the most readily understood aspects of this body of evidence involves differences within pairs of identical twins. Because identical twins are genetically identical, any differences within pairs must be due to environment. More specifically, such environmental influences must be nonshared in the sense that they make siblings (in this case, twins) growing up in the same family different from one another. Thus, the findings that identical twin correlations for personality rarely exceed .50 and that identical twin concordance for schizophrenia is less than 50% indicate that nonshared environment is of paramount importance in the development of personality and psychopathology.

A direct test of the extent to which shared experiences make children in the same family similar is provided by adoptive siblings, genetically unrelated children adopted into the same family early in life. Because these pairs of children are not genetically related, their similarity can be caused only by what is referred to as shared family environment. The correlation between adoptive siblings indexes the total impact of all shared environmental factors that make individuals growing up in the same family similar to one another. Consistently, adoptive sibling studies of personality show negligible influence of shared environment. A possible exception to the rule of the importance of nonshared rather than shared environment is juvenile delinquency, for which concordances for both identical and fraternal twins tend to be very high, suggesting little genetic influence and substantial shared environmental influence (Gottesman, Carey, & Hanson, 1983). However, it has been suggested that this apparent shared environmental effect may be specific to twins because twins may be partners in delinquent acts because they are the same age (Rowe, 1983b). The test of this hypothesis will come when other behavioral genetic designs such as adoption studies are applied.

The conclusion that environmental factors affecting personality operate primarily in a nonshared manner suggests that instead of thinking about environmental influences on a family-by-family basis, we need to think on an individual-by-individual basis. The message is not that family experiences are unimportant; rather, the argument is that environmental influences in individual development are specific to each child, rather than general to an entire family.

The evidence for the importance of nonshared environment comes from analyses of components of variance in behavioral genetic research. These components of variance are anonymous in the sense that neither specific DNA nor specific environmental variables are assessed. The next step for research on nonshared environment is to assess the extent to which specific measures of the environment are shared or nonshared. The key is to study more than one child per family. Any environmental variable that has been investigated on a family-by-family basis in studies of one child per family can be extended to consider nonshared environment if two criteria are fulfilled: The measure must be specific to each child and the environment of more than one child must be assessed in each family. Even prototypical between-family variables such as socioeconomic status can be studied in terms of differences from one sibling to the next as family fortunes go up and down. However, the point is that environmental factors will make a difference in the long run only to the extent that they are not shared by children growing up in the same family. Within the family, likely candidates for nonshared environment are differential parental treatment and differential sibling interactions, in addition to the well-studied static family structure variables such as family size and composition. Differential experiences beyond the family also need to be examined, including relationships with teachers, friends, and peers. It is also possible that nonsystematic factors such as accidents or illnesses initiate differences between siblings that, when compounded over time, make children in the same family different in unpredictable ways.

So far, the answer to this first question appears to be that siblings growing up in the "same" family live remarkably separate lives (Dunn & Plomin, 1990). The second step in this program of research is to identify specific measures of nonshared environment that address the question, Why are siblings in the same family so different? That is, instead of asking the extent of differences in the environments of siblings, we can search for nonshared experiences that relate to sibling outcomes. Progress is being made in beginning to address this issue (Dunn & Plomin, 1990). The ongoing Nonshared Environment in Adolescent Development Project mentioned earlier is focused on this question, although it is too early to report its results (Reiss et al., in press). A third question involves possible genetic mediation of associations between nonshared environment and outcomes, which brings together the two topics discussed in this chapter. The Nonshared Environment in Adolescent Development Project is imbedded in a behavioral genetic design so that it can disentangle genetic sources of sibling experiential differences from nonshared environment.

CONCLUSIONS

Chess and Thomas promoted research on temperament in part as a reaction against the extreme environmentalism that was prominent in the 1950s. This work has led to a more sophisticated approach to environmental influences on development in which children are viewed not merely as passive receptacles for environmental influences but as active participants who select, modify, and even create their experiences.

Behavioral genetic research has provided a unique perspective on these issues. In addition to documenting the importance of genetic factors, this research has produced two challenges to traditional thinking about environmental influences in development. First, genetic factors are enmeshed with traditional measures of the environment. Second, environmental influences salient to most domains of development are not shared by children growing up in the same family.

REFERENCES

Baker, L. A., & Clark, R. (1990). Genetic origins of behavior: Implications for counselors [Introduction to special feature]. *Journal of Counseling and Development, 68,* 597–600.

Bouchard, T. J., Jr., & McGue, M. (1990). Genetic and rearing environmental influences on adult personality: An analysis of adopted twins reared apart. *Journal of Personality, 58,* 263–292.

Braungart, J. M., Plomin, R., Fulker, D. W., & DeFries, J. C. (1992). Genetic influence of the home environment during infancy: A sibling adoption study of the HOME. *Development Psychology, 28,* 1048–1055.

Buss, A. H., & Plomin, R. (1984). *Temperament: Early developing personality traits.* Hillsdale, NJ: Lawrence Erlbaum.

Chess, S., & Thomas, A. (1984). *Origins and evolution of behavior disorders.* New York: Brunner/Mazel.

Chipuer, H. M., Plomin, R., Pedersen, N. L., McClearn, G. E., & Nesselroade, J. R. (1992). Genetic influence on family environment: The role of personality. *Developmental Psychology, 29,* 110–118.

Dunn, J., & Plomin, R. (1986). Determinants of maternal behaviour toward three-year-old siblings. *British Journal of Developmental Psychology, 57,* 348–356.

Dunn, J., & Plomin, R. (1990). *Separate lives: Why siblings are so different.* New York: Basic Books.

Dunn, J., & Plomin, R. (in press). Why are siblings so different? The significance of differences in sibling experiences within the family. *Family Process.*

Eaves, L. J., Eysenck, H. J., & Martin, N. (1989). *Genes, culture and personality.* New York: Academic Press.

Gottesman, I. I., Carey, G., & Hanson, D. R. (1983). Pearls and perils in epigenetic psychopathology. In S. B. Guze, E. J. Earls, & J. E. Barrett (Eds.), *Childhood psychopathology and development* (pp. 287–300). New York: Raven Press.

Lerner, R. M., Lerner, J. V., Windle, M., Hooker, K., Lenerz, K., & East, P. L. (1986). Children and adolescents in their contexts: Tests of a goodness of fit model. In R. Plomin & J. Dunn (Eds.), *The study of temperament: Changes, continuities, and challenges* (pp. 99–114). Hillsdale, NJ: Lawrence Erlbaum.

Loehlin, J. C. (1992). *Genes and environment in personality development.* Newbury Park, CA: Sage.

Loehlin, J. C., & Nichols, R. C. (1976). *Heredity, environment, and personality.* Austin: University of Texas Press.

Plomin, R. (1986). *Development, genetics, and psychology.* Hillsdale, NJ: Lawrence Erlbaum.

Plomin, R., & Bergeman, C. S. (1991a). The nature of nurture: Genetic influence on "environmental" measures. *Behavioral and Brain Sciences, 14,* 373–385.

Plomin, R., & Bergeman, C. S. (1991b). Nature and nurture. *Behavioral and Brain Sciences, 14,* 414–424.

Plomin, R., Chipuer, H. M., & Loehlin, J. C. (1990). Behavioral genetics and personality. In L. A. Pervin (Ed.), *Handbook of personality theory and research* (pp. 225–243). New York: Guilford Press.

Plomin, R., Chipuer, H. M., & Neiderhiser, J. M. (in press). Behavioral genetic evidence for the importance of nonshared environment. In E. M. Hetherington, D. Reiss, & R. Plomin (Eds.), *Separate social worlds of siblings: Impact of nonshared environment on development.* Hillsdale, NJ: Lawrence Erlbaum.

Plomin, R., & Daniels, D. (1987a). Why are children in the same family so different from each other? *Behavioral and Brain Sciences, 10,* 1–16.

Plomin, R., & Daniels, D. (1987b). Children in the same family are very different from each other, but why? *Behavioral and Brain Sciences, 10,* 44–54.

Plomin, R., DeFries, J. C., & Fulker, D. W. (1988). *Nature and nurture in infancy and early childhood.* New York: Cambridge University Press.

Plomin, R., DeFries, J. C., & Loehlin, J. C. (1977). Genotype-environment interaction and correlation in the analysis of human behavior. *Psychological Bulletin, 84,* 309–322.

Plomin, R., & Hershberger, S. (1991). Genotype-environment interaction. In T. D. Wachs & R. Plomin (Eds.), *Conceptualization and measurement of organism-environment interaction* (pp. 29–43). Washington, DC: American Psychological Association.

Plomin, R., Lichtenstein, P., Pedersen, N. L., McClearn, G. E., & Nesselroade, J. R.

(1990). Genetic influence on life events during the last half of the life span. *Psychology and Aging, 5,* 25–30.

Plomin, R., Loehlin, J. C., & DeFries, J. C. (1985). Genetic and environmental components of "environmental" influences. *Developmental Psychology, 21,* 391–402.

Plomin, R., McClearn, G. E., Pedersen, N. L., Nesselroade, J. R., & Bergeman, C. S. (1988). Genetic influence on childhood family environment perceived retrospectively from the last half of the life span. *Developmental Psychology, 24,* 738–745.

Plomin, R., Reiss, D., Hetherington, E. M., & Howe, G. (1992). Nature and nurture: Genetic influence on measures of the social environment. Manuscript submitted for publication.

Reiss, D., Plomin, R., Hetherington, E. M., Howe, G., Rovine, M., Tryon, A., & Stanley, M. (in press). The separate worlds of teenage siblings: An introduction to the study of the nonshared environment and adolescent development. In E. M. Hetherington, D. Reiss, & R. Plomin (Eds.), *Separate social worlds of siblings: Importance of non-shared environment on development.* Hillsdale, NJ: Lawrence Erlbaum.

Rowe, D. C. (1981). Environmental and genetic influences on dimensions of perceived parenting: A twin study. *Developmental Psychology, 17,* 203–208.

Rowe, D. C. (1983a). A biometrical analysis of perceptions of family environment: A study of twin and singleton sibling kinships. *Child Development, 54,* 416–423.

Rowe, D. C. (1983b). Biometrical genetic model of self-reported delinquent behavior: A twin study. *Behavior Genetics, 13,* 473–489.

Rutter, M., & Pickles, A. (1991). Person-environment interactions: Concepts, mechanisms, and implications for data analysis. In T. D. Wachs & R. Plomin (Eds.), *Conceptualization and measurement of organism-environment interaction* (pp. 105–136). Washington, DC: American Psychological Association.

Scarr, S. (1992). Developmental theories for the 1990s: Development and individual differences. *Child Development, 63,* 1–19.

Thomas, A., & Chess, S. (1977). *Temperament and development.* New York: Brunner/Mazel.

Thomas, A., & Chess, S. (1980). *The dynamics of psychological development.* New York: Brunner/Mazel.

Thomas, A., Chess, S., & Birch, H. (1968). *Temperament and behavior disorders in children.* New York: New York University Press.

Thomas, A., Chess, S., & Birch, H. (1970). The origin of personality. *Scientific American, 223,* 102–109.

Thomas, A., Chess, S., Birch, H., Hertzig, M., & Korn, S. (1963). *Behavioral individuality in early childhood.* New York: New York University Press.

Windle, J., & Lerner, R. M. (1986). The "goodness of fit" model of temperament-context relations: Interaction or correlation? In J. V. Lerner & R. M. Lerner (Eds.), *Temperament and social interaction during infancy and childhood* (pp. 109–119). San Francisco: Jossey-Bass.

PART VI

ISSUES IN ASSESSMENT
OF INDIVIDUAL DIFFERENCES

19

Assessment of Individual Differences in the Temperament of Children: Evaluation of Interactions

Sean C. McDevitt

The importance of the work of Alex Thomas and Stella Chess lies in its understanding of the evolution of child–environment interaction. Outcome for children appears to emerge from the dynamic interplay between parent and child and between child and environment, and in the multiple experiences that occur from before birth onward. The richness and complexity in the volumes that emanated from the New York Longitudinal Study (NYLS), starting with *Behavioral Individuality in Early Childhood* (Thomas, Chess, Birch, Hertzig, & Korn, 1963), convinced many child development researchers and clinicians that this seminal contribution ought to be followed by confirmation and validation of the NYLS findings by further empirical research. Because the NYLS was a pioneering anterospective effort, much of its quantitative and methodological decision making admittedly was based on improvisation and intuition rather than on detached, calculated proven research strategies. Even with the limitations inherent in research design, the import of the NYLS findings demanded replication and validation. Certainly the essence of what the NYLS team was observing and recording could be reduced to objective, empirically based fact!

In the early 1970s it seemed simple enough to do just that. Collaborating with William Carey, who had already begun work on this topic (Carey, 1970), and others in the Philadelphia area (Robin Hegvik, William Fullard, and Barbara Medoff-Cooper), we embarked on the process of constructing a series of parent rating instruments for measuring the nine NYLS temperament characteristics. Now nearly 20 years later, five parent report scales are available for assessing temperament from 1 month until 12 years of age (McDevitt & Carey, 1978; Carey & McDevitt, 1978; Hegvik, McDevitt, & Carey, 1982; Fullard, McDevitt, & Carey, 1984; Medoff-Cooper, Carey, & McDevitt, 1993). In the meantime, literally dozens of others have also emerged, measuring temperament or some variant of the original concept throughout the life span, from many different theoretical perspectives and in many different cultures. What seemed like such a simple task has provoked controversy and critical discussion of basic issues of definition, concept, stability, and utility of temperament. We are still far from objectively assessing the complexity of the phenomenon that was recorded in the NYLS, in spite of the great strides that have been made toward that goal.

The purpose of this chapter is to review the problems with and obstacles to measuring individual differences in children's personality given the experience of research on temperament. Improvement in the assessment enterprise will ultimately benefit those whose task it is to optimize growth and development of children in primary care and clinical settings and to conduct effective prevention and intervention. Although several methods exist for assessing temperament through interview and behavioral observation, a detailed analysis of these measures would be beyond the scope of this chapter. The following discussion will focus on the most commonly employed technique, the questionnaire.

ASSESSMENT ISSUES

Temperament scales have many commonalities, and it would be hazardous to overemphasize the differences. As with individuality in personality, individual instruments can have characteristics that make them more functional in some settings than other scales or than in other settings. However, little attention has been given to looking systematically at differences in the elements of temperament assessment techniques in order to understand their major strengths and weaknesses. In general the major differences between assessment instruments occur in the following areas: (1) concepts of temperament (purpose), (2) environmental context (role of specific situations), (3) parental/rater bias (or inclusion), and (4) developmental level.

These differences may lead the potential user to select an instrument for a specific use, or expect a result that is consistent with the characteristics of the scale. Although reviews of the comparative psychometric properties of temperament questionnaires have been published (Hubert, Wachs, Peters-Martin, & Gandour,

1982; Slabach, Morrow, & Wachs, 1991), little effort has been made to analyze what effect differences in questionnaire construction and content might have on the phenomenon being assessed. Secondarily, the usefulness of a temperament assessment technique for prevention or intervention may be somewhat dependent upon the manner in which the technique was developed.

CONCEPTS OF TEMPERAMENT: HOW MANY DIMENSIONS TO ASSESS

In the NYLS the concept of temperament began with the notion of "primary reaction patterns" (Thomas, Chess, Birch, & Hertzig, 1960), which were thought to be internal, biologically determined behavioral dispositions. The phenomenon was clearly "within the child," and the original measurement technique, a semistructured interview, was designed to elicit observational descriptions of these dispositions. In fact the original 10 dimensions were identified through an analysis of the content of the answers given to open-ended questions about the infant's behavior. The inability to distinguish between Attention Span and Persistence behaviorally led to the revision of the dimensions to the current nine. However, the fact that these characteristics were distinguishable did not make them independent statistically, nor did it limit the number of dimensions that could be determined to nine. It was thought that these were the most accessible in infancy for longitudinal study, and may be useful in demonstrating the origins of behavioral individuality. The beginnings of the NYLS concept of temperament were empirical, not intuitive as some have argued to justify redefining them.

Much has been made by factor analytic researchers about the lack of independence of the nine NYLS dimensions (Buss & Plomin, 1975), with the concurrent recommendation that the number of dimensions be reduced through statistical means. Clinicians who value the NYLS constructs because of their demonstrated utility disagree and argue that refinement of measurement technique should be the main purpose of further assessment improvements (Carey, 1983). Academicians, whose focus is on parsimoniously describing an object of analysis, wish to simplify the nine dimensions to fewer "purer" temperaments. While utility is ultimately the final evaluation criterion, the alteration of these characteristics imposes the burden of demonstrating utility all over again, since the variables measured have been changed in some unknown degree.

Since the late 1950s, numerous alternative schemes for conceptualizing temperament have been proposed. The concepts of childhood temperament largely follow from the original NYLS dimensions and their factorial derivatives, though there are some models that stem from the clinical and research literature on activity level, impulsivity, and introversion-extroversion (see Buss & Plomin, 1975).

As with the study of intellectual functioning, temperament characteristics have unitary concepts such as general intelligence (Bates's difficultness factor) (Bates, Olson, Pettit, & Bayles, 1982), clinical scales that are intercorrelated like the Wechsler series (Carey & McDevitt, 1978), and factorial dimensions like the Primary Mental Ability scales (Rothbart's IBQ). A better scholar than I could make a longer list of comparisons. In contrast to the situation with intelligence, however, with temperament there are instruments that purport to measure the phenomenon throughout the life span from infancy to adulthood (Buss & Plomin, 1975; Windle & Lerner, 1986). Alternatively, there are questionnaires designed for time spans as short as 3 months (EITQ) (Medoff-Cooper et al., 1991).

One of the most important distinctions in the assessment of temperament stems from the underlying purpose of the concept. While clinicians measure temperament to provide prevention and intervention services to children and their care givers undergoing stressful interactions, researchers seek to identify and measure the basic or fundamental aspects of temperament as an overall dimension of personality.

THE EFFECT OF CONTEXT ON ASSESSMENT:
WHAT CONTEXTS TO CONSIDER

As it became clear empirically over time that the cross-situational consistency of these dispositions was moderate at best, an interactional viewpoint evolved wherein temperamental styles were seen as having a range of specific expressions, with the "real" temperament being some midpoint or most frequently expressed value around which the majority of typical situations tended to cluster (Thomas & Chess, 1981). The interactional concept, while less definitive, fit the data better and allowed researchers to maintain at least a modicum of generality to their concepts. This was so since cross-situational consistency could be maintained only with very narrow dimensions such as "activity while sleeping," which included both a behavioral disposition and a context. Some factorial studies in fact narrowed scales with large numbers of items down to such dimensions until they contained only two or three similar questions. From an assessment perspective, the interactional approach results in the rater responding to a series of context-specific items that are "averaged" over all of the situations included in a questionnaire. The degree to which the ratings are similar over all the items is the internal consistency of the questionnaire (sometimes called internal validity), and it indicates its integrity (and that of the concept) for that dimension. If the items in a scale cannot reach an acceptable level of internal validity, it may indicate that the concept is not viable for the dimension or the contexts being considered. Such was the case with the physiological rhythmicity dimension of the Middle

Childhood Temperament Questionnaire (Hegvik et al., 1982), which, in spite of several pretests, never reached an internal consistency above .40. A conceptually related dimension, predictability, was substituted and appeared to have acceptable internal validity.

The behavioral geneticists, studying an internal genetically determined concept, chose to reduce cross-situational inconsistency by having the rater respond to items with no context included at all, such as "the child is intense" (Buss & Plomin, 1975). This "in the child" concept requires the rater to sum over all observations of intensity and select a score that reflects their experiences with the individual being rated. When this summative rating is repeated over similarly worded items, a homogeneous scale results. Temperament questionnaires that utilize noncontextual items may demonstrate factorial validity, but so may context-specific ones if other aspects of questionnaire design are engineered appropriately (see the next section).

DEALING WITH PARENTAL/RATER BIAS

Almost as controversial as the issues regarding the concept of temperament and its stability are the debates surrounding the ability of a care giver to objectively observe and rate the behavioral style of an infant or child. Questionnaires completed by parents fell into disrepute after the work of Sears and others indicated little correlation between questionnaire results and the findings of researchers observing similar situations or behaviors. Debate regarding the advisability of assessing temperament by questionnaire led to the revision of the concept in some circles to "perceptions" of temperament, the perceptions being those of the rater. There are fundamental differences between those who believe that temperament as a concept includes so much rater bias that it is partially (or largely) defined by a measurement artifact, whether intentionally or not, and those who believe that scores on temperament measures may contain a certain amount of error attributable to inaccuracies by the individual rating the infant or child. In fact, some perception-oriented measures ask the rater to describe how the infant's behavior makes the *rater* feel in order to assess the "difficultness" of the *infant* (Bates et al., 1982).

The perceptions approach deals with the rater influence in two ways. Some conservative researchers argue that it is more accurate to label temperament ratings as perceptions because this significant source of bias can't be eliminated, especially in interviews and questionnaires, and it would be misleading to talk about the measures without reference to bias (Wolk, Zeanah, Coll, & Carr, 1992). Other more clinically oriented researchers feel that the perception of the care giver is important and colors the way in which the interaction occurs with the child. In this view, the perception rating may be the more accurate predictor of later status since both sides of the interaction are being included in the assessment. The work of Bates on predicted coercive behavioral control by mothers and the teachability dimension of Keogh and colleagues (this volume) fall into this latter category. In either case, the perceptions approach assumes a less clearly accessible concept of temperament for measurement by either clinicians or researchers.

A third approach, measuring both specific ratings and general impressions (perceptions), distinguishes between the two and attempts to utilize them both clinically. Carey (1989) has described this process and given specific case examples where an "easy" child by rating is perceived by general impression as "difficult" and vice versa.

There appears to be some evidence that raters who are suffering from emotional problems such as depression may rate their infants less accurately than mothers who are not depressed (Whiffen, 1990). However, little other evidence pro or con exists.

Methodologically, it is difficult to estimate bias by inference, that is, the lack of correlation between observations and ratings. Interpreting the absence of significant relationships runs the risk of trying to prove a null hypothesis. One of the problems in estimating bias may be the absence of objective observational measures of temperament that could serve as a benchmark for determining the validity of ratings by care givers. Presently there exists no validated observational measure of temperament from which a reliable estimate of bias could be made. One of the difficulties appears to be that behavioral observations in naturalistic settings are not highly replicable, and studies with few observations to aggregate may not even be as reliable as the questionnaires they presume to evaluate.

Another source of rater bias, less frequently discussed, has to do with the placement of the items within the questionnaire. Some instruments cluster items that will be scored on the same dimension together in the questionnaire, while others randomize or block randomize the presentation to the rater. Students of psychometrics know that adjacent presentation of similar items tends to inflate their intercorrelation with one another, which will influence both factorial and internal consistency estimates. Moreover, some scales categorize items into sections that contain the name of the category or dimension as the subheading. Comparative analysis of these indices should include consideration of whether the instrument design maximizes or minimizes bias as a source of potential error.

Another technique for reducing rater bias, reversing items, so that high scores indicate the presence of a characteristic on some items but low scores do on others in the same dimension, also tends to minimize inappropriate inflation of intercorrelation. In some characteristics, such as Emotionality, there appear to be two separate components in some measures and item reversal may not be feasible (Goldsmith, 1987). But other temperamental characteristics do seem to have measurable aspects on both sides of the dimension, which could be assessed to minimize distortion. It may be prudent to consider factorial validation of unipolar item-adjacent questionnaires critically and determine empirically whether the results are robust enough to withstand removal of these two inflationary practices.

CHANGES DUE TO DEVELOPMENTAL LEVEL

Age and/or developmental level also have an important effect on measurement of temperament, especially for the context-specific instruments. In addition to the developmental changes described above in regard to characteristics such as rhythmicity, there are no doubt other changes in overt behavior that can change the expression of temperament over time. Cognitive suppression, development of new physical capabilities, such as walking and running in the second year, and changes in the environments children inhabit (such as school entrance) can have a major impact on the behavioral topography of temperament. These events represent a major challenge to measurement devices that attempt to assess temperament through overt behavior. In questionnaires that use a sample of behavioral items, there is no certainty that the new contexts that are selected in the next developmental period are equally representative of the temperament as the items selected in the previous period.

The opposite measurement strategy, using items that are applicable over the life span, has been employed by Windle and Lerner (1986), and by Buss and Plomin (1975), in the DOTS-R and EASI (now EAS) respectively. Factorial validation over the life span can provide evidence of continuity in the temperament dimensions assessed. Stability estimates over time should also be maximized by these instruments. However, it may be that these measures are less sensitive to concurrent events than those that assess age-contextual items. This is an empirical issue, and one that could lead to some interesting research. A second type of age-related change, increases or decreases in mean score over time, can be measured only "within instrument" unless one is willing to assume that behavioral contexts between age periods are equivalent.

SUMMARY AND CONCLUSIONS

In spite of the importance of the concept, the assessment of temperament has proved to be a complex and difficult task. Researchers have employed a variety of strategies to measure one of a number of objective coherent concepts of temperament, including variations in definition such as the number of dimensions, different considerations of environmental context, contrasting handling of rater bias, and diverse approaches to behavioral changes at later developmental levels. While great strides have been made in reliable measurement, no objective method for determining temperamental status is as yet accepted as the benchmark for comparison of validity with other measures. Until such measures are developed, temperament scales, observations, and interviews will be judged by a variety of validity criteria, including factorial integrity; construct validity; and clinical correlations with important indices of physical health, development, and behavioral adjustment.

Ultimately, it may prove difficult to capture completely the essence of the interaction between the behavioral style of the child and the environment in a way that represents temperamental individuality in a single test score. It seems likely that the usefulness of temperament in clinical prevention and intervention and in research settings will be demonstrated increasingly as the sophistication of the assessment enterprise increases. As it increases our ability to match the long-term observations of the rich, complex phenomena delineated by Thomas, Chess, and colleagues in the NYLS, the importance of their contribution to the study of personality development will be more fully understood.

REFERENCES

Bates, J., Olson, S. L., Pettit, G. S., & Bayles, K. (1982). Dimensions of individuality in the mother infant relationship at 6 months of age. *Child Development, 53*, 446–461.

Buss, A. H., & Plomin, R. (1975). *A temperament theory of personality development*. New York: John Wiley.

Carey, W. B. (1970). A simplified method for measuring infant temperament. *Journal of Pediatrics, 77*, 188–194.

Carey, W. B. (1983). Some pitfalls in infant temperament research. *Infant Behavior and Development, 6*, 247.

Carey, W. B. (1989). Clinical use of temperament data in pediatrics. In W. B. Carey & S. C. McDevitt (Eds.), *Clinical and educational applications of temperament research*. Amsterdam/ Lisse, The Netherlands: Swets and Zeitlinger.

Carey, W. B., & McDevitt, S. C. (1978). Revision of the Infant Temperament Questionnaire. *Pediatrics, 61*, 735–739.

Fullard, W., McDevitt, S. C., & Carey, W. B. (1984). Assessing temperament in one to three year old children. *Journal of Pediatric Psychology, 9*, 205–216.

Goldsmith, H. H. (1987). *The Toddler Behavior Assessment Questionnaire manual*. Eugene Department of Psychology, University of Oregon.

Hegvik, R., McDevitt, S. C., & Carey, W. B. (1982). The Middle Childhood Temperament Questionnaire. *Journal of Developmental and Behavioral Pediatrics, 3*, 197–200.

Hubert, N. C., Wachs, T. D., Peters-Martin, P., & Gandour, M. (1982). The study of early temperament: Measurement and conceptual issues. *Child Development, 53*, 571–600.

McDevitt, S. C., & Carey, W. B. (1978). The measurement of temperament in 3 to 7 year old children. *Journal of Child Psychology and Psychiatry, 19*(3), 245–253.

Medoff-Cooper, B., Carey, W. B., & McDevitt, S. (1991). EITQ: The Early Infancy Temperament Questionnaire. *Journal of Developmental and Behavioral Pediatrics*, in press.

Slabach, E. H., Morrow, J., & Wachs, T. D. (1991). Questionnaire measurement of infant and child temperament. In J. Strelau & A. Angleitner (Eds.), *Explorations in temperament: International perspectives on theory and measurement*. New York: Plenum Press.

Thomas, A., & Chess, S. (1981). The role of temperament in the contributions of individuals to their development. In R. M. Lerner & N. A. Busch-Rossnagel (Eds.), *Individuals as producers of their development*. New York: Academic Press.

Thomas, A., Chess, S., Birch, H., & Hertzig, M. (1960). A longitudinal study of primary reaction patterns in children. *Comprehensive Psychiatry, 1*(8), 103–112.

Thomas, A., Chess, S., Birch, H. G., Hertzig, M. E., & Korn, S. (1963). *Behavioral individuality in early childhood*. New York: New York University Press.

Whiffen, V. E. (1990). Maternal depressed mood and perception of child temperament. *Journal of Genetic Psychology, 15*(3), 329–339.

Windle, M., & Lerner, R. M. (1986). Reassessing the dimensions of temperamental individuality across the life span: The Revised Dimensions of Temperament Survey (DOTS-R). *Journal of Adolescent Research, 1*, 213–230.

Wolk, S., Zeanah, C. H., Coll, C. T. G., & Carr, S. (1992). Factors affecting parents perceptions of temperament in early infancy. *American Journal of Orthopsychiatry, 62*(1), 71–77.

PART VII

PREVENTION AND INTERVENTION STRATEGIES IN THE MEDICAL SETTING

20

Specific Prevention and Intervention Strategies Used to Accommodate Individual Needs of Newborn Infants

Barbara Medoff-Cooper

Because I was a doctoral student in a university that was and continues to be committed to temperament research, it is not surprising that the work of Alexander Thomas and Stella Chess became a central theme of my research. The expression of temperament as a dynamic interactional phenomenon, as well as a "goodness-of-fit" model, has continued to be the guiding force in my clinical practice with healthy as well as high-risk infants. Although Thomas and Chess's New York Longitudinal Study (NYLS) (Thomas & Chess, 1977) began when the infants were 3 months of age, mostly because of the relative instability of temperament characteristics in the early weeks of life, I believe that it is our responsibility to begin anticipatory guidance concerning individual differences on the first day of life. It is with this in mind that I have structured this article in honor of Thomas and Chess. This chapter explores factors contributing to behavioral individuality in the neonatal period for both full-term and preterm babies. It discusses how parents can be helped by clinicians to understand the particular behavioral styles of their infants in order to accommodate their individual needs. Although this chapter has some material overlapping with Dr. Hertzig's excellent presentation in this same collection, the difference is that my emphasis is a primary care, anticipatory guidance perspective.

Individual differences in behavioral style are readily demonstrated as early as the first hours of life. For example, there are some infants with lusty intense cries who are difficult to soothe, and others with mild cries who are easy to soothe. These differences are influenced by multiple factors, are evidently transient, and may or may not reflect the temperament characteristics that emerge in the coming months. However, despite the lack of extensive research correlating early behaviors with later temperament, it is important to understand the gamut of individual styles parents encounter in newborns. These are the varied behaviors with which the parents must deal then and there, whether they will prove to be enduring characteristics or not.

RESEARCH FINDINGS

Individual Differences: Full-Term Infants

What factors contribute to the individual behavioral differences in term neonates such as being easier to handle or more irritable and difficult to soothe?

Birth Weight. For one thing, there are differences as measured by the Neonatal Behavioral Assessment Scale (NBAS) (Brazelton, 1973) between normal- and low- or large-birth-weight infants. Normal-weight infants are those infants who are of an appropriate weight for gestational age compared to standardized norms. (For term infants that usually means between 5 1/2 lb and 10 lb.). Low birth weight or small size for gestational age may be caused by a variety of factors such as poor maternal nutrition or smoking. Infants who are large for their gestational age are often the product of a mother with diabetes. Both the low-birth-weight or small-for-gestational-age (Scarr & Williams, 1973) and the large-for-gestational-age groups (Chase, 1974) can be considered groups at risk for a variety of physical or developmental complications.

Normal-weight infants were found to have higher attention-orientation scores than the other two groups (Riese, 1986). This means that they displayed greater auditory and visual alertness. Infants in the two extreme groups had higher scores on measures of irritability, rapidity of buildup, activity, and peak of excitement, making them likely to be harder to manage.

Sex. In addition to birth weight, sex seems to be a significant factor in determining behavioral differences. In studying individual differences in 30 full-term opposite-sex twins with a mean chronological age of 4.5 days, Riese (1986) found female neonates to be more irritable than males. No other behavioral differences were noted, except that female neonates were more difficult to soothe than males.

The differences in arousal level (irritability) may be related to maturity since girls at birth are more mature (Stratton, 1982). It may be that maturity (in the sense of being aware enough of the environment to react to it) affects performance in the areas of soothability and irritability and mood. These differences were revealed by a five-category observation assessment scale that included irritability, resistance to soothing, reactivity, reinforcement value, and activity (Riese, 1982). Many of the measures are similar to those of the NBAS.

Genetic, Intrauterine, and Perinatal Factors. Although there is much support in the literature for a genetic influence on behavioral style in infancy and childhood (Torgersen & Kringlen, 1978), this does not yet seem to be expressed in the neonatal period (Riese, 1990). Riese suggests that the individual differences in the newborn are more influenced by intrauterine and perinatal factors. It is safe to say that perinatal factors are probably stronger than any other factors during this early newborn period. Genetic influences will become more evident beyond the newborn period in infancy.

Preterm Infants—Uncomplicated

Even though increasing technological advances in life-support systems in neonatal intensive care units (NICU) have greatly decreased mortality and morbidity in the preterm infant (U.S. Congress, 1989), there remains fairly consistent reporting of difficult temperament or behavioral style for preterm infants during hospitalization (Medoff-Cooper, 1988) and for at least the first 6 months of life (Medoff-Cooper & Schraeder, 1982; Medoff-Cooper, 1986; Washington, Minde, & Goldberg, 1986). In the early months of life, preterm infants are often described by their parents as being difficult to soothe, arrhythmical in body functions, and negative in mood.

Despite these reports from parents, Hertzig and Mittleman (1984) did not find preterm infants to be more difficult as defined by the constellation of characteristics that includes irregularity in bodily functions, withdrawing behaviors in new situations, nonadaptability to change, and negative expression of mood over the first 3 years of life. However, the low-birth-weight infants were less adaptable, less distractible, and more intense, and had a higher threshold of responsiveness to sensory stimuli than full-term infants, which may be just as troublesome to parents as some of the characteristics that make up the typical "difficult temperament" cluster. In contrast, Oberklaid, Prior, and Sanson (1986) and Ross (1987) did not find any significant differences in temperament ratings between preterm and full-term infants at, respectively, 4 to 8 months and 12 months of age. One problem in comparing all of the results is the differences in the study designs. These include varying methods and/or instruments for assessing temperament and ages at which the testing was completed, as well as differences in gestational ages at birth. For example, Oberklaid and colleagues included all infants below 37 weeks gestational age in the preterm group, which is different from the Ross and Medoff-Cooper and Schraeder studies, in that they included only infants with a gestational age below 32 weeks.

The age at which an infant is assessed for individual differences is important. It appears that the difficult behavioral style of the preterm infant moderates with increasing age. In one study of 41 very-low-birth-weight (VLBW) infants, 31.7% of the group were found to be difficult as compared to 10% in the standardization group at 6 months as measured by the Infant Temperament Questionnaire. At 1 year of age, there was great moderation in the amount of difficultness, in that only half that number of infants were still rated as difficult, which is now approaching the norm of 12.3% (Medoff-Cooper, 1986).

Preterm Infants—Complicated

Research has explored perinatal risk factors such as gestational age at birth, birth weight, severity of medical complications, and incidence of intraventricular hemorrhage as possible contributors to the manifestation of difficult behavioral style of the preterm infant. Yet no one perinatal or postnatal complication has so far proved to be a strong predictor of behavioral style.

There has been some evidence to suggest that infants who have experienced a neurological insult are more likely to be "difficult" to manage by displaying poorly adaptive characteristics (Rutter, 1977). Similarly, Hertzig (1983) reports that although the temperament profile for all low-birth-weight infants was not more "difficult" than that for full-term ones, neurologically impaired premature infants were more likely to display the five difficult temperament characteristics. They may exhibit irregular biological functions, adapt slowly to change, withdraw in new situations, and exhibit intense and negative moods. Infants in the Hertzig study were assessed with the NYLS interview at 6-month intervals during the first 2 years of life and at 3 years of age (see her chapter in this volume).

After assessing a group of 67 preterm infants at 3 months (corrected for gestational age) with the Bates Infant Characteristics Questionnaire, Garcia-Coll and colleagues (1988) reported that regardless of the presence or severity of intraventricular hemorrhage (IVH), preterm infants demonstrate fewer positive responses and less overall activity than full-term infants do. Preterm infants with small intraventricular hemorrhage (grade I to II) were significantly less sociable and more difficult to soothe than full-term infants. Unexpectedly, they were also more difficult to soothe than preterm infants with more serious intraventricular hemorrhages (grade III to IV). One explanation may be that infants with serious IVHs may have impaired sensory motor responses.

Nonetheless, two infants of the same premature gestational age may exhibit very different responses to a particular procedure or medical complication. For example, clinical evidence indicates clearly that some preterm infants, especially the medically fragile, are more physiologically stressed by handling and environmental stimuli than are others of the same gestational age (Als et al., 1986; Gorski, 1983). Some preterm infants may be able to maintain normal physiological status when handled, while others may become bradycardic or tachycardic. Therefore, factors other than distinct genetic makeup must contribute as well to behavioral response.

In an attempt to assess the individuality of such behaviors, Gorski (1983) describes a set of physiological distress signals (PDS) that seem to differentiate a preterm infant's behavioral style in response to the noisy, overstimulating environment of the neonatal intensive care unit. Subtle signs of distress include hiccuping, grimaced face, avoidance gazing, and mottling. The gross signs of distress are temperature instability, tachycardia, apnea, bradycardia, and vomiting. Thus Gorski is suggesting that the degree to which an infant responds to the environment could be viewed as his or her reaction to environmental overload and as a precursor to differences among individuals. For example, a preterm infant who has a dramatic increase in heart rate when being handled may also in later months be the infant who is unadaptable and withdrawing in new situations.

Of all the infants in the intensive care nursery, it is the infants with bronchopulmonary dysplasia (BPD) who are most likely to display PDS. Long after other preterm infants have been able to maintain their physiological stability when being handled, the infant with BPD continues to have an elevated heart and respiratory rate, as well as the chronic facial grimace (Medoff-Cooper, 1988).

Drug Abuse—Influences on Neonatal Temperament

Although there remains a great deal of controversy about the relationship of prenatal drug exposure, and more specifically cocaine abuse, on newborn behavior, it does appear that some exposed infants are at greater risk for neurobehavioral sequelae, including behavioral abnormalities. These infants often display low thresholds for overstimulation and require a great deal of assistance to maintain control of their hyperexcitable nervous system (Griffith, 1988). When assessed on the NBAS, neonates exposed to cocaine showed a decrease in interactive abilities and state organization as compared to nonexposed infants (Chasnoff, Burns, Schnoll, et al., 1985). The most symptomatic infants are often described as being extremely irritable by the nursery staff. Their low sensory threshold for environmental stimuli, intense cry, and low soothability, in addition to a diminished ability for attention (Zuckerman & Frank, 1992), present a unique set of challenges for parents who may be the least able to cope with a less than ideal infant. However, it is not clear how long this difficult behavioral style persists.

CLINICAL INTERVENTION

Newborns' individual behavioral responses are highly varied, and many different factors—age, sex, neurological development, genes, and so on—contribute to the manifestations of the behaviors. Therefore, it is important to know what medical care givers can do to recognize them and help parents of infants with a more difficult behavioral style. Both general information and individual guidance can assist parents to understand their particular baby's behavioral style.

Over the past few decades, the length of time a woman stays in the hospital after the delivery of an infant has decreased dramatically. It is not uncommon for a full-term infant and mother to be discharged within 36 hours of the vaginal birth and only 72 hours after a cesarean delivery. This short hospital stay leaves little time for appropriate teaching, with much to be accomplished. Teaching should include information not only on bathing, feeding, and dressing, but also on infant temperament and its variations.

Full-Term Infants

Although we know that there may be little stability of behavioral style over the first weeks of life, helping parents get a clear understanding of how their particular baby responds to the nursery environment aids in the establishment of a "good fit" between the parents' expectations of the infant and the infant's behavior.

General Advice. New parents are seldom consciously aware of the tension that arises from the discrepancy between an idealized view of an infant who cries little, comforts easily, is responsive to parental care giving, and quickly begins to sleep through the night, and the reality that many babies behave quite differently. In fact, parents are quick to judge their success in parenting by the length of time an infant cries or how long it takes to soothe the distressed infant. Seldom is a new parent told that how much an infant cries throughout a day may vary from 1 to 8 hours and that the intensity may vary as well (Brazelton, 1962). Parents can be informed and their task lightened by experienced health care professionals (nursery nurse, neonatal nurse clinician/practitioner, physician) with good clinical acumen and an interest in being helpful.

Specific Advice. These healthcare professional persons can identify easily those infants who have intense cries and are difficult to soothe. With the knowledge that these characteristics may have little to do with their child's future performance, the parents will be less likely to be overcome with guilt and tension in their interactions with the child. In addition to identifying these behaviors, the health care professional could help the mother provide care more compatible with the infant's individual needs. For example, the physician or nurse might help parents understand that crying may be a result of an infant's inability to get oriented to stimuli or inability to move adequately through various awake-sleep states. Thus, she or he might suggest that parents of those infants present fewer stimuli or make modifications in the feeding, nap, and sleeping schedules of their babies. Likewise, care givers might suggest that some infants need to be handled with greater consistency, since they do not tolerate a variety of people caring for them, are unable to sleep in new places, or do not adapt readily to new schedules. Although these troublesome individual characteristics may be present in only a small percentage of young infants, this type of information should be provided during discharge planning as anticipatory guidance for in the first month of life.

Preterm Infants—More Intensive Instruction

The behavioral difficulties faced by parents of preterm infants are usually considered even greater than those of parents of full-term infants. In the first few weeks to months of life the very-low-birth-weight infant is even less responsive to parental care giving than is the full-term infant (Field, 1979). Parents of a full-term infant can usually enjoy a sense of reciprocity between their smiling and talking and the infant's positive regard. Even in the first weeks of life, the full-term infant is able to look at the parent for increasing periods of time, begin cooing back to the parents, and even begin to imitate mouthing movements (Bandura, 1962). Parents of VLBW infants frequently do not receive this positive reinforcement from their infants. Instead, many preterm infants provide their parents with few cues concerning their needs and spend most of their waking hours fussing. In addition, many preterm infants tend to be arrhythmical in their bodily functions, and difficult to soothe (Hermans, Cats, & Ouden, 1985).

It was explained earlier that these behaviors may not be enduring temperament differences; they result from an immature neurological system. Nevertheless, parents will need help in adapting to their infant's behavior. The best possible way to assist parents of preterm infants to appreciate their particular infant's behavioral style is to encourage them to take part in care procedures in the neonatal intensive care nursery (NICU). If parents learn how their infant responds to handling, what the best techniques for cuddling are, and which modes of soothing are most effective (music vs. a voice, stroking vs. rocking), then they are better prepared for discharge.

Parenting a preterm infant in the early weeks after discharge is not an easy task. Mothers frequently report that the PDS continue for several weeks. Too often these infants continue to avoid eye contact, have a grimace on their face, and have skin mottling when they are touched, all of which may help to create a less than ideal parent-child relationship. These behaviors are a source of frustration for a parent who is trying to engage the infant's attention. Therefore, it is essential that parents comprehend that the behaviors demonstrated by their infant are not in response to the quality of their parenting. Rather, they are evidence of a temporarily immature neurological system (Medoff-Cooper, 1988). The physiological signals of distress reflect disorganization and the infant's ability to cope with stimuli in the environment at that time. However, during the next few weeks infants will have matured enough to lose these behaviors (Washington et al., 1986). Rather than feeling guilty about their children's behavior, parents can be more tolerant, knowing that they are not responsible. They should be aware that aversive behaviors will not necessarily continue.

Thus, health care professionals have two major tasks in helping parents of preterm infants establish a meaningful and rewarding parent-child relationship. The first task is to ensure that parents are able to have physical contact with the infant as soon as the infant is medically stable. Only with contact will the parent learn how the infant responds to environmental stimuli. The second task involves anticipatory guidance. So often parents return to the 1-month pediatric visit feeling as if they are not doing a good job. If they knew prior to discharge that the infant's difficult behavioral style is not a function of poor parenting, they would be much more confident and reassured. Removing this burden of guilt is probably the best thing that child-health professionals can do to assist parents and infants to establish a healthy relationship. More positive interactional patterns will do much to ensure the development of the infant into a well-adjusted child and adult.

CONCLUSIONS

Although behavioral characteristics in the neonatal period may not demonstrate the level of continuity they do in later childhood, child-health professionals can help parents to understand the individual differences of the particular child at that time. Who is responsible to do this teaching? Certainly in the hospital setting most of the newborn teaching is provided by the nursery nursing staff. In addition, during daily newborn rounds, the physician or nurse practitioner can and should supply the parents with the appropriate anticipatory guidance. In the intensive care nursery, the primary nurse bears the main responsibility to plan and carry out the discharge teaching for families.

Once the infant is discharged from the hospital, the primary health care provider (physician or nurse practitioner) should assume the role of helping parents to understand the specific behavioral characteristics of their infant and to be able to respond to them appropriately. Parenting a newborn who is perceived to be difficult is a particularly frustrating experience, which can be made easier by informed, sensitive health care professionals.

REFERENCES

Als, H., Lawhon, G., Brown, E., Gibes, R., Duffy, F., McAnulty, G., & Bickman, J. (1986). Individualized behavioral and environmental care for the very low birth weight infant at high risk for bronchopulmonary dysplasia: Neonatal intensive care unit and developmental outcome. *Pediatrics, 78*, 1123–1132.

Bandura, A. (1962). Social learning through imitation. In M. R. Jones (Ed.), *Nebraska Symposium on Motivation* (pp. 211–269). Lincoln: University of Nebraska Press.

Brazelton, T. B. (1962). Crying in infancy. *Pediatrics, 29*, 579–588.

Brazelton, T. B. (1973). *Neonatal Behavioral Assessment Scale.* Philadelphia: J.B. Lippincott.

Chase, H. (1974). Perinatal mortality: Overview and current trends. *Clinics in Perinatal Medicine, 1*(1), 3–18.

Chasnoff, I., Burns, W., Schnoll, S., et al. (1985). Cocaine use in pregnancy. *New England Journal of Medicine, 313*, 666–669.

Field, T. (1979). Interaction patterns of preterm and term infants. In T. Field (Ed.), *Infants born at risk* (pp. 33–356). New York: Spectrum.

Garcia-Coll, C., Emmons, L., Vohr, B., Ward, A., Brann, B., Shaul, P., Mayfield, S., & Oh, W. (1988). Behavioral responsiveness in preterm infants with intraventricular hemorrhage. *Pediatrics, 81*(3), 412–418.

Gorski, P. (1983). Premature infant behavior and physiologic responses to care giving intervention in the intensive care nursery. In J. Call, E. Galenson, & R. Tyson (Eds.), *Frontiers of infant psychiatry.* New York: Basic Books.

Griffith, D. (1988). The effects of perinatal cocaine exposure on infant neurobehavior and early-infant interaction. In I. Chasnoff (Ed.), *Drugs, alcohol, pregnancy and parenting.* Boston: Kluwer Academic Publishers.

Hermans, J., Cats, B., & Ouden, L. (1985). The development of temperament in very low birth weight children. In W. Frankenberg, R. Emde, & J. Sullivan (Eds.), *Early identification of children at risk* (pp. 279–285). New York: Plenum Press.

Hertzig, M. (1983). Temperament and neurological status. In M. Rutter (Ed.), *Developmental neuropsychiatry* (pp. 164–176). New York: Guilford Press.

Hertzig, M., & Mittleman, M. (1984). Temperament in low birthweight children. *Merrill-Palmer Quarterly, 30*, 201–211.

Medoff-Cooper, B. (1986). Temperament in very low birth weight infants. *Nursing Research, 35*, 139–143.

Medoff-Cooper, B. (1988). The effects of handling on preterm infants with bronchopulmonary dysplasia. *Image: Journal of Nursing Scholarship, 20*, 132–134.

Medoff-Cooper, B., & Schraeder, B. (1982). Developmental trends and behavioral styles in very low birthweight infants. *Nursing Research, 31*, 69–72.

Oberklaid, F., Prior, M., & Sanson, A. (1986). Temperament of preterm versus full-term infants. *Developmental and Behavioral Pediatrics, 7,* 159–162.

Riese, M. L. (1982) Procedures and norms for assessing behavioral patterns in full-terms and stable pre-term neonates. *JSAS Catalog Selected Documents of Psychology, 12*(6). (Ms. No. 2415)

Riese, M. L. (1986). Implications of sex differences in neonatal temperament for early risk and developmental/environmental interactions. *The Journal of Genetic Psychology, 147*(4), 507–513.

Riese, M. L. (1990). Neonatal temperament in monozygotic and dizygotic twin pairs. *Child Development, 61,* 1230–1237.

Ross, G. (1987). Temperament of preterm infants: Its relationship to perinatal factors and one-year outcome. *Developmental and Behavioral Pediatrics, 8,* 106–110.

Rutter, M. (1977). Brain damage syndromes in childhood: Concepts and findings. *Journal of Child Psychology and Psychiatry, 18,* 1–21.

Scarr, S., & Williams, M. (1973). The effects of early stimulation on low birthweight infants. *Child Development, 46,* 94–101.

Stratton, P. (1982). Newborn individuality. In P. Stratton (Ed.), *Psychobiology of the human newborn* (pp. 221–261). New York: John Wiley.

Thomas, A., & Chess, S. (1977). *Temperament and development.* New York: Brunner/Mazel.

Torgersen, A. M., & Kringlen, B. (1978). Genetic aspects of temperamental differences in infants. *Journal of the American Academy of Child Psychiatry, 17,* 433–444.

U. S. Congress, Office of Technology Assessment, 1989.

Washington, J., Minde, K., & Goldberg, S. (1986). Temperament in preterm infants: Style and stability. *Journal of the American Academy of Child Psychiatry, 25*(4), 493–502.

Zuckerman, B., & Frank, D. (1992). "Crack kids": Not broken. *Pediatrics, 89,* 337–339.

21

Specific Uses of Temperament Data in Pediatric Behavioral Interventions

William B. Carey

Despite the rapidly growing body of research literature on temperament, only a few articles and two books (Carey & McDevitt, 1989; Chess & Thomas, 1986) have been published suggesting practical ways that clinicians might use the concept in behavioral interventions. I have previously proposed that there are three principal uses of temperament concepts and data in pediatric practice (Carey, 1981, 1982): (1) general educational discussions with parents to increase their awareness and understanding, (2) identification of the particular child's temperament profile to provide a more organized and objective picture, and (3) interventions that influence the temperament–environment interaction when its dissonance is leading to reactive symptoms. These possibilities were illustrated with readily available examples but without a systematic review of all possible records to develop a more complete view of all the variations on these main themes.

This report presents a more detailed analysis of these specific opportunities for pediatric intervention. During a period of 2 years, I have had the burdensome but interesting task of reviewing practically all the active charts (perhaps 1,200) in my general pediatrics practice as I have prepared individual transcripts to send to other physicians after the termination of that practice in September of 1989. Such an analysis cannot be regarded as truly quantitative in that processes of selection have operated at several points: the parents' decision to participate in the practice, their presentation of their problems to the physician, the variable recording of these discussions by the physician, and the fact that even after 2 years not all records have been requested. However, the several reaction patterns reported here turned up with such frequency that they would surely stand out in a more rigorous cross-sectional study. We should stress that these are concerns encountered in pediatric care, not just psychiatric diagnoses.

The principal findings of this survey are as follows: When parents are concerned about their children's behavior, temperament data are usually helpful. If there is a mild or moderately severe behavioral adjustment problem, information on the child's temperament may clarify the diagnosis and guide the management. When there is parental concern about behavior but no adjustment problem (involving social competence, task performance, or self-assurance), the temperament itself may be the source of the concern. The remainder of this report will be largely a development of these points.

What about using temperament data to predict problems in the child? Despite the enthusiasm of researchers, the attempt to use temperament data alone to predict clinical problems has been disappointing. Although a number of such predictions have been demonstrated, few of them are sufficiently strong to make them clinically useful with such issues as accidents and child abuse. We should remember, however, that making predictions about forthcoming problems is not what is expected of us in primary medical care. Our main job is to understand and attempt to solve current problems brought to us for our help. Routine temperament determinations in the general population have not yet been shown to be of value for prevention (Carey & McDevitt, 1989).

BEHAVIOR PROBLEM PRESENT, TEMPERAMENT APPARENTLY INVOLVED

The earlier reports concluded that the clinician may attempt to influence the temperament–environment interaction when its dissonance is leading to reactive symptoms by suggesting alternative methods of parental management (Carey, 1981, 1982; Chess & Thomas, 1986). If this method is successful, the reactive symptoms should disappear and the parents learn to live in greater harmony with the temperament. The recent chart review reported here has elaborated on this by showing that there are three principal situations in which this advice applies: (1) acute social behavior problems, (2) recurrent behavior problems, and (3) school problems.

Acute Behavior Problems

By acute behavior problems we mean problems of at least moderate severity and of fairly abrupt onset. These are frequently found in children with difficult temperaments who have been doing satisfactorily under normal circumstances with competent parental handling, but who have reacted to heightened stress more dramatically than others (siblings or classmates) who have tolerated it without such a disruption. In these instances the presence and magnitude of these symptoms may be attributable more to the reactivity of the child's temperament than to the pathogenicity of the events or the biological vulnerability of the child. Some examples will illustrate this process:

Three-year-old George was a temperamentally difficult child about whom the parents had offered no previous complaints. With the arrival of a younger sister, he became hostile toward his parents and fought with and injured a younger child in the neighborhood. The concerned professional parents asked about a psychiatric consultation. Pediatric management, however, consisted of reframing the problem as an overreaction to stress rather than a larger problem in the child or the parents, and of some simple suggestions on child management (limits, time alone with the parents, etc.). The behavior problem abated rapidly, and family harmony was restored.

Seven-year-old Walter had always been relatively difficult temperamentally, but his parents had handled him so well that no previous behavioral problems had emerged. In the fall of his second-grade year, his mother returned to work full-time, his father needed a surgical operation, and two close grandparents died. His slightly older and much more flexible brother took all this in stride, but Walter was overwhelmed by the stress and developed a school phobia and sleep problems. Unfortunately, the psychiatrist whom the family consulted directly did not believe in temperament. She diagnosed him with a panic disorder with some underlying neurological defect and wanted to use a new psychotropic drug not yet approved for children. Belatedly sought pediatric advice revised the diagnosis to an overreaction to stress in a relatively inflexible but neurologically intact child, vetoed the use of any drugs, and supported brief psychotherapy aimed at assuaging upset feelings from the extraordinary stress and building self-confidence for the handling of stresses in the future. The behavior problems disappeared rapidly and did not return. The whole problem could have been handled in the pediatric setting.

Sixteen-year-old Barbara was a shy person (slow-to-warm-up traits on the Middle Childhood Temperament Questionnaire 4 years before). In her junior year of high school, she expressed distress and doubts about her abilities and great indecision about her future plans despite her more than adequate school record and her good social relations. With pediatric counseling the parents were able to see this situation as a shy person feeling temporarily overwhelmed by the impending separation from the family. They helped her with her self-esteem and gave her opportunities to discuss uncomfortable feelings. She made the necessary decisions for herself and eventually left for college timidly but confidently. Consultation with a mental health specialist was not needed.

The lesson to be learned from these cases and many others like them is that knowing about a child's temperament often helps one to understand the origins of behavior problems and leads to more appropriate management. A poor fit may be the explanation rather than preexisting pathology. When there is an acute behavior problem, we should consider the possibility of an overreaction to stress due to the child's temperament. Such a conclusion must, of course, be supported by an investigation of various possible contributory factors, including a full assessment of the temperament characteristics. This can usually be done comfortably in the primary medical care setting without referral. It may even be accomplished there better and faster because of the existing professional relationship and the extensive information about the child already on hand.

The experienced clinician may find a parallel between this situation of behavioral overreaction and that in which an intense, negative child always screams about any pain. Such a child may alarm the unprepared caretaker or medical person because of the magnitude of the complaints. Successful management must include recognition of the child's temperament in order to avoid an unnecessary, expensive, and traumatic search for serious problems.

Recurring Behavior Problems

For some children the behavioral symptoms and the parental concerns about them are not so sudden and dramatic but are rather of a more chronic or recurrent nature. The child's temperament is likely to remain somewhat stable, but because of shifting combinations of developmental status and environmental factors, the child may have separate periods of behavioral dysfunction related to the temperament–environment interaction.

Kelly was a somewhat irritable, inflexible, and sensitive child who presented a series of behavioral concerns for her attentive parents. She was quite colicky in the early weeks of life until her parents learned not to be overresponsive to her. Subsequently she had problems with night waking, not staying in bed when put there, and changing from one activity to another. All of these problems required, and quickly responded to, the parents' understanding that they were temperamentally based and their learning a few simple techniques such as ignoring tantrums and using suitable warnings and limits. When she was last seen at age 5 years, her social relationships were cordial both at home and at school, although she was still temperamentally difficult.

Sam was a similarly negative, unadaptable, and sensitive child who had produced a series of behavioral concerns related to these characteristics. In his first few weeks he was colicky, and in the next several months he had a problem with night waking. At 4 years, he repeatedly and firmly resisted going to nursery school, although he was happy once there. When he was 6, his mother was still dressing him, complaining that it would not get done otherwise. At age 8 there were complaints of aggressiveness toward peers at school because he wanted to do things his way. All these problems improved or disappeared with pediatric counseling dealing with the temperamental factors.

Jim was a 12-year-old boy who was difficult as an infant and continued to be low in adaptability on subsequent determinations. As an infant he sustained a laceration of his scalp, which is common among difficult infants. As his parents' marriage deteriorated, Jim first experienced functional abdominal pain at age 6 to 7 years and later worsening school performance. Meanwhile, his more pleasant and flexible sister continued to perform well physically and scholastically. It seems that Jim's sequence of clinical conditions was related to his more intense style of reacting to the shared stresses.

Thus, the child's temperament furnishes a somewhat consistent style of reacting to stresses. As new environmental challenges arise, the resulting stress may evoke varied episodes of behavioral dysfunction.

School Performance Problems

School problems present a somewhat different picture. Schools do not refer for evaluation by physicians all children with scholastic function problems. Among the factors determining such referrals are local school policies and expectations that the physician has something to offer. Children who do not adapt themselves to school routines and pay attention to their work are apparently those most commonly sent for consultation, usually with the expectation that some drug such as methylphenidate will be prescribed and will prove helpful.

It was no surprise that the charts reviewed for this report invariably showed that children referred from schools had either difficult temperament or "low task orientation" (low persistence/attention span, high distractibility, and high activity) or some combination of these features. This experience is congruent with a study published several years ago (Carey, McDevitt, & Baker, 1979) of 61 children referred by their teachers to a pediatric neurologist for problems in behavior and learning. Regardless of the diagnosis ultimately applied, these children were consistently low in adaptability and persistence/attention span as rated by their mothers.

The school complained that 6-year-old Vince could not sit still and pay attention. By temperament questionnaire he was found to be inattentive and low in adaptability, but psychological testing added that he also had difficulties with visual-motor and spatial perceptions that were interfering with his performance. He responded to a combination of educational, psychological, and pharmacological interventions.

Seven-year-old Ralph was diagnosed by his teacher, the school psychologist, and the consultant neurologist as having attention deficit hyperactivity disorder. The Middle Childhood Temperament Questionnaire (MCTQ) showed him to be low in task orientation and in adaptability. He was also a rather unpredictable child, was inappropriately dependent on his mother, and had a delay in visual-motor skills. He too improved with a combination of therapies.

A significant and possibly surprising finding of this survey is that many children who had these same temperamental characteristics of low task orientation and difficulty not only did not have significant academic problems but were even doing well scholastically. A review of the 36 children who had very low adaptability and persistence/attention span (scores greater than one standard deviation) in the standardization samples of the Behavioral Style Questionnaire (BSQ) or the MCTQ or both supported this view. Although these children probably had a higher rate of academic problems than the general population, many of them had acceptable or outstanding academic records. (A precise tabulation was not possible.)

An illustration of this situation was Clara, who showed a low task orientation temperament at 6 on the BSQ and at 10 on the MCTQ standardization samples, along with elements of difficult temperament at both times. Through high school her academic career was one of high scores on aptitude tests but only average results in achievement. She had no learning disabilities and no known behavior problems. For her level of abilities she was underachieving, but she did earn Bs and Cs. Her parents were disappointed but not worried; no abnormality was diagnosed. By sophomore year in college her motivation to study had become activated. She forced herself to overcome her poor work habits and won high scholastic honors.

Consultant specialists, who examine only children having troubles in school, have formulated the concept of attention deficit hyperactivity disorder (ADHD). They believe that certain behavioral traits virtually identical to the temperament cluster of low task orientation constitute the "disorder" of ADHD. In the light of the evidence presented here, it would seem better to think of the behavioral traits as risk factors rather than as the whole problem, just as we regard difficult temperament as a risk factor for behavior problems rather than as the clinical diagnosis itself. The outcome in school performance appears to depend not simply on the presence of certain behavioral characteristics but also on (1) the strength and durability of the characteristics, (2) other factors in the child such as learning problems and motivation, (3) the quality of the school environment, and (4) the role of the family. This promising hypothesis is ready for more rigorous exploration.

Other Clinical Problems with Involvement of Temperament

In addition to problems in social behavior and school function, temperament has been found to contribute to a variety of other clinical conditions, largely in the area of physical function (Carey, 1985). Besides the colic, sleep disturbances, functional abdominal pain, and accidents in the anecdotes just mentioned, there is the possibility of such involvement also in other conditions such as child abuse, failure to thrive, obesity, and reactions to physical illness. These important clinical interactions are the subject of studies elsewhere and will not be considered further here (Carey & McDevitt, 1989).

PARENTAL CONCERN ABOUT BEHAVIOR, BUT NO ADJUSTMENT PROBLEM

When the parents are concerned about the child's behavior but there is no adjustment problem present (no deviations in social competence, task performance, and self-assurance), the two principal explanations to consider are that there is a "poor fit" between the child's temperament and the environment or that there is a parental perception problem. Our attention at this point is focused on the first of these two possibilities. By poor fit we mean varying degrees of misunderstanding or intolerance of the temperament that make for an incompatible relationship. The charts reviewed for this report support the conclusion that almost any characteristics can evoke perplexity or concern in parents but that the most common ones are those usually identified as temperament risk factors: difficult characteristics, slow-to-warm-up ones, and low task orientation. Other concerns mentioned were high and low activity, high persistence, low soothability (distractibility in infants), and high sensitivity. These were all normal variations in behavioral style without resulting behavioral or functional problems, although they were accompanied in some cases by environmental challenges or parental misperceptions.

Sarah was an intense, irritable infant and continued to be difficult to manage through the next several years. However, aside from some intensely expressed rivalry with her younger sister, she had shown no behavior adjustment problem by the time she was last seen at age 5. The parents frequently complained about the difficulties of rearing this child, but the outcome was good because of their superior understanding, tolerance, sense of humor, and skill.

Harry's parents worried about him when he was about 2 years old because of his slow acceptance of novelty, such as with his new day-care arrangements. His mother was concerned that he was "insecure" and that it was all her fault for returning to work. A slow-to-warm-up profile at 6 months and again at 2 years demonstrated a continuing pattern of shyness that they could, and subsequently did, handle successfully without guilt.

Three-year-old Peter's mother complained that she had great trouble getting him to stop activities of which she disapproved, such as climbing on the furniture. Further questioning revealed that he had no real behavior problems and that he persisted also at activities she favored, such as drawing. She was relieved to realize that high persistence, though sometimes a trial in toddlers, also has a positive side and is a characteristic of great potential adaptational value as the child grows older.

Parent counseling in these situations consists of helping them to understand and tolerate better these variations of normal. As the children mature, they can share in these insights about their temperaments.

OTHER DIAGNOSES

Two major behavioral diagnostic classifications that do not involve participation of the child's temperament are mentioned here briefly for completeness: (1) behavioral problems related to purely environmental factors and (2) parental concern when there is no behavior problem or temperament risk factor. Severe problems are mentioned in the next section.

Behavior problems involving purely environmental factors with negligible participation of the child's temperament do not require much elaboration. These well-known etiologic factors include (a) parental handling-marital conflict, over- and undercontrol, unrealistic expectations, inconsistencies, abuse, (b) other environmental factors like separations from and deaths of significant persons, and (c) physical illness in the child and its management. In these instances cause and effect are usually clear in the parents' minds. A pediatrician may be asked for help, but parents are more likely to go directly to mental health specialists for consultation.

Parental concerns about children's behavior when there is neither an adjustment problem nor a temperament risk factor apparently arise from two main sources. The parents may be inexperienced or misinformed about what normal behavior is like in children, or there may be psychosocial disturbances in the parents that prevent them from appreciating the normality of the child or that promote projection of their problems onto the child. Supplying parents with correct information is easy, but dealing with their personal problems may be beyond the capacities of the primary care clinician.

MANAGEMENT

This review demonstrates once again that temperament plays an important role in a wide variety of behavioral concerns of parents. Clear understanding and sound management of these issues must include some assessment of temperament. Major problems like anorexia nervosa or conduct disorders appear to have negligible contributions from the child's temperament and should be referred to the psychiatrist or other mental health specialist. Most of the mild and moderate behavioral concerns of parents can and should be handled by the primary medical clinician, whether pediatrician, family physician, or nurse practitioner.

Whatever else is called for by the clinical condition, a basic step possible for all of us is helping the parents to understand the child's temperament and to tolerate and deal with it more effectively. Techniques for doing this have been described more fully elsewhere (Carey, 1986; Chess & Thomas, 1986; Turecki & Tonner, 1989). Other elements of the management program embrace correction of parental misperceptions, revision of parental handling and other aspects of the environment, behavioral therapy for the child, and reassurance.

With issues of school function, the temperamental characteristics associated are likely to be only part of the etiology of the problem, just as they are with social behavior abnormalities. Primary care medical persons should not presume that these behaviors are the whole "disorder" and prescribe on that basis. Collaboration with an educational psychologist and school personnel is absolutely essential for comprehensive evaluation and management.

If an adjustment of the caretakers' handling of the child's capacities and characteristics is not effective, or if the behavioral deviations are severe, chronic, or multiple, referral for psychotherapy or family therapy is indicated.

SUMMARY

Previous publications have reported clinical usefulness of temperament measurements in three general ways: (1) educational discussions with parents, (2) identification of the particular child's temperament profile to clarify understanding of it, and (3) intervention when dissonances in the temperament–environment interaction have produced reactive symptoms.

A recent review of the active office records in a general pediatrics practice provided the occasion for a more detailed elaboration of these specific opportunities for intervention. This survey includes a broader range of parental concerns than those identified in the NYLS.

When a behavior problem is present, temperament data are likely to explain why and how the symptoms arose and to affect the management as follows: (1) Acute social behavior problems are frequently found in difficult children who have been doing satisfactorily under normal circumstances but who have overreacted to suddenly heightened stress that other children have tolerated without such disruption. (2) Recurring behavioral problems may involve difficult temperament or other temperament risk factors that periodically generate stress from shifting interactions of developmental status, physical health, environmental challenges, and parental problems. (3) Children referred for school problems are likely to have elements of low task orientation, difficult temperament, or both. However, these are only behavioral predispositions rather than the whole "disorder" since some children with these same behavioral traits do adequately or even quite well in school.

When parents are concerned about behavior but no adjustment problem is present, temperament may be the source of the concern. Almost any characteristics may be involved, but most commonly they are difficult traits, the slow-to-warm-up pattern, or low task orientation.

Unless the problems are severe, chronic, or multiple and require immediate referral to mental health specialists, the primary medical care clinician can offer the first line of intervention. By helping the caretakers adjust their expectations and demands to the capacities and characteristics of the child, the clinician can handle successfully most of the parental concerns presented. Useful techniques include teaching better understanding of and responses to temperament, correcting parental misperceptions, environmental manipulations, behavioral management of the child, and reassurance. School performance problems, however, require interdisciplinary collaboration with educators and educational psychologists. Only when this method proves to be ineffective need there be a referral for care by a mental health specialist. This is usually when there are significant pre-existing problems in the child or caretaker.

These conclusions await replication and amplification by more rigorous study.

REFERENCES

Carey, W. B. (1981). Intervention strategies using temperament data. In C. C. Brown (Ed.), *Infants at risk: Assessment and intervention. An update for health care professionals and parents* (pp. 96–106). Piscataway, NJ: Johnson & Johnson.

Carey, W. B. (1982). Clinical use of temperament data in pediatrics. In R. Porter & G. M. Collins (Eds.), *Temperamental differences in infants and young children* (pp. 191–205). London: Pitman.

Carey, W. B. (1985). Interactions of temperament and clinical conditions. In M. Wolraich & D. K. Routh (Eds.), *Advances in developmental and behavioral pediatrics* (pp. 83–115). Greenwich, CT: JAI Press.

25

Carey, W. B. (1986). The difficult child. *Pediatrics in Review, 8*, 39–45.

Carey, W. B., & McDevitt, S. C. (Eds.). (1989). *Clinical and educational applications of temperament research.* Amsterdam/Lisse, The Netherlands: Swets & Zeitlinger, and Berwyn, PA: Swets North America.

Carey, W. B., McDevitt, S. C., & Baker, D. (1979). Differentiating minimal brain dysfunction and temperament. *Developmental Medicine & Child Neurology, 21*, 765–772.

Chess, S., & Thomas, A. (1986). *Temperament in clinical practice.* New York: Guilford Press.

Turecki, S., & Tonner, L. (1989). *The difficult child* (rev. ed.). New York: Bantam Books.

22

Developing Temperament Guidance Programs Within Pediatric Practice

James R. Cameron, David Rice, Robin Hansen, and David Rosen

When Stella Chess and Alexander Thomas published *Temperament and Behavior Disorders in Children* (Thomas, Chess, & Birch, 1968), they focused attention on the role of the child's temperament, as well as its "goodness of fit" with the environment, in the etiology of behavioral problems. In the process, they brought more balance to our understanding of these problems and took some of the blame away from parents. They also underscored the need for parents to understand the individuality of each child and to adapt their parenting accordingly. On the premise that such understanding is not innate, they subsequently published a variety of articles and books (e.g., *Know Your Child*, 1989) to help parents discover their child's unique behavioral style.

Others have followed their lead. William Carey, in particular, has called on pediatricians to incorporate temperament concepts into their well-baby programs and to look to temperament as a contributing factor to a number of common parental complaints: sleep problems, weight gain, and the like (Carey, 1974, 1985). Despite these efforts, however, temperament counseling is still not a standard component of pediatric practice.

WIDGET PHILOSOPHY AND THE UNEVEN PLAYING FIELD

The principal reason is that the "widget" philosophy still prevails; most clinicians still believe (and implicitly are taught) that all children are built on the same standard model in terms of their given behavioral style and that all children go through a universal, developmental sequence. Standard treatments and interventions exist for developmental and behavioral problems, should they occur. If individual differences are recognized, they are seen as insignificant or environmentally induced, except in unusual or extreme circumstances (hyperactivity, attention deficit, etc.). As a result, parents are likely to hear more from their local auto dealer about the handling characteristics of the car they buy ("Excellent gas mileage. Goes all day." "Great acceleration. Takes turns with ease") than they are from their doctor about how to handle their child's unique temperament.

With the widget philosophy in place, building and testing demonstration programs to show the utility and cost-effectiveness of temperament guidance have been extremely difficult. The playing field has been uneven. Those of us who have managed to sustain temperament guidance programs for significant periods of time (Cameron & Rice, 1986; Cameron, Hansen, & Rosen, 1989; Cameron, Hansen, & Rosen, 1991) can attest to the constant uphill struggle against the continuing environmental bias that still seeks to explain most behavioral problems as a function of trauma or stress at home.

In this struggle, Chess and Thomas have been our alchemists, turning our frustration back into persistence. In the early 1980s, with their support, we recognized we had to provide strong evidence of concurrent and predictive validity from measures of temperament to behavioral concerns described by parents. We had to solve the problem of how to provide anticipatory guidance, gather outcome data, and rule out self-fulfilling prophecy effects. We also had to show the clinical utility of our interventions and their cost-effectiveness. All of these tasks had to be accomplished before we could launch widespread temperament-based programs. But how could we collect such evidence without first building and running such a program? And how could we launch even a pilot program in the face of the prevailing environmental bias?

The answer to our "catch-22" problem was a spiral model: Start with a small demonstration program, focusing *both* on sound research criteria (particularly predictive validity) and on indices of user satisfaction. Use those results to gain knowledge and support for a larger pilot program, with more parents, in a variety of pediatric settings, with a wider age range of children. Gradually expand in both directions: stronger statistics showing the predictive validity from temperament assessments to behavioral issues and more detailed evaluation data from parents *and* pediatricians using these programs.

We were aware, of course, of the many unanswered research and clinical questions in the field of temperament: for example, questionnaire reliability, potential biases in using parent questionnaires, and the dangers of pejorative labels. At first, we wondered if a formal program of anticipatory and concurrent guidance would be premature. Gradually we realized, however, that Piaget was right: Past a certain developmental age, the human mind *needs* to impose causality on experience—to make attributions and to find causes for effects. This basic principle meant that we would not be the first "program" to provide temperament guidance. Since time began, parents have undoubtedly sought guidance for temperament-related concerns from a variety of formal and informal sources: family, relatives, friends, neighbors, and, more recently, physicians, popular child care books, advice in the newspapers, and in one instance in our experience, an exorcist (!). Given this inherent need for understanding, we felt the question was not how high our alpha or beta coefficients had to be before we could jump in, but could we do better *now*, with what we knew about temperament, than other practitioners could, particularly those operating from the widget model?

MOVING BEYOND THE PUBLIC HEALTH MODEL

When we began to offer all parents in pediatric clinics an opportunity to fill out a temperament questionnaire and receive feedback, however, we met with resistance from many clinical colleagues. They saw our program as being in the public health model of screening, risk assignment, and preventive treatment, with all the attendant problems of wasted effort in identifying true negatives, false positives, and false negatives, along with the problem of pejorative labeling. Repeatedly, we had to remind our colleagues that screening for "temperamentally difficult" infants and children (whoever they might be) was never our intent. Instead, our goal was to support parents in following Chess and Thomas's exhortation to "know your child!" Whether an infant was temperamentally extreme or near the average, our purpose was the same: to help parents develop a more accurate image of their child's temperament and share with them the experience of other parents whose children had similarly described temperaments.

FUNDAMENTAL PRINCIPLES

The responsibility to "know your child" that Chess and Thomas placed upon parents was liberating. Parents were no longer to be merely the passive recipients of professional (or amateur) advice; parents had something to do and something to contribute. Their diligence in spotting signs of their child's emerging temperament and reporting such signs through temperament questionnaires was essential for accurate temperament assessment. They also had a responsibility to contribute, since by recycling their experience through follow-up questionnaires (What issues actually occurred? What guidance proved effective?), they provided the information that allowed the guidance system to grow and improve.

In accepting this responsibility, however, parents also had a right to expect support: guidance in understanding where to look for signs of their child's emerging temperament, help in integrating this collection of signs into a coherent picture, and information (systematically collected from other parents who had developed similar pictures of their child's temperament) telling them what issues were more likely to occur and, should they occur, what practical approaches seemed to work best.

The admonition to parents to "know your child" meant that pediatricians also had work to do and the right to expect support. We have found that few pediatricians in group or health maintenance organization (HMO) practices would routinely use temperament concepts without a supportive, systematic program in place. From their perspective, the key to such a program was a staff member in their practice or department who had been fully trained to understand temperament, who could help them identify the contributions of temperament to a particular problem during a corridor conference, and who was available to accept referrals as needed.

In more successful programs, we found these parental and professional responsibilities and supports interconnected. Parents who were more systematic in looking for and reporting their child's temperament gave their pediatrician more useful temperament information. Pediatricians who treated temperament awareness as a standard component of their well-baby program (like DPT shots), and who talked positively to parents about the guidance program, received more differentiated information from the parents.

THE PROGRAM

In building this program, we have been fortunate in working with a variety of health maintenance organizations and, for the last 6 years, with the oldest and largest HMO in northern California, Kaiser Permanente. An HMO has important advantages when trying to implement such a program: large numbers of subscribers, practitioners who can easily pass information back and forth through a shared data base, and support services that are more extensive than those of small clinics or private practices. HMOs have a more-than-academic interest in the cost-effectiveness of such programs, their ability to attract and retain new clients, and the willingness of their physicians to adopt and use them.

At the present time, 13 hospitals and their satellite pediatric clinics in the northern California, Kaiser Permanente organization are using this program. Various components of the program have been adapted for use by other HMOs and smaller, group pediatric practices in California and Arizona.

In most facilities, the program begins with a health education manual, available in the third trimester to all prospective parents through ob-gyn departments. The manual explains the importance of differences in temperament, shows how infants with different temperaments move through the early developmental stages, and indicates where parents should look for signs of their child's emerging temperament. The manual also contains a 4-month temperament questionnaire for the collection of these temperament perceptions. Additional temperament questionnaires are also available as handouts at well-baby visits and in a 5-month health education mail-out to parents who have not yet returned a questionnaire.

Returned questionnaires are scored by a computer program that looks first for biases in the rater's response pattern (perseveration, use of extreme scores), then integrates the child's temperament from three levels of abstraction: (1) the rater's general impressions in the nine temperament areas, (2) temperament scale scores in these nine areas, and (3) an analysis of the questionnaire items themselves, showing what items contributed to high or low scale scores. The program also generates a temperament profile and written, anticipatory guidance to parents.

ANTICIPATORY GUIDANCE

At the core of the infancy program is the anticipatory guidance component that lets parents know what temperament-related behavioral issues are likely to occur for their infant in the 5-to 16-month period . . . and what are *not* likely to occur. For example, first-time mothers who are trying to decide when to go back to work find it just as helpful (and reassuring) to know that their infant is *un*likely to develop sleep or separation issues as to know that their infant is likely to battle for control at mealtimes.

The anticipatory guidance letter begins with a discussion of temperament and the purpose of our program: to help parents integrate their perceptions of their infant's temperament and to know what other parents with similar perceptions have encountered in the months ahead. The letter then discusses the significant aspects of the infant's profile, focusing particularly on those areas of temperament that predict to issue occurrence *and* management difficulty in the 5- to 16-month period: energy level (Activity and Intensity) and adjustability (Adaptability, Approach-Withdrawal, Persistence, and Mood). Finally, the letter discusses the likelihood of specific issues in the areas of Separation, Sleep, Assertiveness, Mealtime, Accident Risk, and Sensitivity in the 5- to 8-, 9- to 12-, and 13- to

16-month periods. All likelihood statements are based on probability calculations, derived from a data base of over 1,000 HMO infants followed from 5 to 16 months in our Kaiser research program.

Parents of moderate temperament infants typically choose to receive this information by mail. However, more anxious mothers or those with more temperamentally extreme infants can choose a half-hour appointment with a trained temperament counselor in the pediatric department. And even if parents of high energy and/or low adjustability infants ask for written feedback, they also receive a follow-up telephone call from the temperament counselor. The purpose of this personal contact is to make sure the parents understand the feedback and realize that if any temperament-related behavioral issues are occurring, these issues are normal for their child. During this phone conversation, the temperament counselor can also try to dissolve any denial that parents may develop around their temperamentally extreme infants, raising the probability that such parents will talk with their pediatrician or the temperament counselor if any issues occur in the future that are hard to understand or manage. Future telephone follow-ups are also planned.

Copies of the temperament profile are placed in the infant's medical chart, along with any telephone notes. At the next well-baby visit, the doctor or nurse can compare the questionnaire results to office impressions and, where needed, discuss those topics raised by written feedback or telephone follow-ups.

GUIDANCE FOR EXISTING TEMPERAMENT-RELATED PROBLEMS

In addition to this proactive, anticipatory service, pediatricians can also ask the temperament counselor (typically a nurse or child development specialist) to mail out questionnaires to children aged 1½ to 12 if they identify possible temperament-related issues in routine clinic visits. In addition to completing the temperament questionnaire, parents are asked to list current behavioral problems. In many cases, both parents or different caretakers are asked to complete separate questionnaires.

The profiles generated by each of these questionnaires for older children are routinely reviewed by a pediatric psychologist in the central offices of the Temperament Project. A short, written report explaining possible temperament origins to the behavioral problems listed by the parents is prepared and mailed to the facility's temperament counselor. Each temperament counselor also has a file of written health education advice sheets for the common, temperament-related issues the Temperament Project has encountered over the past 6 years; a list of the more appropriate issue sheets is included. Follow-up phone discussions with the temperament counselor provide the necessary backup support as the temperament counselor and pediatric staff work with the parents or schools to resolve these temperament-related issues.

IMPLEMENTING THE PROGRAM

Evidence of predictive validity, cost-effectiveness, and consumer satisfaction is not enough to convince a new medical facility to adopt such a program. In each new setting, we have learned that we also need to find at least one person, typically a pediatrician with seniority and/or rank in the department, who would act as an advocate. These advocates, when trained, serve as Temperament Program coordinators at their facility. Most such advocates have personally coped with a temperamentally extreme child and are quite willing to mobilize other health care workers, champion for funds and other resources, and ensure that the support system for parents and for the pediatric department as a whole runs smoothly.

Trained temperament counselors within each pediatric facility are also necessary. They not only make follow-up phone calls and see parents, they also continually receive information from our program about how temperament "works" and pass that information along to interested members of the pediatric department or clinic. The background or training of the temperament counselor may vary, but for this informational osmosis to work, he or she must be a member of the pediatric department staff.

EVALUATION

If HMO program managers and pediatricians are going to adopt and continue to invest in such temperament guidance programs, they want concrete evidence of cost-effectiveness. To that end we have used a variety of evaluation methods.

1. *Predictive validity.* Parents' reports of their child's temperament are necessarily subjective, as are subsequent parental reports of issues and problems that later occurred. However, any significant statistical relationship between these two subjective realms is an *objective* reality. Our follow-up studies have documented such predictive validity in the six content areas covered by our anticipatory guidance letter.

2. *Experimental versus control group comparisons.* Our follow-up studies have also demonstrated that parents who have a temperamentally extreme child and receive anticipatory guidance are significantly *less* likely to experience difficulty in understanding or managing later temperament-related issues than are parents of infants with similar temperament in a no-guidance control group.

3. *Consumer satisfaction surveys and videotaped testimonials from parents.*

While survey numbers are useful, interviews with parents who have a temperamentally extreme child and have participated in the program are particularly impressive in demonstrating precisely where such programs are effective.

4. *Videotaped interviews with pediatricians who have used the service for 2 or more years.* Pediatricians in facilities that have not yet adopted this program are interested in hearing from their peers how this program has affected their peers, particularly with respect to additional workloads or loss of involvement with and control over their patients.

5. *Case studies where funds have been saved, by avoiding costly referrals to other HMO departments.* For example, parents with an unexpected temperamentally extreme child often attribute their difficulties to some yet undiagnosed medical problem and insist on a series of expensive diagnostic evaluations. Cases where these unneeded evaluations have been avoided through work with the temperament counselor and referring pediatrician have an influence on cost-conscious HMO administrations.

CONCLUSION

When Moses received the Ten Commandments, he was reported (by knowledgeable humorists) to have grumbled, "But where's the funding?" Raising expectations without raising support has always proved risky.

If the widget model were true, there would be no need to provide support for parents to help them understand their child's unique behavioral style more accurately. If you have seen one widget, you have seen them all. The genius of Chess and Thomas is that they started an avalanche of research that has proved the widget model wrong. Inertia being what it is, however, that model still prevails in most pediatric clinics.

The task we have accepted has been to create programs that support both parents and their health care providers, so that the commandment "Know Your Child" and the corollary, "Know Your Patient," can be fulfilled. Instituting information systems that combine written and personal temperament guidance in a cost-effective fashion into pediatric settings is one way to see that the widget model is finally laid to rest.

REFERENCES

Cameron, J. R., Hansen, R., & Rosen, D. (1989). Preventing behavioral problems in infancy through temperament assessment and parental support programs. In W. B. Carey & S. C. McDevitt (Eds.), *Clinical and educational applications of temperament research* (pp. 155–165). Amsterdam/Lisse, The Netherlands: Swets & Zeitlinger.

Cameron, J. R., Hansen, R., & Rosen, D. (1991). Preventing behavioral problems in infancy through temperament assessment and parental support programs within health maintenance organizations. In J. H. Johnson & S. B. Johnson (Eds.), *Advances in child health psychology* (pp. 127–139). Gainsville: University of Florida Press.

Cameron, J. R., & Rice, D. C. (1986). Developing anticipatory guidance programs based on early assessment of infant temperament: Two tests of a prevention model. *Journal of Pediatric Psychology, 11*(2), 221–234.

Carey, W. B. (1974). Night waking and temperament in infancy. *Journal of Pediatrics, 84*, 756–758.

Carey, W. B. (1985). Temperament and increased weight gain in infants. *Journal of Developmental and Behavioral Pediatrics, 6*, 128–131.

Chess, S., & Thomas, A. (1989). *Know your child: An authoritative guide to today's parents.* New York: Basic Books.

Thomas, A., Chess, S., & Birch, H. (1968). *Temperament and behavior disorders in childhood.* New York: New York University Press.

PART VIII

PREVENTION AND INTERVENTION STRATEGIES IN THE DAY CARE AND SCHOOL SETTING

23

Seeing the Child in Child Care: Day Care, Individual Differences, and Social Policy

Edward Zigler and Nancy W. Hall

Rapid social change is a fact of family life in the United States today. Demographic changes in the makeup of the work force, shifts in traditional roles and values, pervasive economic pressures, and changes in childbearing patterns have all served to redefine the American family and its needs (Blankenhorn, Bayme, & Elshtain, 1990). No one has been more profoundly affected by work force, political, and economic changes in the past three decades than our nation's children. Basic needs of families and children are going unmet, unaddressed by political programs and legislation that have failed to keep pace with the essential changes taking place in family and community structures.

Among the most striking of these changes is the explosive increase in the percentage of women participating in the out-of-home work force. A consequence of both escalating economic pressures affecting two-parent families and the increase in the number of single-parent (typically female-headed) households, this phenomenon has brought about a rise in the number of children experiencing substitute child care. Even before the end of the 1980s, over 50% of the mothers of infants under 1 year of age were working outside the home (Bureau of Labor Statistics, 1987). Experts estimate that this figure will reach at least 66% before the year 2000 (Zigler, Hopper, & Hall, in press). Nearly half of these women are single heads of households and the sole supporters of their children (Kamerman, Kahn, & Kingston, 1983).

As we have discussed at length elsewhere (see, for example, Zigler & Gilman, 1990; Zigler & Hall, 1988; Zigler & Lang, 1991; Zigler et al., in press), one of the most immediate crises presented by these demographic changes concerns the short- and long-term sequelae of day care for child development. We will not review in detail here the concerns that have been expressed by many regarding this phenomenon, or the debates raised by research and theory about day care and its outcomes (the interested reader is referred to Zigler & Lang, 1991, for a review of these issues).

SEEING THE CHILD IN CHILD CARE

It has long been our contention that it is too simplistic to ask, "How does day care affect children?" Instead, we ought to be asking, "How do different types and conditions of day care affect different types of children?" (Gamble & Zigler, 1986; Zigler & Freedman, 1990; Zigler & Gordon, 1982; Zigler & Hall, 1988; see also Rutter, 1982). Identifying and researching each of the variables that mediate child care outcomes and fitting it into its proper place in the complex day-care equation may seem like a Herculean task. We do, however, have at our immediate disposal today enough information that we can identify the *major* factors that influence child care outcomes. Moreover, we should be able to use this information to begin to fashion and mount effective legislation to *improve* these outcomes and to address the needs of today's families.

We will not attempt within the boundaries of this chapter to address all of these variables; we—and others—have done this elsewhere. The question at hand concerns the nature of the child, and how the individual child's characteristics and personality figure into this equation. Decades of child development research have given us the theoretical underpinnings that permit us to pose such a question; those of us for whom children and their welfare are our central focus no longer think twice about assuming that even the youngest infants are active participants in their own socialization, or that they bring to any social situation elements that change that situation and that prime the situation to affect them in turn. And yet, day-care research has only recently begun to include characteristics of individual children as independent variables. Among the most important of these characteristics are individual expressions of variation in behavioral style, referred to as temperament (Chess & Thomas, 1983; Thomas & Chess, 1977; Thomas & Chess, 1980)

This approach is consonant with Thomas and Chess's own, which emphasizes "that temperament is likely to affect personality outcomes . . . by affecting the social relationships that produce personality" (Bates, 1987, p. 1103). Bates goes on to ask about how temperament might influence social development, and asserts that it must be, in the day-care setting, through interaction with other variables.

TEMPERAMENT AND THE DAY-CARE DECISION

Even before reviewing the effect of the child's temperament on child-care giver interactions in the day-care setting, let us consider how temperament might influence parental decisions to use other-than-mother care in the first place. Several workers have speculated on the effect that the child's behavioral style might have on the mother's decision to seek or return to employment outside the home during the child's infancy or toddlerhood (e.g., Lamb, Chase-Lansdale, & Owen, 1979; McBride & Belsky, 1985; Melhuish, 1987).

Lamb and his colleagues (1979), for instance, theorized that difficult temperament in an infant might contribute to the likelihood that the mother would enter or reenter the out-of-home labor force. Mothers of easy babies, they suggested, might be equally likely to be employed for pay or be full-time homemakers, as their babies' adaptability ought to enable the mothers to select either option with good results.

The findings of Lerner and Galambos's (1986) studies of temperament and its association with differential levels of maternal participation in the labor force only partially bear out this supposition, however. Interviews with mothers who participated in the New York Longitudinal Study (Thomas & Chess, 1977) revealed instead that mothers who reported that their children were temperamentally difficult were more likely to be homemakers. Consistent with Lamb and colleagues' speculation, though, paid-employed mothers *were* more likely to rate their children as easy. In a later study, Galambos and Lerner (1988) found that the only variable that was significantly related to the mother's participation in the labor force during infancy was temperament during toddlerhood, such that mothers of toddlers rated as difficult were significantly less likely to have been working for pay when their children were infants.

This research, and similar studies yielding similar findings (e.g., Hock, Christman, & Hock, 1980; Lerner & Galambos, 1988; McBride & Belsky, 1985; Morgan & Hock, 1984), are important not just for the value they may have in helping us to understand the variables relevant to decisions regarding work force participation among the mothers of young children. Beyond this, they point to the need to employ a process model (Lerner & Galambos, 1985) in calculating the respective contributions and mutual influences of maternal and child characteristics on women's decisions regarding paid employment. Such variables must be included in any comprehensive studies of both child care and maternal employment.

IN THE DAY-CARE SETTING

To what extent can day-care personnel fill a mental health role by recognizing individual differences among their charges and responding to them appropriately? How does day care of different types and quality affect children of different temperaments? Although there are few data that address these questions, the empirical findings available support three relevant points: that day-care workers appear to evaluate and interact with children on the basis of temperament in much the same way that parents do, that children of different temperaments appear to be differentially affected by substitute child care, and that future research in this area should assess the differential effects of day care by type of care and child temperament concurrently.

Temperament and the Day-Care Provider

A small but theoretically important body of research (see Bates, 1987, for a complete discussion of the implications of this type of research) compares parents' and care givers' perceptions and reports of child temperament. One study characteristic of this group (Northam, Prior, Sanson, & Oberklaid, 1987) examined the convergence between mother and care giver temperament ratings of the same toddlers, and found these ratings to be significantly positively correlated by the time the children were 2 to 3 years old.

Research on the relationship between child temperament and maternal behaviors (Bates, Olson, Pettit, & Bayles, 1982; Hildebrandt & Cannan, 1985; Milliones, 1978) has established that difficulty in the child's behavior may lead to attenuated maternal responsiveness and other interactional problems. In other research (Fagan, 1990; Gamble & Zigler, 1986; Maccoby, Snow, & Jacklin, 1984), the complex relationships among temperament, behavior problems, and gender are noted.

In the absence of a comparable body of work on child temperament and day-care provider behaviors, we will have to draw our best hypotheses for day care based on the maternal-child literature. In support of this assumption, Griffin and Thornburg (1985), Hildebrandt and Cannan (1985), and Bates and colleagues (1982) all find that day-care provider responsiveness is affected by interactions with children rated as being of difficult temperament. One may assume that many of the same mechanisms at work in the home are also at work in the day-care setting. Since so many children now enter substitute care very early (often as young as 2 weeks of age) and spend a large portion of their time in this environment, further study specifically focusing on the dynamics of the day-care setting is essential.

Temperament and Day-Care Type

To date, the vast majority of data that are gathered in the child care setting are obtained from relatively high-quality center-based child care facilities. The scarcity of empirical findings based on a broad selection of child care settings (with respect to both type—that is, home-based vs. family vs. center care—and quality of care) hinders our ability to make generalizations about the differential effects of child care settings and quality levels on children of different temperaments.

Melhuish (1987), in a longitudinal study of Swedish firstborn children, did find significant associations among nursery (center) care, difficult temperament, and increased child concern at separation from the mother in the presence of a stranger. Griffin and Thornburg (1985) found that center care givers were significantly more likely than care givers from family day-care homes to perceive the temperament of the children in their care as being difficult, even when no differences among parental ratings from these groups were found. Center care children were also rated by their care givers as less compliant and less likable than children in family day care. This lends support to the authors' suggestions that the demands placed on care givers by the larger number of children in day-care center groupings negatively affect care giver perception of child characteristics. Only further research will bear out or challenge these findings.

In summing up the importance of studying temperament in the child care setting and the ways in which temperament affects and is affected by day care, Anderson-Goetz and Worobey (1984) note that the construct of temperament might be viewed as a tool for gaining insight into a child's behavior and interactions with others. Attention to temperament, they write, improves the accuracy of observations of children in day care, and is invaluable in planning programs and activities. Brazelton (1983), in advising parents, emphasizes the need to consider each child's individual temperament when selecting child care and interviewing potential care givers.

IMPLICATIONS FOR SOCIAL POLICY

The more we know about child care and the variables that influence its outcomes, the more complex the picture becomes. We do not feel sanguine about the potential effects of substitute child care in its present state in the United States, particularly where infants and toddlers are concerned (Zigler et al., in press).

If we adhere to a cumulative stress model of social development, it is reasonable to hypothesize that poor day-care quality and expression of certain temperament characteristics (such as being low on approach/avoidance, or high on distractibility or intensity) can contribute to a poor day-care outcome. The converse of this hypothesis would be that appropriate day-care environments can help children who might be classified as temperamentally difficult to avoid developing behavior problems that might arise were these children to be placed in environmentally stressful substitute care settings.

As we have noted elsewhere (Zigler, 1989; Zigler & Lang, 1991), the potential problems described here *can* be prevented. We have at our immediate disposal the information and tools needed to develop family support and child care programs that are responsive to the very real and demonstrable needs of communities, families, and individual children. In short, we know what works. Decades of research and program development have prepared us for the task at hand.

What is missing is the involvement and commitment of the federal government, which has abdicated its responsibility to children and families. Yet the tide may be turning. Government leaders are becoming increasingly aware that they can no longer ignore the pressing needs of families. Parents are becoming savvy consumers of child care, and are not happy with the options presently available to them, or with the lack of government involvement in child care issues (Zinsser; 1989).

As we move forward toward the 21st century, we offer a few basic recommendations for improving child care in the United States for all children, especially those whose economic status, age, or personal characteristics place them at a potentially high risk for poor social and cognitive development outcomes. Our plan, the details of which we have elaborated before (Zigler, 1989; Zigler & Lang, 1991; Zigler et al., in press), includes several components.

First, a continuation and expansion of research on child care and the variables that mediate its effects, with particular emphasis on both individual child characteristics and a wider variety of child care settings and degrees of quality of care.

Second, a nationwide, federally mandated set of standards for child care quality. We know that good quality child care is characterized by low child-to-staff ratios, appropriate care giver training (including that which enables staff to recognize, appreciate, and work with children of different temperaments as individuals), low staff turnover, decent wages, small group size, and safe and appropriate physical environments (Child Care Employee Project, 1989; Ruopp, Travers, Glantz, & Coelen, 1979).

Next, a national parental care leave law to broaden parents' options and address the growing concern that many children are being placed in day care at too young an age (Early Childhood Research Quarterly, 1988; Hopper & Zigler, 1987). The United States is presently the only industrialized nation in the world with no paid parental leave policy.

Fourth, implementation of a child or family allowance policy similar to that currently in place in Canada and many European nations. We propose an expansion of the Social Security system (see Zigler & Lang, 1991, for a detailed proposal) that would provide an annual stipend of approximately $5,000 per family during the child's first year.

Finally, an integrated network of child care services through the School of the 21st Century model already in place in some states (Zigler, 1989; Zigler & Lang, 1991). A broadly based, prevention-oriented model, the School of the 21st Century provides communities with a cohesive system of preschool and school-aged child care that makes use of existing school facilities, resource and referral services to locate infant care, education and support services to family day-care providers, parent education and support programs, and preventive health screening during the first 3 years of life.

It may seem like a long way from child temperament to child care policy. But the more we learn about the links among child development, family support, and child care, the clearer it becomes that basic developmental research must inform legislation and program development. These programs, if formulated on sound principles that take into account both broad laws and individual nuances of development, will produce demonstrable, long-lasting, cost-effective results for children and families. The knowledge to enact such family support measures is at our disposal.

REFERENCES

Anderson-Goetz, D., & Worobey, J. (1984). The young child's temperament: Implications for child care. *Childhood Education*, *61*, 134–140.

Bates, J. E. (1987). Temperament in infancy. In J. D. Osofsky (Ed.), *Handbook of infant development*. New York: John Wiley.

Bates, J. E., Olson, S. L., Pettit, G. S., & Bayles, K. (1982). Dimensions of individuality in the mother-infant relationship at 6 months of age. *Child Development*, *53*, 446–461.

Blankenhorn, D., Bayme, S. & Elshtain, J. B. (1990). *Rebuilding the nest: A new commitment to the American family*. Milwaukee: Family Service America.

Brazelton, T. B. (1983). *Infants and mothers: Differences in development*. New York: Delta.

Bureau of Labor Statistics, U. S. Department of Labor. (1987). *Employment perspectives: Women in the labor force* (Fourth quarter, Report No. 749). Washington, DC: U.S. Government Printing Office.

Chess, S., & Thomas, A. (1983). Dynamics of individual behavioral development. In M. D. Levine, W. B. Carey, A. C. Crocker, & R. T. Gross (Eds.), *Developmental-behavioral pediatrics* (pp. 158– 175). Philadelphia: W. B. Saunders.

Child Care Employee Project. (1989). *Who cares: Child care teachers and the quality of care in America; Executive summary, National Child Care Staffing Study.* Oakland, CA: Author.

Early Childhood Research Quarterly. (1988). *Infant day care: A special issue, 3*(3).

Fagan, J. (1990). The interaction between child sex and temperament in predicting behavior problems of preschool age children in day care. *Early Child Development and Care, 59*, 1–9.

Galambos, N., & Lerner, J. V. (1988). Child characteristics and the employment of mothers with young children: A longitudinal study. *Annual Progress in Child Psychiatry and Child Development*, 177–193.

Gamble, T. J., & Zigler, E. (1986). Effects of infant day care: Another look at the evidence. *American Journal of Orthopsychiatry, 56*, 26–42.

Griffin, S., & Thornburg, K. R. (1985). Perceptions of infant/toddler temperament in three child care settings. *Early Childhood Development and Care, 18*, 151–160.

Hildebrandt, K. A., & Cannan, T. (1985). The distribution of caregiver attention in a group program for young children. *Child Study Journal, 15*, 43–55.

Hock, E., Christman, K., & Hock, M. (1980). Factors associated with decisions about return to work in mothers of infants. *Developmental Psychology, 16*, 535–536.

Hopper, P., & Zigler, E. (1987, May). Center care: How soon is too soon? *Child Care Center*, 7–9.

Kamerman, S., Kahn, A. J., & Kingston, P. (1983). *Maternity policies and working women.* New York: Columbia University Press.

Lamb, M. E., Chase-Lansdale, L., & Owen, M. T. (1979). The changing American family and its implications for infant social development: The sample case of maternal employment. In M. Lewis & A. Rosenblum (Eds.), *The child and its family* (pp. 267–291). New York: Plenum Press.

Lerner, J. V., & Galambos, N. (1985). Mother role satisfaction, mother-child interaction, and child temperament: A process model. *Developmental Psychology, 21*, 1157–1164.

Lerner, J. V., & Galambos, N. (1986). Temperament and maternal employment. *New Directions for Child Development, 31*, 75–88.

Maccoby, E. E., Snow, M. E., & Jacklin, C. N. (1984). Children's dispositions and mother-child interaction at 12 and 18 months: A short-term longitudinal study. *Developmental Psychology, 20*, 459–472.

McBride, S. L., & Belsky, J. (1985, April). *Maternal work plans, actual employment and infant temperament.* Paper presented at the Biennial Meeting of the Society for Research in Child Development, Toronto, Canada.

Melhuish, E. C. (1987). Socio-emotional behavior at 18 months as a function of daycare experience, temperament, and gender. *Infant Mental Health Journal, 8*, 364–373.

Milliones, J. (1978). Relationship between perceived child temperament and maternal behaviors. *Child Development, 49*, 1255–1257.

Morgan, K. C., & Hock, E. (1984). A longitudinal study of psychosocial variables affecting the career patterns of women with young children. *Journal of Marriage and the Family, 46*, 383–390.

Northam, E., Prior, M., Sanson, A., & Oberklaid, F. (1987). Toddler temperament as perceived by mothers versus day care givers. *Merrill-Palmer Quarterly, 33*, 213–229.

Ruopp, R., Travers, J., Glantz, F., & Coelen, C. (1979). *Children at the center.* Cambridge, MA: Abt Books.

Rutter, M. (1982). Social-emotional consequences of day care for preschool children. In E. F. Zigler & E. W. Gordon (Eds.), *Day care: Scientific and social policy issues*. Boston: Auburn House.

Thomas, A., & Chess, S. (1977). *Temperament and development*. New York: Brunner-Mazel.

Thomas, A., & Chess, S. (1980). *Dynamics of psychological development*. New York: Brunner/Mazel.

Zigler, E. (1989). Addressing the nation's child care crisis: The School of the 21st Century. *American Journal of Orthopsychiatry, 59*, 484–491.

Zigler, E. F., & Freedman, J. (1990). Psychological-developmental implications of current patterns of early child care. In S. Chehrazi (Ed.), *Psychological issues in day care*. Washington, DC: American Psychiatric Press.

Zigler, E., & Gilman, E. P. (1990). An agenda for the 1990s: Supporting families. In D. Blankenhorn, S. Bayme, & J. B. Elshtain (Eds.), *Rebuilding the nest*. Milwaukee: Family Service America.

Zigler, E. F., & Gordon, E. W. (1982). *Day care: Scientific and social policy issues*. Boston: Auburn House.

Zigler, E., & Hall, N. W. (1988). Day care and its effect on children: An overview for pediatric health professionals. *Journal of Developmental and Behavioral Pediatrics, 9*, 38–46.

Zigler, E., Hopper, P., & Hall, N. W. (in press). Infant mental health and social policy. In C. Zeanah (Ed.), *Handbook of infant mental health*. New York: Guilford Press.

Zigler, E., & Lang, M. (1991). *Child care choices*. New York: Free Press.

Zinsser, C. (1989, July). Special survey results: Your message to the president on child care. *Working Mother*, 36.

24

Temperament and Teachers' Views of Teachability

Barbara K. Keogh

Educators, as well as other professionals who work with children, owe thanks to Stella Chess and Alex Thomas for reaffirming the importance of temperament in children's experiences and development. The contributions of temperament to children's adjustment and behavior have been well documented by Thomas and Chess (1977) and by others (see Kohnstamm, Bates, & Rothbart, 1989). For the most part, the emphasis has been on temperament within the family context, particularly during infancy and the early years, but increasing evidence suggests that temperament also describes individual differences that contribute to children's school experiences (Hegvik, 1986; Keogh, 1982, 1989; Lerner, Lerner, & Zabski, 1985; Martin, 1989). After the family, school is the most powerful formal socialization influence in children's lives. Thus, the study of temperament and schooling is particularly important, as argued by Thomas and Chess in a number of their publications.

The contribution of individual differences in children's temperament to their behavior and adjustment in school has been the focus of an ongoing program of research at UCLA. Our work has been carried out within the conceptual framework of temperament proposed by Thomas and Chess, and we have used their idea of "goodness of fit" as a way to capture the interactions of individual differences and classroom experiences (Keogh, 1986). Applying the notion of goodness of fit to the classroom, we emphasize that teachers are key players in child-school

Preparation of this chapter was supported in part by a grant from the National Institute of Child Health and Human Development to the Sociobehavioral Research Group of the UCLA Mental Retardation Center.

interactions. We suggest that understanding children's school adjustment and achievement requires, in addition to recognition of differences in children's characteristics, recognition of differences in teachers' beliefs and attributions about schooling (Keogh, 1982, 1986), and their perceptions of individual students. We view teachers as active decision makers (Shavelson, 1976), and suggest that their instructional and management decisions about students are based on a composite of selected information that has been filtered through and integrated with the teachers' beliefs about what pupils "ought" to be like, that is, about the characteristics of teachable children. We have found that teachers have consensual ideas about the attributes that define teachability, and that it is possible to assess these views reliably (Kornblau, 1982; Kornblau & Keogh, 1980). The focus in the present chapter, thus, is on the role of teachers in the goodness-of-fit paradigm, using examples of research with normally developing children and children with developmental and learning problems.

CONTEXT AND GOODNESS OF FIT

Thomas and Chess (1977) defined goodness of fit in terms of consonance or dissonance between an individual's "capacities, characteristics, and style of behaving" and the "properties of the environment and its expectations and demands" (p. 11). It is clear that children differ in how well or how poorly their personal characteristics match the demands and constraints of home and family interactions, and how compatible they are with parents and siblings. It is also clear that children bring real differences in cognitive skills and behavioral styles to school, some constellations of attributes being more compatible than others with school demands. For example, activity level, persistence, flexibility, and quality of mood are important ingredients in the classroom "mix," and differences on these dimensions may or may not be compatible with teacher and classroom demands. Schools and classrooms are complex social systems with particular constraints and requirements that interact with a range of individual abilities and characteristics. Therefore, both contextual and individual difference variables must be considered when assessing goodness of fit in school.

The bulk of research on temperament in schools has been focused on pupil characteristics, although there is increasing recognition of situational or contextual influences. Lerner and colleagues (1985), for example, distinguish between physical and social characteristics of an environment or context. Applied to school, this distinction suggests that some demands and some constraints have to do with the physical or structural characteristics of the classroom (e.g., space, number of pupils in classroom, crowdedness), others with interpersonal demands such as getting along with peers, functioning in a group, or dealing with the attitudes or expectations of others. It is reasonable that highly active, intense, and reactive children are likely to have more difficulty adjusting to crowded, poorly organized classrooms than to orderly classrooms with adequate physical space. Slow-to-warm-up and low-activity children may be more comfortable in quiet and well-routinized classrooms than they are in classrooms that are fastpaced and changing.

Other demands relate to the instructional program and to the content of a curriculum. For example, Hall and Cadwell (1984) found that children's temperamental variations were more highly correlated with instructional tasks that demanded sustained performance than with tasks that required the generation of new learning. Hegvik (1986) reported higher correlations between temperamental variants and arithmetic performance than between temperament and reading, a finding consistent with those of Maziade, Côté, Boutin, Boudreault, and Thivierge (1986) in a longitudinal study of French-Canadian children. In summary, there is emerging evidence that understanding the role of temperament in children's schooling requires consideration of both individual and contextual variables, including the physical characteristics of the classroom and the content of instruction.

TEMPERAMENT AND TEACHABILITY

At UCLA work on temperament in schooling has been directed at still another component of the classroom context, the teacher. We have proposed "teachability" as a synthesizing construct to get at teachers' views of individual children and their ideas and beliefs about desirable attributes. To operationalize the idea of teachability, Kornblau (1982) developed a 33-item teachability scale based on teacher-generated descriptors of model or ideal students. The items define three major factors: Cognitive/Motivational Characteristics, School Appropriate Behaviors, and Personal/Social Skills. Included in the Cognitive/ Motivational component are items such as the following: clear thinking-logical-rational, insightful-perceptive, bright. The component of School Appropriate Behaviors includes these descriptors: follows directions, completes work on time, is attentive to classroom proceedings. The Personal/Social component captures characteristics such as: friendly, sense of humor, sincere. The weighting of items and factors has been found to vary slightly according to grade level and according to teacher, but overall agreement about the characteristics of model or ideal pupils is striking. Importantly, despite the obvious importance of intelligence or cognition in schooling, we have found that teachers' views of children's teachability are not a function of cognitive strengths alone. Rather, individual differences in children's behavioral styles or temperaments have been identified as important contributors to teachers' perceptions of teachability, and thus to their instructional and management decisions (see Keogh, 1982, 1986, 1989, for review).

In a series of studies of teachability, we have used a short form of the Teacher Temperament Questionnaire (TTQ) (Keogh, Pullis, & Cadwell, 1982) to assess behavioral style. This scale is a 23-item form of the 64-item TTQ developed by Thomas and Chess. Psychometric work identified three factors: Task Orientation (activity, persistence, and distractibility), Personal/Social Flexibility (adaptability, approach-withdrawal, and positive mood), and Reactivity (intensity, threshold, and negative mood). It is important to note that, using this form of the TTQ, individual differences in children's temperament may be reliably identified in groups of children across a broad age range and within groups of handicapped as well as nonhandicapped children. In recent work, Ratekin (1990) found that the range of scores for mothers' ratings of Down's syndrome and non-Down syndrome children were similar, although there were significant differences between groups on some temperament dimensions. Ratings of approach-withdrawal, distractibility, and mood favored the Down's syndrome group; ratings of persistence favored the non-Down's syndrome children. Supanchek (1989) also found a wide range of temperament ratings by teachers within a group of developmentally delayed children, and Pullis (1985) and Keogh (1983) have documented variations in temperamental characteristics within groups of children identified as learning disabled. These individual differences in temperament are of particular interest, as a major hypothesis guiding our research is that within any classroom, teachers' perceptions of children's teachability are influenced by temperamental differences.

ILLUSTRATIVE FINDINGS

In an extension of our initial work on teachability, we (Keogh & Kornblau) asked teachers to rate children in their classrooms using the Teachable Pupil Survey and the short-form TTQ. The 360 children rated came from four groups: regular elementary ($N = 168$), regular preschool ($N = 82$), special education preschool ($N = 73$), and elementary special education ($N = 38$). Multivariate analysis of variance (MANOVA) techniques identified significant differences among the four groups on all three temperament factors, and gender differences on Task Orientation. All differences favored regular over special education groups, and girls over boys. Significant differences between regular and special education groups were also found for the three Teachability dimensions; the regular education children were rated higher in all comparisons. Girls were rated more positively than boys on School Appropriate Behaviors and on Personal/Social Characteristics.

The strength of association between the temperament factors and the teachability dimensions was estimated with correlation techniques. Not surprisingly, the consistently highest value of *r* was between temperament Task Orientation and School Appropriate Behaviors ($r = .72, .71, .58$, and $.78$ for the four groups, respectively). Temperament ratings of Reactivity were also significantly associated with Teachability scores for Personal/Social Characteristics for both regular education groups and the elementary school special education sample. Examination of the items and dimensions making up the Reactivity factor suggested that positive mood and moderate intensity are important contributors to teachers' views of children's teachability, especially to the Personal Social dimension. It was not just extremes of intensity, but the combination of intensity and quality of mood, that related to the Teachability score.

Before rating individual children, the teachers in the regular education programs had been asked to rate the 33 items in the teachability scale as if they were describing a model or ideal pupil. By comparing the idealized rating with the ratings of actual children, it was possible to derive a discrepancy score for each child. Although similar to their classmates in ability, children with negative discrepancy scores were found to differ from their more positively rated classmates in temperament patterns but not in cognitive characteristics; they were low on Task Orientation and on Personal/Social Flexibility, and high in Reactivity.

The findings of strong relationships between children's temperament and teachers' views of their teachability were corroborated in a study of 59 learning-disabled children (12 girls and 47 boys) by Keogh and Porter[1]. For the group as a whole, Task Orientation was significantly associated with the teachability dimensions tapping School Appropriate Behaviors ($r = .69$) and Personal/Social Characteristics ($r = .50$); temperament Flexibility was correlated significantly with the Cognitive/Motivational dimension of teachability ($r = .55$). Similar patterns of association were found for groups of boys and girls separately and across grade levels. In this study we also assessed teachers' views of children's adjustment and behavior problems using the Child Behavior Checklist-Teachers' Report Form (CBL) (Achenbach & Edelbrock, 1986). For purposes of this study, scores for number of problems, intensity of problems, and externalizing and internalizing problems were analyzed. The strongest relationships were between the CBL scores and temperament ratings of Task Orientation; values of *r* were $-.68$ for Number of problems, $-.64$ for Intensity of problems, and $r = .66$ for Externalizing problems. Scores on the CBL and teachability were also strongly and negatively correlated, values of *r* ranging from $-.61$ to $-.80$. These findings were replicated by Supanchek (1989) in a recent study of developmentally delayed children.

---

[1]We wish to thank the students, teachers, and administrators of the Frostig Center in Pasadena, California, for their participation in this study.

DISCUSSION AND IMPLICATIONS

Our work to date has consistently documented relationships between teachers' views of children's temperament and their views of their teachability. Two points deserve emphasis if we are to understand the interactions of temperament and teachability. First, it should be noted that temperament and teachability are not synonymous, that the correlations between the two are significant but do not approach unity. In our model, teachability is the more encompassing construct, and temperamental variation is a major contributor. Empirical support for this interpretation is illustrated by the results of a regression analysis of temperament and teachability in a study of learning-disabled children; the three temperament factors, IQ, and gender accounted for 61% of the variance in teachability ratings, the temperament factor of Task Orientation being the most powerful contributor (Keogh, 1983). Clearly, individual differences in behavioral styles are important, but not exclusive, influences on teachers' perceptions of children in school.

Second, although the notion of teachability is appealing, the ties between teachers' perceptions and their behaviors are still being explored. In earlier studies in the UCLA program, we found through observations in elementary school classrooms that the frequency of interactions between teachers and pupils viewed as high or low in teachability was similar. However, the interactions with low-teachable pupils tended to be limited to management and instruction, whereas there was considerable positive social interchange between teachers and high-teachable children. Differences in teacher-pupil interactions have also been observed in preschool settings. As an example, Keogh and Burstein (1988) found that nonhandicapped children with positive temperaments had the most interactions with teachers, whereas handicapped children with positive temperaments had the least. In recent work, Siegel (1991) described associations between teachers' attitudes of attachment or rejection and their views of learning-handicapped and nonlearning-handicapped children. Although pupils' achievement level contributed to teachers' attitudes about particular children, behavior and personal characteristics were also important. Teachers used a wide range of descriptors when talking about children in both the learning-handicapped and the nonlearning-handicapped groups. Many of these descriptors tapped aspects of behavioral style, for example, good at staying on task, attentive, social, tough, bossy, easily distracted.

In summary, in a program of work stimulated by the Thomas and Chess conceptualization of temperament, we have found that individual differences in behavioral styles may be reliably identified within groups of handicapped as well as normally developing children. We have found also that these differences are important contributors to teachers' views of children's teachability and to the nature of teacher-child interactions within classrooms. Life in the classroom is not the same for all children, and teachers' time and attention are not necessarily evenly distributed. More importantly, perhaps, the affective nature of teacher-pupil interactions varies, some children finding the classroom a comfortable and accepting environment, others feeling less valued, even rejected. Few teachers are aware of possible inequities in their interactions with children, yet it is clear that there are real differences in teachers' behaviors and in their affect.

Despite methodological and statistical problems in empirical demonstration of goodness of fit, observational research and findings derived from interviews with teachers support the idea that goodness of fit is a useful construct that captures an important aspect of the teacher-child relationship. Thus, it may help us understand some of the differences in teachers' decisions and behaviors as they interact with individual children. The traditional emphasis in schooling has been on cognitive characteristics, yet findings from a number of research programs argue for the importance of temperamental variation as a major contributor in the goodness-of-fit equation.

STRATEGIES FOR PREVENTION AND INTERVENTION

On an applied, clinical level we suggest that teacher-pupil interactions may be improved by increasing teachers' sensitivity to individual differences in children's temperamental characteristics, and by making teachers more aware of their own reactions to these differences. An interesting and serendipitous finding in a number of our studies has been the teachers' spontaneous comments about the helpfulness of temperament as a way of thinking about children's behavior. In a sense, acceptance of the reality of temperamental individuality frees teachers from traditional cognitive or motivational explanations for children's behavior in school: High-activity, intense children are not necessarily purposefully misbehaving; slow-to-warm-up children are not necessarily dull or unmotivated. Awareness of temperamental differences also provides a more positive framework for classroom organization and behavior management: Slow-to-warm-up children need time to anticipate changes in routines and schedules; high-activity, intense children are likely to have problems in crowded situations.

Bates (1989) has articulated the usefulness of temperament as a way of reframing problems in the family context, noting that "'temperament' is one way of escaping from a framework of blame, thereby reducing resistance to change" (p 348). His idea is equally relevant to the classroom. Educators, counselors, and psychologists who work in schools have been greatly helped by the pioneering work of Thomas and Chess, but in the long run it will be the children who benefit the most.

REFERENCES

Achenbach, T. M., & Edelbrock, C. S. (1986). *Manual for the teacher's report form and teacher version of the child behavior profile.* Burlington: University of Vermont, Department of Psychiatry.

Bates, J. E. (1989). Applications of temperament concepts. In G. A. Kohnstamm, J. E. Bates, & M. K. Rothbart (Eds.), *Temperament in childhood.* Chichester, England: John Wiley.

Hall, R. J., & Cadwell, J. (1984, April). *Temperament influences on cognition and achievement in children with learning disabilities.* Paper presented at the Annual Conference of the American Educational Research Association, New Orleans.

Hegvik, R. L. (1986, May). *Temperament and achievement in school.* Paper presented at the Sixth Occasional Temperament Conference, Pennsylvania State University.

Keogh, B. K. (1982). Children's temperament and teachers' decisions. In R. Porter & G. M. Collins (Eds.), *Temperamental differences in infants and young children* (pp. 269–279). CIBA Foundation Symposium 89. London: Pitman.

Keogh, B. K. (1983). Individual differences in temperament: A contribution to the personal-social and educational competence of learning disabled children. In J. D. McKinney & L. Feagens (Eds.), *Current topics in learning disabilities* (pp. 33–55). Norwood, NJ: Ablex.

Keogh, B. K. (1986). Temperament and schooling: Meaning of goodness of fit? In J. V. Lerner & R. M. Lerner (Eds.), *New directions for child development: Temperament and social interaction in infants and children* (pp. 89–108). San Francisco: Jossey-Bass.

Keogh, B. K. (1989). Applying temperament research to school. In G. A. Kohnstamm; J. E. Bates, & M. K. Rothbart (Eds.), *Temperament in childhood.* Chichester, England: John Wiley.

Keogh, B. K., & Burstein, N. D. (1988). Relationship of temperament to preschoolers' interactions with peers and teachers. *Exceptional Children, 54*(5), 69–73.

Keogh, B. K., Pullis, M. E., & Cadwell, J. (1982). A short form of the Teacher Temperament Questionnaire. *Journal of Educational Measurement, 29*(4), 323–329.

Kohnstamm, G. A., Bates, J. E., & Rothbart, M. K. (Eds.). (1989). *Temperament in childhood.* Chichester, England: John Wiley.

Kornblau, B. W. (1982). The Teachable Pupil Survey: A technique for assessing teachers' perceptions of pupil attributes. *Psychology in the Schools, 19,* 170–174.

Kornblau, B. W., & Keogh, B. K. (1980). Teachers' perceptions and educational decisions. In J. J. Gallagher (Ed.), *New directions for exceptional children: No. 1. The ecology of exceptional children* (pp. 87–101). San Francisco: Jossey-Bass.

Lerner, J. V., & Lerner, R. M. (Eds.). (1986). *Temperament and social interaction in infants and childhood. New directions for child development series,* No. 31. San Francisco: Jossey-Bass.

Lerner, J. V., Lerner, R. M., & Zabski, S. (1985). Temperament and elementary school children's actual and rated academic performance: A test of a "goodness of fit" model. *Journal of Child Psychology and Psychiatry, 26*(1), 125–136.

Martin, R. P. (1989). Activity level, distractibility, and persistence: Critical characteristics of early schooling. In G. A. Kohnstamm, J. E. Bates, & M. K. Rothbart (Eds.), *Temperament in childhood.* Chichester, England: John Wiley.

Maziade, M., Côté, R., Boutin, P., Boudreault, M. D., & Thivierge, J. (1986). The effect of temperament on longitudinal academic achievement in primary school. *Journal of the American Academy of Child Psychiatry, 25*(5), 692–696.

Pullis, M. E. (1985). LD students' temperament characteristics and their impact on decisions by resource and mainstream teachers. *Learning Disabilities Quarterly, 8,* 109–122.

Ratekin, C. (1990). *Temperament in children with Down Syndrome.* Doctoral dissertation, University of California, Los Angeles.

Shavelson, R. J. (1976). The psychology of teaching methods. In N. Gage (Ed.), *Yearbook of the National Society for the Study of Education.* Chicago: University of Chicago Press.

Siegel, J. (1991). *Regular education teachers' attitudes and behaviors toward mainstreamed learning handicapped students.* Doctoral dissertation, University of California, Los Angeles.

Supanchek, P. (1989). *Effects of a dynamic assessment approach with developmentally delayed children.* Doctoral dissertation, University of California, Los Angeles.

Thomas, A., & Chess, S. (1977). *Temperament and development.* New York: Brunner/Mazel.

PART IX

PREVENTION AND INTERVENTION STRATEGIES IN THE COMMUNITY SETTING

25

The Temperament Program: Community-Based Prevention of Behavior Disorders in Children

Bill Smith

Located in a county-run human service agency in rural eastern Oregon, the Temperament Program offers parenting advice tailored to the individual needs of each child and family. The program's unique intervention model has been created in consultation with temperament researchers including Stella Chess and Alexander Thomas, the project's primary advisers. Since its start in 1988, the program has rapidly evolved into a comprehensive service capable of meeting a wide variety of needs.

Parents enter the Temperament Program for many different reasons but with the common theme of concern about the behavior of a particular child. The program's services are provided by specially trained parents, called temperament specialists, who are supervised by a mental health professional. Because individualized parenting advice can be beneficial to any parent, no restrictions are placed on the types of behavioral concerns addressed by the program. Parents leave the Temperament Program with a better understanding of their child, many effective parenting strategies, a plan for the future, and a resource book of parenting information geared to their particular needs.

The Temperament Program is often the first involvement families have in social services. It may be the only service needed by a particular family, or it may be included alongside others. The Temperament Program has been found to complement mental health counseling, psychiatric services, day treatment, special education, medical care, foster and adoptive child services, juvenile corrections, and child protection services.

Client Population

A scholarship program funded by the Oregon Mental Health Division has made it possible for parents from all income levels to participate. Participants have resembled local demographics in terms of income, occupation, family configuration, and geographic location. While the program's emphasis is on helping parents with temperament issues, nontemperament issues affecting child development are also addressed. Examples include behavior disorders, physical and sexual abuse, developmental disorders, chronic and severe medical conditions, school issues, and family disruptions such as divorce or the death of a loved one. Temperament theory makes up the core of the service by providing the context within which these other issues are understood.

Psychiatric diagnoses can be established for most children whose parents participate in the program. Common categories include attention deficit hyperactivity disorder, oppositional-defiant disorder, conduct disorder, adjustment disorder, various academic skill disorders, and post-traumatic stress disorder. Other represented categories include mental retardation, autism, separation anxiety disorder, overanxious disorder, and psychological factors affecting physical condition.

Community Outreach

The Temperament Program offers a free service called a "Child Behavior Screening" to organizations that serve children and families. The service is flexible and can usually be incorporated into one of the organization's normal activities. For example, the local education service district has included this screening in their annual efforts to identify preschool-aged children in need of special education services. Over the past four years, they have helped us to screen more than 350 children. Smaller screenings have also been conducted with Headstart programs, church groups, support groups, and other existing groups.

Parents complete the 36-item Eyberg Child Behavior Inventory (Eyberg & Ross, 1978) and 52 additional items that help in determining the child's temperament. The screening is optional, but few parents refuse to participate. The questionnaire is scored on a variety of scales including eight temperament dimensions. Based on these findings, temperament specialists spend about 15 minutes with each parent asking additional questions and discussing results. The Temperament Program is recommended to about 40% of parents who attend such screenings.

An impressive amount of community outreach also occurs informally via word-of-mouth referral by parents in the program. More than half of the program's participants enter as a result of the screenings or informal outreach. The remainder enter through referrals from other service providers.

INTERVENTION MODEL

Theory

The Temperament Program was based on the research and theories of Chess and Thomas. Temperament is assessed using their nine categories, and the principle of "goodness of fit" provides the basis for the intervention approach. Additionally, concepts from the book *The Difficult Child* (Turecki, 1985) have been very helpful, especially in earlier versions of the program.

Children's difficulties are understood within the context of (1) temperament, (2) other prominent individual differences such as intelligence or learning disabilities, (3) past history of uncommon childhood experiences such as abuse or chronic illness, and (4) current life experience including family and school variables. This detailed understanding of the child permits an analysis of the child's prominent *talents* and most needed *skills*. Talents are defined as attributes or abilities arising out of the child's temperament, intellect, and other inborn characteristics. Skills are defined as attributes or abilities that are acquired through practice. Within this framework, talents result from "nature" and skills are "nurtured" until they become "second nature."

The behaviors that parents are most often concerned about in their children tend to be those that have persisted despite repeated efforts to help. Behaviors of this type can usually be traced to lacking or underdeveloped skills. Because each child is born with a unique set of talents and needed skills, the process of parenting is different for every child. Parenting provides a "good fit" when it is appropriately tailored to the child's unique needs and abilities. Viewing a child's behavior in this way makes it possible to normalize what is happening and quickly move to practical solutions.

Temperament provides an excellent example of how normal children vary in terms of how easy or difficult they are to raise. Children rated high or low on a given temperament dimension present more challenges to their parents than children rated in the moderate range. This is because the extremes of temperament always produce combinations of talents and needed skills. For example, withdrawing children are naturally cautious, but lack risk-taking skills. They also tend to enjoy solitary activities, but may have difficulties developing social skills. Even temperament characteristics that might seem to be purely beneficial can produce challenges. For example, children with extremely positive moods often lack skills for knowing when and how to express seriousness or concern.

Generally, the more temperament characteristics rate either high or low for a child, the more challenging he or she will be to raise. Even though these qualities bring with them many inborn talents, the talents quickly become overused when needed skills are not developed. For example, a withdrawing child's cautiousness might drift toward fear and seclusion as the child continues to struggle with life's increasing demands for instantaneous involvement in new experiences.

Once a child's challenging behaviors are traced to lacking or underdeveloped skills, the solution involves helping the child develop the needed skills by providing experiences appropriate to his or her individual style, potential, and level of development. Parents can provide these experiences by creating and using "learning strategies." Learning strategies are parenting techniques that promote skill development within the context of a patient, understanding, and supportive parental relationship.

This emphasis on skill building also makes it possible for parents to become more accepting of traditional forms of intervention, including counseling, special education, and medication. Additionally, activities not normally thought of as forms of intervention become important options. Examples include karate classes for children with anger-control problems, scouting for shy children, and gymnastics classes for accident-prone active children.

A case example is included to illustrate these concepts.

Case Example

Andy was 5 years old when his parents entered the Temperament Program, concerned about his defiant, argumentative behavior at home. Outside the home Andy was reported to be a well-behaved and generally quiet child. His parents were extremely confused by the dramatic contrast between his home and nonhome behavior. They were also concerned about his steadfast refusal to separate from them for any appreciable length of time. Having refused to attend preschool and kindergarten, Andy was now refusing to start the first grade.

Andy's temperament assessment indicated that he was very withdrawing, slow in adjusting to change, emotionally intense, and highly active. His other temperament characteristics were all in the moderate range. From his history, Andy appeared to be a normal child raised in a normal family. Still, it was easy to understand why his parents were concerned. Not only did he constantly demand that they play with him, he always wanted to be in charge, could not sit still, and was prone to having rageful tantrums lasting up to an hour each.

Because their attitudes toward him had become increasingly negative, Andy's parents found it helpful to make a list of his many talents. The talents stemming mostly from his temperament included his cautiousness, enthusiasm, and unlimited energy, and the fact that he was often headstrong and willing to express his opinions. It was also learned that Andy had musical talent, an excellent memory, and above average intelligence.

The reasons for Andy's behavior problems were relatively easy to understand because they stemmed so directly from his temperament. Andy was a very shy child who behaved shyly in any environment that was the least bit unfamiliar. Thus, Andy was in many ways a model child when he went places with his parents. At home he was more comfortable, and the full expression of his temperament became possible. Not only did Andy prefer his home environment, he ruled it actively and loudly with tantrums occurring regularly when he didn't get his own way.

Although it was easy to understand Andy's behavior, changing it was another thing entirely. A temperament specialist helped Andy's parents understand that the most crucial skill he needed to develop was the ability to accept influence over his behavior. In fact, Andy had overused his talent for being headstrong, and now it was going to be doubly hard for him to learn to accept the influence of his parents. Many learning strategies were created to help Andy develop this skill. In one strategy a small battery-powered clock was used to help Andy adjust to changes requested by his parents. For example, when his parents wanted him to stop playing and get ready for dinner, they would say, "I know it's sometimes hard for you to change what you are doing. I want you to start getting ready for dinner. You can use your clock if you want. We'll be starting when the big hand reaches the 5."

Andy's parents gradually helped him develop skills for accepting their influence. They were then able to start focusing on other needed skills. Although they still felt he needed home schooling, midway through the year it became possible for Andy's parents to start transitioning him to regular school. They teamed up with another family that was home schooling a boy Andy's age, and the two boys "attended school" together, alternating weeks at each other's home. As the "fit" improved, Andy's tantrums gradually decreased in both frequency and intensity. His parents are now helping him develop skills for containing his emotional intensity by practicing his "inside voice" and "outside voice."

Service Providers

We are often asked how parents without professional training can be so successful in providing this service to other parents. This is not an easy question to answer. Our response has as much to do with the limitations of professional help as it does with the advantages of having parents help parents.

Because it is impossible for anyone to understand a child in the complex way the parent understands the child, professionals will always be limited in their ability to tailor their interventions to the individual needs of children. This issue is compounded by the fact that most professionals are still trained in traditional theories of child development that do not take into account inborn individual differences. But even when professionals include temperament and other inborn characteristics in their assessments, much of the child's individuality remains untapped simply because there is no substitute for getting to know a child through the parenting process.

So parents and professionals must, to a large degree, create their interventions based on different viewpoints and different ways of understanding the child. Professionals tend to construct more general interventions that rely on techniques and strategies designed to produce positive change under widely varied circumstances. Parents tend to evolve specific interventions that rely on a more detailed understanding of the child and the power of a loving relationship. When viewed this way, it becomes clear that parents and professionals make different contributions to a child's development. The obvious goal becomes a partnership between parents and professionals that draws upon the unique contributions of all parties involved.

While most parents are appreciative of professional services, the vast majority of them are highly skeptical of professional advice about parenting. We have found this to be especially true for parents who have difficult children. As these parents enroll in the Temperament Program, many say the same thing, "Don't talk to me about *time out* or *star charts*—punishments and rewards do not work for my child." Collectively, these parents have found that much of the advice available for parents is overly simplistic. To be fair, it is not so much that these parenting strategies don't work, but that these strategies (a) do not take advantage of the strengths of the parent-child relationship and (b) are too general to bring about appreciable changes in the behaviors that are of most concern to most parents.

One unfortunate outcome of the clash that sometimes occurs between parents and professionals regarding parenting issues is that many parents feel unappreciated or even blamed for the dedicated efforts they have made in raising their children. Again, parents of difficult children seem especially susceptible to these feelings. Our view is that much of this lack of appreciation stems from (a) a lack of understanding of the complex nature of the parenting process and (b) the often unwarranted assumption that techniques and strategies that are effective within the context of professional services will also be effective within the context of the parenting relationship.

The Temperament Program essentially provides a bridge between the efforts of the parents, which are highly individualized to the child's needs, and professional efforts, which are necessarily less individualized but also very helpful. The bridge is the temperament specialist who (a) has the ability to fully understand the parents' world, (b) helps the parents build their parenting approach around their understanding of their child, and (c) can make effective referrals to other community resources as needed.

When the role of the temperament specialist is viewed in this way, parents become the most qualified individuals for the job. We hire on two criteria: parenting experience and the ability to be helpful to others. We also try to hire parents who are raising one or more difficult children of their own. Training is accomplished in a relatively short amount of time using a process that builds upon the parents' natural abilities. The temperament specialist is conceptualized as an "ideal neighbor"—that is, someone who is accepting of the parent's values and who offers only advice that is likely to help. This role requires a working knowledge of temperament theory, the ability to collect information efficiently, appropriate tools and references, a process for problem solving, appropriate consultants, and time to apply these supports to meet the needs of each parent served. It is a complex role but not any more complex than the role of being a parent. In fact, the temperament specialist's training is simply an extension of things already learned as a parent.

Intervention Process

A temperament specialist meets weekly with one or both parents. These meetings are informal (i.e., neighborly) and last about 45 minutes each. The length of the program varies for each family with some parents completing it in as few as 4 weeks and others needing up to a year or longer. Services are organized into a four-phase intervention model providing a structured approach while permitting flexibility to accommodate individual needs.

Phase One: Assessment

The temperament specialist conducts a detailed assessment with the child's parents, which includes a child behavior inventory, a semistructured interview, many exercises completed by the parents between sessions, and optional assessment strategies for specific issues. This core process is sometimes extended to include professional services such as mental health assessment for the child, consultation with a child psychiatrist, educational assessments conducted by school personnel, and/or consultation or evaluation by other appropriate experts. The assessment phase does not end until the parent and the temperament specialist reach agreement about the issues involved in the child's behavior.

Phase Two: Parent-Child Relationship Strengthening

Because stresses in the parent-child relationship can undercut even the most appropriate parenting strategies for a particular child, parents are helped to strengthen their relationship with their child by (a) listing the child's talents and (b) examining their own temperaments, values, and expectations in relation to their child's individual needs. In the process, parents gain a greater acceptance of the child's individuality and become even more motivated to make changes in their parenting. This shift in the parent's perception of the child invariably reduces parent-child stress and is a crucial step in the process of achieving a "good fit."

Phase Three: Specific Parenting Advice and Support

The temperament specialist helps the child's parents develop a plan for resolving some or all of the concerns that brought them into the program. Learning strategies are created, and the parents are supported as they begin implementing the plan. As the parents gain confidence in their new approach, suggestions are made for elements that might be added in the future as their child progresses. The program typically ends at this point, but only if the parents decide they are ready.

Parents are also helped in other ways during this phase. For example, temperament specialists often (a) make referrals to other services, (b) provide consultation to professionals involved in the child's education, (c) provide a forum for couples to work out differing opinions about their child, (d) help adolescents understand their temperaments and/or advocate for them within their family system, and/or (e) provide long-term emotional support to parents who have extremely difficult children.

Phase Four: Continued Availability

Parents are encouraged to return to the program when new issues arise or old issues resurface. Follow-up contacts with parents who have completed the program indicate that parents are generally effective in responding to new problem behaviors without further help. Still, many parents do return, and most often their needs are met in just one or two sessions.

PROGRAM OUTCOMES

The development of the Temperament Program has been tracked by the Regional Research Institute for Human Services at Portland State University

(Koroloff, 1989, 1990, 1991, 1992). More extensive analysis of outcome data can be found in these reports.

To date, parents of 230 children ranging in age from 6 months to 18 years have enrolled in the Temperament Program. Most parents complete the program (74%). The most common reason given for not finishing is that the program is more time-consuming than was anticipated. Brief follow-up surveys are mailed about once each year to parents who have completed the program. Of 118 surveys mailed to date, 80 (68%) have been returned.

Parents have been generally satisfied with the program's services. On a five-point scale, 79% have indicated that they have been helped either "much" or "very much" by the program. Ninety-three percent have reported that meetings with their temperament specialists were either "helpful" or "very helpful." A similar percentage (86%) have found the written materials either "helpful" or "very help-ful." Parents have been most likely to say that they were using the concepts they learned "sometimes" or "often" (88%). They have tended to report "some" or "much" improvement (79%) in their child's behavior as a result of their involve-ment in the program. Additionally, 13% have reported that their child's behavior had improved "very much."

In one question parents are asked to list the three most important things they learned in the program. Analysis of these written responses indicates that parents on the whole are (a) becoming more confident in their parenting abilities, (b) developing effective parenting techniques, (c) becoming more understanding and accepting of their children, (d) becoming more optimistic about their children's futures, and (e) generalizing the concepts they learn to influence the way they think about and respond to other children.

In response to a request for at least one suggestion for improving the program, most parents have requested additional services and information. Specifically, they wanted (a) more opportunities for long-term contact with the program, (b) written materials on a variety of topics not covered, (c) support groups, (d) ser-vices their children could participate in, including group experiences and counsel-ing, and (e) ways to get information about temperament into the schools.

CONCLUSIONS

It was no accident that the Temperament Program so quickly evolved into such a popular, comprehensive service. There is a "good fit" between temperament theory and the views of most parents. Parents know that kids are different from the start, and most do an excellent job of meeting the individual needs of their children despite a lack of information to show them how. But when parents run into difficulties, where do they turn for the answers they need? Sadly, there is often no place to turn. Everyone suffers when this happens—the child, the parents, the family, and society as a whole.

It is a tribute to Chess and Thomas that their concepts were so readily adapted to create this successful community-based early intervention program. The ease with which parents from all walks of life are able to understand and use their concepts supports the importance and relevance of temperament theory. The desire of most of our participants for more information and services underscores the need for other efforts to apply these concepts. The many examples of specific prevention and intervention approaches contained in this book highlight the fact that this work has begun. As these efforts continue, and are expanded by others, much will be learned about child development and the difficult job of parenting may become easier.

REFERENCES

Eyberg, S. M., & Ross, A. W. (1978). Assessment of child behavior problems: The validation of a new inventory. *Journal of Clinical and Child Psychology, 7*(2), 113–116.

Koroloff, N. (1989, February). *Getting a great start: Early intervention demonstration projects (interim report).*[1]

Koroloff, N. (1990, March). *Getting a great start: Part II. Early intervention demonstration projects—January 1988 to June 1989.*[1]

Koroloff, N. (1991, March). *Starting right: An interim report on early identification and prevention services for children at risk of mental or emotional disorders demonstration project—July 1989 to December 1990.*[1]

Koroloff, N. (1992, February). *Starting right: Part II. A final report on early identification and prevention services for children at risk of mental or emotional disorders demonstration project—July 1989 to June 1991.*[1]

Turecki, S. (1985). *The Difficult Child.* New York: Bantam Books. (Revised 1989)

---

1. Available from the Regional Research Institute for Human Services, Portland State University, Portland, OR 97207.

26

Parent Support Groups

Catherine J. Andersen

As described in earlier chapters in this volume, individual differences in children's characteristics may constitute risk factors in specific environments. Several authors have described pioneering prevention programs incorporating knowledge about individual differences, which show considerable promise. In the previous chapter, Smith demonstrated the value of a community-based and professionally run program that uses parent counselors in a preventive role. This chapter describes a small, western Canadian, parent-run support program with a similar theoretical framework. It differs from the Temperament Program in that it is run by parents with minimal professional supervision and no direct professional involvement with participating families.

The value of parent support groups in reducing stress in raising children with disabilities and chronic illnesses is well-known. As well, support groups have been recommended for families of children diagnosed with attention deficit hyperactivity disorder (Barkley, 1990). On the basis of his clinical experience, Turecki (1989) has recommended support groups for families of children with temperament risk factors and describes briefly how such groups have been run in the Difficult Child Program at Beth Israel Hospital in New York City.

Support groups offer families opportunities to ventilate their feelings, to reduce their isolation, and to acquire information and education. Parent-run support groups have two appealing features: low cost, and no less important, the active involvement of families in their own treatment. The second feature, providing opportunities for families to develop their own solutions, is increasingly being recognized as a critical factor for change in families in situations where external rewards are low, as is often the case when they have very difficult children (Cunningham, 1988). It must be recognized, however, that the self-help program to be described here has not been subjected to rigorous evaluation, although plans

267

for its systematic study are under way. The purpose of this chapter, then, considering that extravagant claims about success cannot be made, is to suggest possibilities to others involved in prevention and intervention.

I. BACKGROUND AND STRUCTURE OF THE PROGRAM

The Difficult Child Support Association of British Columbia (DCSA) was founded in 1988 by two mothers who were informally introduced by a social service agency because they had independently commented on how valuable the work of Chess and Thomas, as applied by Turecki and Tonner (1985), had been to them in understanding and managing their temperamentally difficult sons.

After the two mothers made contact with other families of similar preschool-aged children, a core group of families approached prominent professionals in the community for help in the development of an organization with a mandate to develop support for families of children with temperament risk factors.

The DCSA is an incorporated nonprofit society, run by a board of parent directors with the assistance of a professional advisory board. The advisers donate their time and expertise to reviewing parent education literature, including the newsletter, and to providing general guidelines. However, the association does not provide screening, diagnosis, testing, or treatment to participating families. We do not make referrals or recommendations, but we provide information about appropriate services available.

The DCSA currently supports itself entirely with membership fees and small private donations. Membership fees are very low (currently, $10 per year per family) and are waived for families on social assistance. It is our conviction that those interested in providing such support services to families should not feel helpless to run such programs during times of governmental restraints. Because we use parent volunteer group leaders and make use of free community facilities, our costs have been very low. This is not to say that we endorse widespread cutbacks in essential social services; of course, these services must be maintained. Self-help support programs cannot be substitutes for professionally run programs, but may be valuable adjuncts to them, and can be run at very low cost with a great deal of volunteer effort.

Families of children under 12 can refer themselves directly to the organization. Many learn about its existence from newspaper stories, community announcements, or social service agencies. Increasingly, families are being referred by physicians and mental health professionals who recognize the value of our programs. The development of a screening procedure to ensure that referrals and self-referrals to our groups are appropriate is a critical issue that we will be addressing over the next few years, and one about which we will be seeking guidance from temperament researchers and clinicians. (The very unsatisfactory compromise we have made until now has been to ask families to read *The Difficult Child* [Turecki & Tonner, 1989], to see if the program seems appropriate for them.)

Our support groups currently meet in the evenings, although we have had requests for daytime groups. The frequency of the meetings is determined by the core members. Often they settle on twice a month. Groups usually meet in facilities such as preschools, and we find it very helpful if we can have access to coffee-making, video, and photocopying equipment. Child care centers have been very generous in permitting us to use their facilities and equipment free of charge.

In the early years of our program, we tried a number of ways to recruit and educate group leaders, but are now considering developing a specific training program for them. My own view is that people from a wide range of backgrounds can be good leaders. A background in early childhood education, nursing, social work, or psychology can be very helpful. However, I think most parents in our programs believe that the leader must have had personal experience with a temperamentally difficult child. Our current parent leaders work closely with the board of directors, who in turn refer many questions to the professional advisory board.

II. EDUCATIONAL COMPONENT OF SUPPORT PROGRAM

The DCSA's support program places a great deal of emphasis on parent education. Although we recognize the value of support groups as places where parents can ventilate their feelings, we also believe that our programs will not have much preventive effect if they offer this type of support alone. In addressing temperamental differences in children as risk factors, we are necessarily trying to improve temperament–environment fit, family functioning, and behavior management as each individual circumstance dictates (Chess & Thomas, 1984; Maziade et al., 1990).

Although professionals are involved in the production and delivery of some aspects of our parent education program—for example, by offering guest lectures and by screening parenting books and videotapes—support group leaders also play an educational role by helping to focus discussion at meetings without claiming to be experts. They do try to help parents with practical problem solving, however, making frequent references to the key principles of our educational programs and referring parents to our recommended literature. Leaders also show videotapes on specific topics as they arise. (Each support group maintains a library of our recommended literature and audiovisual materials, and these are regularly borrowed by parents and professionals, and are much appreciated.)

We have also experimented recently with more structured study groups, also parent led, where participants work through Turecki and Tonner's (1989) program, and other materials, and report back their experiences to the group for discussion. More formal parenting courses and talks have been delivered by professionals who are also parents of temperamentally difficult children. All of the educational and support formats we have tried have been extremely well received by parents but remain to be systematically evaluated.

The educational components of our support programs are focused on the following broad range of integrated issues:

A. Understanding Normal Individual Differences

Our approach to temperament-related problems is solidly based on the work of Chess and Thomas (1984), Turecki and Tonner (1989), and Carey and McDevitt (1989). Parent evaluations of our programs suggest that information about temperament increases parents' understanding of their children's behavior and promotes more positive views of the children. We do not find it difficult to avoid simplistic applications of temperament concepts in our support groups where parents feel comfortable and speak freely, perhaps because discussion leaders are seen as sympathetic friends, rather than as critical professionals. Many times an eager group leader or another parent attempting to help has been told that her simple solutions ("give your active child more room to play" or "remove distractions from the child with poor attention") do not work, miss the point, or lead to undesirable consequences.

B. Task Mastery: An Important Goal of Development

Chess and Thomas (1984) have pointed out the crucial role that task mastery plays in development. Kagan also emphasizes the need for parents to understand "that at each stage of development the child needs different resources from the family" (1989, p. 52) in order to master critical developmental tasks. We find it helpful to discuss these ideas with parents. For example, extremely protective parents of highly inhibited preschoolers often need to see that their child needs gradual exposure to social situations, rather than protection from them, at this particular stage of development.

C. Separating Normal from Deviant Behavior

At support groups we provide literature with basic information about normal developmental patterns, about secondary problems in children with temperament–environment conflict, and about developmental disorders such as autism, attention deficit hyperactivity disorder, and learning disabilities. Group leaders and the association's executive director will strongly recommend professional help when families report serious marital or family conflict, fears of abusing their children, seriously aggressive or withdrawn behavior in the children, or major difficulties at preschool, day care, or school, or whenever there is a suggestion that the child is not developing normally (such as severe language delay or bizarre behavior). In this connection, it must be recognized that all children in our community have ready access to family physicians and pediatricians. We find that many parents in our groups have already been informed that their child is essentially normal, and simply want extra help in day-to-day management and coping. Others are waiting to see a child psychiatrist. Many participating families are seeing a mental health professional as well as participating in our support groups.

D. Reducing Stress from the Temperament–Environment Interaction

Most parents who approach DCSA are experiencing considerable stress from the temperament–environment interaction. We find that the majority of parents are not fully aware that their negative attention to problematic behavior— shouting, slapping, and scolding—generally accentuates the problems. Those who are aware nevertheless find it difficult to initiate changes in the interactions. Many parents admit that they do not find their "difficult" children fun to be around, and sometimes avoid their children's company, often for fear of stirring up conflict. Parents are sometimes attracted more to methods of punishment than to strategies for promoting more positive interactions. Although Barkley (1987) and Webster-Stratton (1989) have discussed the difficulties in promoting positive interactions between parents and children with difficult behavior, we are disappointed that there is little practical material addressing this critical matter, although recent work by Strayhorn and Weidman (1991) looks very promising. We look forward to seeing more such efforts from clinicians and researchers, preferably in forms that are suitable for self-help programs.

Our own approach to promoting more positive interactions between parents and children involves several recommendations. We find that treatment of parental depression is often important, as is obtaining relief from full-time parenting (e.g., placing the child in day care or preschool). Reducing stress through participating in our support groups and by making use of other community groups and resources is emphasized. We find, however, that improving parents' interactions with their children nearly always involves their making accommodations to individual differences. For example, although we do recommend a regular, unstructured "play time" between parent and child, and follow the ideas of behavioral therapists such as Barkley (1987) in advising parents not to direct, criticize, or in any way undermine their children's play during these sessions, we also recognize that temperamental characteristics, such as intensity of reaction or distractibility, can greatly influence the nature and quality of these shared times for both parent and child. Clearly, "fit' can be an important issue here.

At group meetings, we invite parents to work together in developing solutions to difficulties related to children's individual response patterns. An example that comes to mind is that of a parent, who was also a teacher, who reported her experiences with an easily stimulated and rather inflexible 3-year-old, the youngest of four children. The mother was a strong believer in letting her children join in the family's domestic activities as a way of strengthening relationships and building competence, but found that her daughter worked herself into such a pitch of excitement while "helping to cook" that the entire family began to dread the child's participation.

Interference from the others, even in the form of mild directions and assistance, only increased the child's arousal and resistance. "Then I bought her a really huge mixing bowl and put a shower curtain on the counter and one on the floor and let her cook to her heart's content. When we stopped bugging her about the mess, she calmed down somewhat," said the mother, with some satisfaction at having found a simple and effective solution, one that did not compromise her own aspirations. After hearing this story, other parents began to discuss how they might structure situations in ways that could reduce conflict between themselves and their children. In these discussions, group leaders encourage families to keep in mind both their children's individual characteristics and their family's specific values and expectations when working out solutions.

E. Understanding the Effects of Marital Discord and Family Stress on Children's Behavior

Chess and Thomas (1984) stated that in the New York Longitudinal Study marital discord was an even stronger predictor of disorders in children than difficult temperament. Yet, as Barkley (1987) and Campbell (1990) point out, many families do not seem to be aware that young children are vulnerable to this particular type of stress. Others seem aware, but have great difficulty in addressing marital conflict. A concern that has arisen at DCSA is the possibility that the mother's participation in the group, in the absence of marital support, might compound a couple's problems. Even when the marriage is stable, we have had little success in persuading fathers to attend support group meetings, although it is noteworthy that both partners tend to sign up for our formal, "paid-for" parenting courses. We are looking hard for ways to encourage fathers to participate in support groups, but we must bear in mind the fact that the father is often the only available babysitter, and in many cases the only person other than the mother willing or able to manage an exceptionally difficult young child.

F. Recognizing the Interaction of Temperament and Clinical Problems

Carey (1986) has pointed out that, although a considerable amount is known already, much more research is needed on the interaction of children's temperaments with clinical problems, such as asthma. Our impression is that DCSA families have disproportionate numbers of children with health problems, notably, frequent respiratory infections and allergies. We hope very much that more research attention will be paid to these problems in relation to temperament and behavior.

A word on the controversial topic of dietary effects on behavior might be useful at this point, since we recognize that many clinicians are fearful of referring families to support groups, because they often have the reputation of promoting fad diets. We feel that it is not enough for clinicians to dismiss the hypotheses of Feingold (1974) and others as premature and poorly supported. Following the suggestions of those who propose a link between dietary ingredients and disordered behavior, parents believe they see a relationship between their children's temperament and the foods they ingest. They quickly lose confidence in professionals who jeer at this notion. Nevertheless, families in our groups have not tended to become involved in fad diets. This may be due, in part, to the open-minded approach we take to this question, but likely also reflects the fact that the few who have tried dietary approaches have reported limited success and increased family stress.

III. OTHER SUPPORT FUNCTIONS OF THE ASSOCIATION

The DCSA also offers indirect support to families by presenting workshops and lectures to teachers, nurses, social workers, and medical students. These programs are offered by either professional or parent speakers, and frequently focus on the role of temperament in development and on practical approaches to temperament-related problems. We also publish a professionally screened quarterly newsletter.

IV. RESEARCH NEEDED ON BENEFITS OF PROGRAM

We recognize that neither the concepts applied in our parent education material nor the principles and processes of self-help can be assumed to have direct benefits to children. Until we have evaluated our programs rigorously, we will not know for certain whether there are significant improvements in our families' perceptions of, relationships with, and management of their children because of their participation in our programs. Nevertheless, families have expressed their enthusiasm for DCSA, and we have witnessed some extremely encouraging outcomes in the short time that we have been in operation.

The families of the Difficult Child Support Association are the direct beneficiaries of the pioneering work of Stella Chess and Alexander Thomas, who brought to light the powerful role of children's individual temperaments in their healthy and unhealthy development. We are inspired by their confidence in ordinary people and by their compassion for the very real difficulties that families face. As a grandfather who attended a DCSA meeting said: "It is so wonderful that there is now so much understanding of these questions. It wasn't so when our son was young, and my wife and I suffered greatly, with great harm to our boy. Now we're going to make sure things work out all right for our grandson, who is also a handful. Let us be thankful, very thankful, to the people who have helped us with their work, their research, and by writing these books."

REFERENCES

Barkley, R. A. (1987). *Defiant children: A clinicians' manual for parent training*. New York: Guilford Press.

Barkley, R. A. (1990). *Attention deficit hyperactivity disorder: A handbook for diagnosis and treatment*. New York: Guilford Press.

Campbell, S. B. (1990). *Behavior problems in preschool children: Clinical and developmental issues*. New York: Guilford Press.

Carey, W. B. (1986). Clinical interactions of temperament. In R. Plomin & J. Dunn (Eds.), *The study of temperament: Changes, continuities and challenges* (pp. 151–162). Hillsdale, NJ: Lawrence Erlbaum.

Carey, W. B., & McDevitt, S. C. (1989). *Clinical and educational applications of temperament research*. Berwyn, PA: Swets North America. Originally published by Swets & Zetlinger, Lisse/Amsterdam, The Netherlands.

Chess, S., & Thomas, A. (1984). *Origins and evolution of behavior disorders: From infancy to early adult life*. New York: Brunner/Mazel.

Cunningham, C. E. (1988). A family systems oriented cognitive-behavioral program for parents of AD-HD children. In R. A. Barkley (Chair), *Treating attention deficit hyperactivity disorder (AD-HD): The state of the art*. Symposium conducted at the meeting of the American Psychological Association, Atlanta.

Feingold, B. F. (1974). *Why your child is hyperactive*. New York: Random House.

Kagan, J. (1989). Stress on and in the family. In M. W. Yogman & T. B. Brazelton (Eds.), *In support of families* (pp. 42–54). Cambridge, MA: Harvard University Press.

Maziade, M., Caron, C., Côté, R., Merette, C., Bernier, H., Laplante, B., Boutin, P., & Thivierge, J. (1990). Psychiatric status of adolescents who had extreme temperaments at age 7. *American Journal of Psychiatry, 147*, 1531–1536.

Strayhorn, J. M., & Weidman, C. S. (1991). Follow-up one year after parent-child interaction training: Effects on behavior of preschool children. *Journal of the American Academy of Child and Adolescent Psychiatry, 30,* 138–143.

Turecki, S. (1989). The difficult child center. In W. B. Carey & S. C. McDevitt (Eds.), *Clinical and educational applications of temperament research* (pp. 142–153). Berwyn, PA: Swets North America.

Turecki, S., & Tonner, L. (1985). *The difficult child.* New York: Bantam Books.

Turecki, S., & Tonner, L. (1989). *The difficult child* (rev. ed.). New York: Bantam Books.

Webster-Stratton, C. (1989). Systematic comparison of consumer satisfaction of three cost-effective parent training programs for conduct problem children. *Behavior Therapy, 20,* 103–115.

PART X

CONCLUSIONS

27

Advocacy for the Health of the Public

Leon Eisenberg

To do well for children, it is not enough to mean well; it is the combination of commitment to their welfare and knowledge of their needs that makes it possible to be effective on their behalf. The careers of Stella Chess and Alex Thomas embody both of those qualities. At a time when the received wisdom depicted the child as a blank slate on which experience wrote the text, Alex and Stella undertook empirical research that proved beyond a doubt that variability in temperamental traits interacted with experience in determining personality and psychopathology. They brought their knowledge to professional and lay groups alike. Throughout their lives, they have consistently supported programs that enhance life opportunities for young people. Their example has inspired others to combine rigorous investigation with passionate commitment to human welfare, both of which are reflected in social activism.

SOCIAL ACTIVISM AND THE PHYSICIAN

Many physicians are uncomfortable with the very idea of social activism. It is enough, they feel, to be helpful to their patients on a case-by-case basis. Speaking out in the public arena is unseemly behavior for a professional, they contend. Indeed, when Benjamin Spock used his public authority as the nation's best-known pediatrician because of his book, the legendary *Baby and Child Care,* to picket against the Vietnam war, and allowed himself to be arrested and put on trial, he was condemned by many colleagues for having violated the canons of professional etiquette (and, not incidentally, their conservative political views).

Yet, what Ben Spock did was in a great medical tradition, one spectacularly exemplified by Rudolf Virchow (1821–1902).

Rudolf Virchow is remembered today as the founder of modern biomedicine. It was he who established cell doctrine in pathology: "Where a cell arises, there a cell must have previously existed, just as an animal can spring only from an animal, a plant only from a plant" (Virchow, 1860, p. 54). It was he who established the pathophysiology of pulmonary embolism, leukemia, abnormal heme pigments, amyloid bodies, and trichinosis, among others. However, the history taught medical students has been silent on Virchow's tireless social activism.

In the summer of 1847, Upper Silesia was devastated by an epidemic of relapsing fever. The public scandal shamed the central government in Berlin into appointing a commission of investigation, with Virchow as a member. He wrote the commission report (Virchow, 1848/1985, pp. 205–319), in which he insisted that the principal causes of the epidemic were the conditions under which the workers were forced to live, notably the bad housing and malnutrition that made them vulnerable to disease. Nothing but universal education, absolute separation of church and school, regional self-government, just taxation, and industrial development could bring about an improvement. For this to happen, "free and unlimited democracy" would be essential!

Virchow's conclusions were based upon close examination of the social factors in the epidemic. He wrote well before the germ theory of disease was formulated. It would be another 20 years before the spirochete *Borrelia recurrentis* was discovered in the blood of relapsing fever patients, and 40 years before the body louse was identified as the vector for the spirochete. Neither of these discoveries has diminished the validity of Virchow's basic conclusions. In our times, no less than in his, relapsing fever is usually seen in epidemics that arise in the wake of large-scale disasters (wars, famine, floods) characterized by overcrowding, poor personal hygiene, and malnutrition (Southern & Sanford, 1969).

In the year of the German revolution of 1848, Virchow and his colleagues called for public provision of medical care for the indigent, prohibition of child labor, protection for pregnant women, a reduced working day in dangerous occupations, adequate ventilation at work sites, and the like. Virchow stated forcefully: "Medical instruction does not exist to provide individuals with an opportunity of learning how to earn a living, but in order to make possible the protection of the public" (Ackerknecht, 1983, p. 140).

Virchow's commitment to the protection of the public led him to seek and win public office. In the Prussian *Landtag* in 1869, he introduced a motion that read, in part:

> Whereas the permanent state of war readiness in almost all the countries of Europe is not the result of enmity between their peoples. . . .

Whereas the reduction in military expenses is absolutely necessary to balance the budget without a further burden on the people. . . . Therefore, we urge the government to reduce military expenses and to use diplomatic means to bring about general disarmament." (Hanauske-Abel, 1981)

Virchow's motion was rejected 215 to 99. Eight months later, in July 1870, the Franco-Prussian War began.

In public health, Virchow's contributions were no less extraordinary than his contributions to basic science. The discoverer of the pathophysiology of trichinosis led a successful 10-year campaign to establish compulsory meat inspection. He designed and supervised a sewage disposal system for Berlin, which became the model for Europe. He was a tireless exponent of health education for the general public; otherwise: "The layman will remain servilely subordinate to medical authority; a resounding title. . . . will constitute a most lucrative shingle for a medical quack." (Virchow, 1848/1985, p. 54).

THE SATISFACTIONS OF PATIENT CARE

However, to demonstrate that social advocacy has a long and honorable history in medicine does not obviate the tension in the practitioner caught between the goals (and satisfactions) of clinical medicine, with its focus on the outcome of the one-to-one patient–physician encounter, and of social medicine, with its primary focus on the health of populations. Consider the vicissitudes in the worlds of practice and advocacy.

Few experiences in medicine are as gratifying as seeing a patient recover from a serious illness, particularly when the care we have provided has contributed to the good outcome. The satisfaction is all the greater when the diagnosis presents an intellectual challenge and the choice of therapy requires nice discrimination, but recovery is a happy experience even when we are mere bystanders. It adds to the pleasure if patient and parents are grateful and if colleagues or students compliment our performance, but those are add-ons; knowing that one has done the right thing and that all has gone well is quite enough. Indeed, doctors need that internal compass because appreciation and good performance don't always go together. We are sometimes praised when our care has been less than optimal and sometimes face criticism when we've done all that could be done but the outcome has not been pleasing. Still, there aren't many things to match the personal satisfactions that come from clinical practice. The problem is there before you, you do what needs to be done, and you see the result, most often with a short turnaround time. Cause and effect seem self-evident, sometimes even when they're not.

Doctoring makes a difference much of the time, the difference is usually apparent within a short time frame, and what the medical care team does matters. Of course, parents may not accept the recommended treatment, fiscal and regulatory mechanisms may make it unavailable, but what has or hasn't happened is up front, feedback is immediate. Moreover, one-on-one care is what our medical training on the wards and in the clinics has taught us to provide. Population medicine, if included in the curriculum at all, is given short shrift.

Contrast all of this with social advocacy. Effective action depends on recruiting support from many others; the feedback loop between initiation and accomplishment is necessarily long and effects on health, even when the program is finally initiated, may be difficult to discern amid other secular trends. Effects may be far larger than those that come from one-on-one care, but they are more uncertain, are not easily attributable to one's own efforts, and may be a long time in coming. None of this diminishes the need for social activism, but it helps to account for the preference of physicians for the clinical arena.

Yet, the clinician must be aware of the limitations imposed on clinical effectiveness by the social context. The very best efforts of doctors may be entirely ineffectual when adverse social conditions overwhelm the very same medical measures that yield good results under better circumstances.

THE EFFECT OF SOCIAL CONTEXT ON THE OUTCOMES OF CARE

The limited ability of medical interventions to overcome the noxious effects of an unhealthy environment is evident from a health care experiment McDermott, Deuschle, and Barnett (1972) conducted from 1956 to 1962 at Many Farms, a Navajo community on a large tribal reservation. The population was nonliterate and non–English speaking, had little cash income, and lived in extended families in one-room, windowless, log and mud dwellings with dirt floors. The infant mortality rate in their community was some three times higher than that for the United States as a whole. There were no physicians in residence, and the nearest hospital services were many miles away. The introduction of a primary health care system was enthusiastically welcomed by the Navajo Tribal Council. Professionals and laypersons alike confidently anticipated significant improvement in community health.

The results fell far short of expectation. Neonatal mortality remained unchanged; at best, there was only a slight reduction in overall mortality. Although the transmission of tuberculosis and the occurrence of otitis media were reduced, there was no change in the prevalence of active trachoma or of the pneumonia-diarrhea complex—the most common causes of illness and death. Each of these microbial diseases is readily transmitted in crowded, poorly ventilated housing; yet differences in pathogenesis among them account for the differential outcomes. Whereas exhaustive case finding followed by effective drug therapy was able to slow the transmission of tuberculosis by reducing the source of bacilli, pneumonia and diarrhea are caused by microorganisms, many of which do not respond to antimicrobial drugs and continuously recirculate among household members. Even though the physician managing the individual child could see improvement in response to medical care, overall rates of morbidity and mortality remained unchanged because transmission continued.

The McDermott health care experiment, despite careful organization and general acceptance by the community, had relatively little influence on health status because of the diseases endemic in the population, the age distribution in the community, and the inability of the medical program to alter living conditions. The most modern technology of the time had relatively little to offer infants living in a vulnerable home environment. In retrospect, McDermott and his colleagues acknowledged that a physician-based system for delivering primary health care was a poor choice, but the Navajo community itself wanted such care. The complexity of the situation is epitomized in the conclusion of McDermott and colleagues' (1972) paper:

> Because of the nature of medicine, as a practical matter its technology has to be deployed irrationally. . . . Who can measure the value obtained by those Many Farms parents who could see obviously expert professionals hovering over their child, desperately ill with pneumonia caused by respiratory syncytial virus? They see someone making a fight. To point out that, in the particular circumstances, the penicillin the child is receiving happens to be valueless, in a technological sense, would seem a petty, if not callous irrelevancy. (p. 30)

The limited effectiveness of medical services in a high-risk environment highlights a central issue: largely preventable medical conditions that stem from social pathology. It illustrates a second point: Whereas the physician can intervene when illness occurs to better the situation of individual patients on a case-by-case basis, improving population health requires measures that extend far beyond the consulting room or the hospital.

BALANCING RESEARCH, SERVICE, AND ACTIVISM

What, then, is the proper role for physicians? To provide the best patient care we know how to deliver? To go well beyond clinical practice to become social activists on behalf of children, many of whom are not our patients and will not need to become patients at all if we are successful? If our role encompasses both of these, how do we partition our time and energy between the two? There are neither simple nor single answers to these questions; how we come to grips with them defines our professional identities.

Clinical practice and social activism do not exhaust the career alternatives for physicians. Rudolf Virchow was also an investigator in the laboratory as well as in the clinic. Research can lead to interventions with an impact far, far greater for health than the accomplishments of the most gifted clinician. It has, however, its own frustrations, highlighted in a commentary (Collins, 1991–1992) by the codiscoverer of the genes for cystic fibrosis and neurofibromatosis:

> . . . the scientist's gratification is the joy of discovery. A key attribute
> of that joy is that it doesn't come along every day. In most laboratories
> like mine, about 75 percent of the experiments are a complete disas-
> ter. If you're not prepared for that, you get frustrated rather quickly.
> It's the 25 percent that partially work that keep you going. If you are
> fortunate, perhaps 1 percent actually makes some new observation,
> and that's what makes it all worthwhile. (p. 7)

Moreover, the translation of basic scientific discoveries into public health measures is, once again, a function of public policy; that is, an outcome of the political process. One of the great scientific advances in pediatrics in our time was the work of John Enders, Thomas Weller, and Frederick Robbins in growing viruses in tissue culture, a contribution that made it possible to develop enormously effective vaccines against poliomyelitis, measles, and German measles (Bloch et al., 1986). Mass immunization against polio reduced cases from an average of 40,000 a year in the early 1950s to less than 10 during the 1980s (Centers for Disease Control, 1991). Similarly, following the introduction of measles vaccine in 1964, case incidence fell from 480,000 in that year to less than 3,000 by 1985; unfortunately, in the years since, there has been a serious recrudescence of cases to more than 27,000 by 1990 (Centers for Disease Control, 1991). Equally distressing upward trends are evident for German measles and pertussis. The reason is quite clear: inadequate immunization rates for low income preschool children and young adults (Markowitz et al., 1989). Our nation has not yet had the political will to assure primary care for all children.

Thus, whether a physician's primary commitment be to clinical practice or to basic research, the effectiveness of her or his efforts is tempered by the social context of that practice or that research. Accordingly, social activism becomes a logical, if not a necessary, extension of one's narrowly professional role in order to enhance its impact on public health. The careers of Stella Chess and Alex Thomas epitomize commitment to the best in all three areas: research, clinical work, and activism, each serving to reinforce the others.

COMMITMENT

Together with their colleagues Herbert Birch, Margaret Hertzig, and Sam Korn, Stella and Alex conceptualized and inaugurated a longitudinal study of temperament as it evolves over the life course (Thomas & Chess, 1957; Chess & Thomas, 1959; Thomas, Birch, Chess, Hertzig, & Korn, 1963). Today, their insights have been so thoroughly incorporated into the mainstream of theory and clinical practice in psychiatry and pediatrics that it may be difficult for students to recognize how revolutionary they were 36 years ago. In those years, Leo Kanner asked me to join him (and later to carry on myself) in preparing the annual reviews of progress in child psychiatry and mental deficiency that appeared in the January issue of the *American Journal of Psychiatry* for many years. In the 1959 review, we commented on the early work by Alex and Stella in the following terms:

[They] have reintroduced the issue of non-motivational factors in behavior, a level of determination somewhat obscured in our contemporary preoccupation with psychodynamic elements. In an effort to assess the extent to which characteristic response patterns may be intrinsically determined, they have launched a much needed longitudinal study of the nature, consistency and modifiability of the response of infants to new stimuli at successive stages of development. (Eisenberg, 1959, p. 609)

In the 1962 review, I noted that their findings:

provide evidence for the existence of "primary reaction patterns" detectable as early as the third month of life. Concurrent information on environmental events (weaning, toileting, etc.) that are conventionally described as "traumatic" revealed far less evidence of behavior disturbed in response to these events than standard theory predicts.

Development is viewed as a transactional process, with individuality of child, parents and life experience determining the resultant personality. (Eisenberg, 1962, p. 601)

No less remarkable is their enduring devotion to their New York Longitudinal

Study—and the loyalty of their "experimental subjects" to them. That study has continued for more than 36 years, leading to a truly unique data set (Chess & Thomas, 1990, 1991). It is typical of Stella, the clinical investigator with a compassionate concern for handicapped children, that she responded to the call of the New York State Health Department to mount a study of the psychiatric problems of children born with congenital rubella after an epidemic rubella year. Among its many products, that study led to her report of the first cases of autism in children so afflicted (Chess, 1977).

Throughout their careers, both Alex and Stella have continued to see patients. Each is a superb clinician and a remarkably effective teacher. Indeed, Stella organized the first systematic child psychiatry liaison program for a pediatric service at New York University (Chess & Lyman, 1969).

From their days in medical school, Alex and Stella have been social activists. Stella was a key figure, along with the psychologists Kenneth and Mamie Clark, in contributing to the excellence of the Northside Center for Child Development, a pioneering clinical service for minority children. Alex's book (Thomas & Sillen, 1972) on racism and psychiatry was an effective weapon in the fight for human rights. In every professional organization they joined, Alex and Stella became activists for human rights and social justice.

Sir Charles Snow (1961), in an address to the annual meeting of the American Association for the Advancement of Science on "The Moral Unneutrality of Science," highlighted the responsibility of scientists in these words:

> Scientists have a moral imperative to say what they know. It is going to make them unpopular in their own nation-states. It may do worse than make them unpopular. That doesn't matter. Or at least, it does matter to you and me, but it must not count in the face of the risks. . . .
>
> There are going to be challenges to our intelligence and to our moral nature as long as man remains man. After all, a challenge is not . . . an excuse for slinking off and doing nothing. A challenge is something to be picked up. . . . (p. 259)

Alex Thomas and Stella Chess have always picked up on challenge—and still do!

REFERENCES

Ackerknecht, E. H. (1983). *Rudolf Virchow: Doctor, statesman, anthropologist.* Madison: University of Wisconsin Press.

Bloch, A. B., Orenstein, W. A., Wassilak, S. G., et al. (1986). Epidemiology of measles and its complications. In E. M. Greenberg, C. Lewis, & S. E. Goldston (Eds.), *Vaccinating against brain syndromes: The campaign against measles and rubella* (pp. 5–20). New York: Oxford University Press.

Centers for Disease Control. (1991). Summary of notifiable diseases, United States, 1990. *Morbidity and Mortality Weekly Reports, 39*(53).

Chess, S. (1977). Follow up report on autism in congenital rubella. *Journal of Autism and Childhood Schizophrenia 7*, 69–81.

Chess, S., & Lyman, M. S. (1969). A psychiatric unit in a general hospital pediatric clinic. *American Journal of Orthopsychiatry, 39*, 77–85.

Chess, S., & Thomas, A. (1959). The importance of non-motivational behavior patterns in psychiatric diagnosis and treatment. *Psychiatric Quarterly, 33*, 326–334.

Chess, S., & Thomas, A. (1990). The New York Longitudinal Study: The young adult period. *Canadian Journal of Psychiatry, 35*, 557–561.

Chess, S., & Thomas, A. (1991). Temperament and the concept of goodness of fit. In J. Strelau & A. Angleitner (Eds.), *Explorations in temperament* (pp. 15–28). New York: Plenum Press.

Collins, F. S. (1991–1992). Physician scientists: A vanishing breed. *Yale Medicine, 26*, 5–8.

Eisenberg, L. (1962). Child psychiatry; mental deficiency. *American Journal of Psychiatry, 118*, 600–604.

Hanauske-Abel, H. M., & Obermair, G. (1981). Zivilisten haben keine Chance. *Die Zeit,* 18 September.

Institute of Medicine. (1985). *Preventing low birth weight.* Washington, DC: National Academy Press.

Kanner, L., & Eisenberg, L. (1959). Review of psychiatric progress: Child psychiatry; mental deficiency. *American Journal of Psychiatry, 115*, 608–611.

Markowitz, L. E., Preblud, S. R., Orenstein, W. A., et al. (1989). Patterns of transmission in measles outbreaks in the United States. *New England Journal of Medicine, 320*, 75–81.

McDermott, W., Deuschle, K. W., & Barnett, C. R. (1972). Health care experiment at Many Farms. *Science, 175*, 23–31.

Snow, C. P. (1961). The moral un-neutrality of science. *Science 133*, 255–259.

Southern, F. M., & Sanford, J. P. (1969). Relapsing fever: A clinical and microbiological review. *Medicine, 48*, 129–149.

Thomas, A., Birch, H. G., Chess, S., Hertzig, M. E., & Korn, S. (1963). *Behavioral individuality in early childhood.* New York: New York University Press.

Thomas, A., & Chess, S. (1957). An approach to the study of sources of individual difference in child behavior. *Journal of Clinical and Experimental Psychopathology, 18*, 347–357.

Thomas, A., & Sillen, S. (1972). *Racism and psychiatry.* New York: Brunner/Mazel.

Virchow, R. (1860). *Cellular pathology.* Translated by F. Chance. New York: Robert M. Dewitt.

Virchow, R. (1985). *Collected essays on public health and epidemiology* (Vol. 1). Edited by L. J. Rather. Canton, MA: Watson Publishing International. (Originally published 1848)

28

Summary and Conclusions: A Promising Opportunity for Better Prevention and Intervention

William B. Carey

In her biographical sketch of Stella Chess and Alexander Thomas, Mahin Hassibi mentioned Stella's maxim about the value of trying to make any important effort serve more than one purpose. In our complex and busy lives, we use our resources wisely if we let any scholarly or practical project perform not only its primary function but also some other useful role. This book is an illustration of that principle. We have assembled an impressive group of experts in the mental health field to pay tribute to two of the truly outstanding leaders of our time. In doing this, we have shaped their contributions around a specific topic so that the book has a second life of its own. The subject is one of special concern to the two people we are honoring—prevention and early intervention in the mental health of children using a "goodness-of-fit" or individual differences model. The authors were allowed greater freedom to discuss subjects of interest to them than they would have been had this been a standard textbook, but they were asked to modify their presentations to make them as pertinent as possible to this central theme. Now, at the conclusion of this work, let us distill from each chapter the elements that bear most directly on that topic.

Current official thinking on prevention and early intervention displays a mixture of discouragement and hope. Such was the tenor of the report of the

American Psychiatric Association's Task Force on Prevention Research of the Council on Research (APA, 1990). This statement described the prevailing skepticism about the efficacy of efforts at prevention as attempted so far. The general lack of success was attributed to the application of measures that were too broad or were not yet sufficiently evaluated. However, the report ended on an optimistic note, urging a concentration on "manipulating specific risk factors in order to significantly decrease the development of major psychopathology (p. 1704)." An example cited was "aggression coupled with shy behavior" in the first grade, which had been found to predict adolescent antisocial behavior. We should note that this seems to be a matter of an early minor deviation of behavior predicting a greater subsequent one. Books on prevention and intervention with children almost always focus on children "at risk" because they are already showing reactive behavior symptoms, or because of physical problems like complications of pregnancy or delivery, or social pathology such as abuse or poverty. The APA report did not mention, as have Chess and Thomas (1986) and Carey and McDevitt (1989), that normal variations of temperament may be risk factors for the mental health of children and a potentially valuable area for prevention and intervention.

INDIVIDUAL DIFFERENCES MODEL

The individual differences or goodness-of-fit model has emerged only recently in modern developmental theory (Thomas, 1981) as a major explanation for children's behavioral, emotional, and functional problems. For centuries tradition has honored theories on constitutional or intrinsic factors, such as humoral imbalance or abnormalities of the brain, in the explanation of these phenomena. In our own century the environmentalist model has dominated, generally finding sufficient cause in the child's milieu to account for all adjustment problems. The more recent interactionist approach looks for an interplay of pathological elements in the individual, the environment, or both. The individual differences or goodness-of-fit model, which is essentially an interactionist one, agrees that there may be pre-existing abnormalities in either the child or the environment, or both but goes beyond that. It supports the view that at times neither the child nor the environment can properly be defined as abnormal but that the abrasive or incompatible relationship between them becomes the source of the conflict and stress in the interaction. The central message of the New York Longitudinal Study (NYLS) of Chess and Thomas (1984) was that normal parents and children can have such a poor fit that the children, the parents, or both can be affected adversely. This valuable insight has not yet been fully appreciated by theorists and practitioners in medicine, psychology, and education. Many still assume that a stressful interaction has to mean pathology in the child or parent.

We hope that this book will help to direct attention to this major area of efforts on behalf of children. The opportunities for effective prevention and intervention are potentially great. Friction between children and their environments because of these poor fits seems to be rather common. When clearly and simply explained, these situations are easily understood by parents, and they can usually be modified successfully even by helpers who do not have extensive professional training. The children who do require professional involvement can usually be aided with relatively brief parent counseling. If the problem is primarily in the incompatibility of the relationship, then usually neither the child nor the caretakers need long and expensive psychotherapy.

Let us now review the chapters of this book to summarize what these individual differences consist of, what range of environmental variables they interact with, and how the two do or do not fit together harmoniously. Then we shall examine the particular strategies appropriate for the various settings where professional persons come in contact with children and their parents.

INDIVIDUAL DIFFERENCES

The individual differences considered here include primarily variations of temperament or behavioral style but also divergences in developmental and physical status. A list of others not explored here would encompass age, gender, race, ethnic group, and talents. Although temperament has been defined in earlier chapters, it is useful to present it again. Thomas and Chess (1977) have described it as the "how" of behavior, as the style or way in which an individual typically behaves. Michael Rutter (1987) has proposed a more extended definition of temperament as

> simple, non-motivational, non-cognitive, stylistic characteristics that represent meaningful ways of describing individual differences between people. For the most part, such differences appear early in childhood, show substantial stability over time after the pre-school years (although the particular behavioural manifestations may change), represent predictable modes of response (although these may require particular situations to bring them out), and possibly have fairly direct neurobiological correlates. (p. 447)

In this volume Professor Rutter suggests some principles for the further clarification of the definition, such as cross-situational pervasiveness and a clear distinction from the behavioral problems to which they may predispose. He proposes that the most likely mechanism for this outcome would be by increasing the susceptibility to environmental adversity or by exercising a direct effect on the interpersonal interaction.

Several authors describe particular dimensions of temperament or their special impact in certain situations. Jerome Kagan elaborates on the consequences of behavioral inhibition, which is similar to the NYLS characteristic of approach/withdrawal. Jan Strelau points to the vulnerability of highly reactive adolescents under social pressure. Judith Dunn describes the considerable impact of temperament differences on sibling relationships, while Roy Martin calls attention to the great and largely unrecognized influence of these behavioral style variations on school performance. Finally, Michel Maziade deplores the lack of attention in psychiatric research to the possibility that normal extremes of temperament may in some cases be strong contributors to major behavioral problems.

Other individual differences in children possibly affecting their mental health include variations and deviations in development and physical health status. Even with such deviations a part of the child's adjustment problems may come about because of the failure of the caretakers to modify their management to the particular requirements of the specific child. Ann and Alan Clarke describe these issues in the area of development. Margaret Hertzig points out how prematurity may be just a variation of normal unless the low-birth-weight infant suffers neurological injury and consequent difficult temperament and behavior problems. Some of these individual differences, such as low IQ and central nervous system damage, are true abnormalities, but most of them that concern us in the goodness-of-fit model are no more than variations of normal. Modern behavioral science has just begun to appreciate the clinical significance of these multiple forms of normal.

Melvin Lewis notes that behavioral problems are substantially more common in children with chronic physical illness, and that requirements for parents and clinicians to achieve a goodness of fit between the child and the caretaking environment are no less important for them. Parental management must be adjusted for both the health problem and the child's temperament. In fact, several studies point to the possibility that the child's temperament may be clinically more significant than the nature or severity of the illness (Carey, 1992).

ENVIRONMENTAL VARIATIONS

In clinical practice it is tempting to simplify the environmental component of the interaction by thinking of it just in terms of the obvious characteristics of the immediate caretaker. However, both the chapter by Charles Super and Sara Harkness and the one by Marten deVries remind us of the other two components of the "developmental niche" in which the child is functioning. Not only do the caretakers themselves have their particular strengths and weaknesses, but also the milieu consists of the cultural structures and practices and the physical setting. Edmund Gordon speculates that the child's cultural surroundings not only are important for the child's behavioral adjustment but may modify or strengthen some temperamental characteristics more than others. The contribution by John McDermott and his associates suggests that the culture's impact on the interaction and on the temperament itself depends also to some extent on the age and sex of the individual.

GOODNESS OF FIT

We do not intend to minimize the variety or strength of the pathological forces that may influence children unfavorably. Prenatal drug exposure and infection with HIV (human immunodeficiency virus) are but some of the physical liabilities confronting today's children; social disorganization and family dysfunction beset them in their living situations. These hazards are well recognized and much discussed. Even in these cases the individual–environment fit is critically important. But what about the pathogenic force of a poor fit between a normal individual and a normal but incompatible environment?

To understand the goodness-of-fit or individual differences model, one must have a clear comprehension of what is meant by the term. Chess and Thomas (1992) have explained that

> goodness of fit results when the properties of the environment and its expectations and demands are in accord with the organism's own capacities, motivations and style of behavior. When this consonance between organism and environment is present, optimal development in a progressive direction is possible. "Poorness of fit" involves discrepancies and dissonances between environmental opportunities and demands and the capacities and characteristics of the organism so that distorted development and maladaptive functioning occur. (p. 84)

This is not meant to imply that all temperaments can easily find congenial niches. Negative and inflexible children are likely to create friction in most settings. Nor does this view hold that normal environments can easily adjust to all behavioral styles. Some situations such as elementary schools have a limited capacity to accommodate the special needs of inattentive and distractible children.

Some examples of goodness of fit may enhance the reader's grasp of the phenomenon. An unusually active child may be variously received in different environments. In a large house in the country with vigorous, athletic parents, this child is likely to fit well. The same child with inactive, quiet parents in a small urban apartment may be so restrained as to develop rebellious behavior. An unusually inactive child would be at home in the second situation but might be coerced by the athletic parents into sports that make the child anxious or angry.

Although the NYLS established goodness of fit as clinically significant mainly in the first decade of life, Richard and Jacqueline Lerner carried their investigation into adolescence. They report that the fit between the adolescent's temperament and the expectation of their teachers was more important for their adjustment than either of the interacting components independently.

Two authors have contributed chapters revealing some of the theoretical and practical complexities of these interactions. Sandra Scarr calls our attention to the considerable degree to which genetically determined characteristics of children influence the surroundings with which they interact. Robert Plomin similarly explains that parent and child are related genetically not only by inheritance but also by the way the parents' genetically determined behavior shapes the child's environment. Nevertheless, he adds that the intrafamilial milieu is not necessarily the same for siblings.

This intricate interplay of a multitude of factors might make it seem that goodness of fit would be vastly too complex for clinicians to untangle at the practical level. However, those of us who have used the individual differences model in our clinical work have found that parents and children fairly readily identify for us the areas in which the dissonance is troublesome. That is where we direct our attention in our efforts to achieve a better accommodation.

CLINICAL ASSESSMENT

Sean McDevitt's contribution provides a sophisticated but practical overview of assessment techniques enabling clinicians to gain a sufficient grasp of the many variables in order to resolve the stressful interaction.

PREVENTION AND INTERVENTION IN VARIOUS SETTINGS

The next seven chapters display some existing attempts at prevention and early intervention in a variety of locations where clinicians, educators, and others come in contact with children and their parents. Throughout these diverse descriptions, one should note the three principle forms taken by this counseling: (1) general educational discussions between the clinicians and parents to provide them with background information; (2) identification of the temperament profile of a particular child to provide a more organized picture of it and of possible parental distortions in their general perceptions of it; and (3) intervention when dissonance in the interaction is leading to reactive symptoms in the child's behavior, feelings, or physical function (Carey, 1982).

Four chapters set forth useful approaches in medical scenes. Barbara Medoff-Cooper reminds us that normal newborn behavior can be perplexing for new parents and that individual differences are present even in the first days of life. Although these early variations of normal may not persist into later months, physicians and nurses should still help parents recognize and deal with them at the time. With prematurity the challenges increase.

William Carey defines primary medical care as the first line of defense in prevention and early intervention. Pediatricians, family doctors, and nurses, who have repeated contacts with children and their parents, can utilize this opportunity to assist parents to adjust their expectations and demands to the capacities and temperaments of their children. He contends that it is within the scope of modern pediatrics to counsel effectively for the great majority of these situations, reserving referral to mental health specialists for the more severe reactive behavior problems or relationship disturbances, not just because of the temperament. This advantageous position has been too little exploited so far.

James Cameron and his associates have evolved a program of education and identification by a team attached to large group medical practices. Their valuable undertaking does not replace similar efforts by the physicians but rather supplements them.

Both in day care and in formal schooling, one discovers great opportunities for teachers to improve the mental health of children by considering their individual differences. Edward Zigler and Nancy Hall comment that day-care workers interact with children much as parents do and can be beneficial in evaluating them and informing parents about their common and unusual features. To this we might add the observation that these early educators are not only more impartial in their judgments than parents but in many cases see a great deal more of the child than the parents do.

Barbara Keogh clarifies the ways in which children's temperament influences teachers' attitudes toward them and affects their instructional and management decisions. Certainly when teachers are trained to be more consciously aware of temperamental differences in their students and their own reactions to them, they will manage their classroom behavior and scholastic performance more effectively.

The last two chapters present examples of useful counseling services that are based in the community, that is, outside the medical and educational systems. In Bill Smith's state-funded Temperament Program in Oregon, mature adults with relatively brief supplementary training have been successful in assisting fellow parents recognize temperament differences and develop patterns of management that fit better with the needs of the children. Across the border in British Columbia, Catherine Andersen's purely voluntary support groups help parents to achieve a better understanding of difficult temperament and its management.

CONCLUSION

In this volume a varied group of authors from Poland to Hawaii has presented a diverse selection of essays. Yet, they agree on three main points: First, all feel admiration and affection for Stella Chess and Alex Thomas and an indebtedness to them for their valuable insights about the behavior of children. Second, all have revealed a commitment to the mental health and welfare of children through research, teaching, and service. Leon Eisenberg has reminded us that at times one must also be a social activist to promote the best interests of children.

Finally, all the authors have in one way or another given a greater depth or breadth of understanding of the goodness-of-fit, or individual differences, model for prevention and early intervention in the mental health of children. None would assert that it is the only approach or that it is even applicable in a majority of instances of cases presenting themselves for professional assistance. It is safe to conclude, however, that a substantial portion of the functional and behavioral problems of children results from situations in which the disharmony between the child and the environment is more pathogenic than either of the two alone.

Just how extensive and how remediable are the interactional problems of this nature? Some observers in primary medical and nursing care suggest that they are quite common and that they improve readily with informed but brief counseling. We shall not be able to answer these questions fully until more studies like the NYLS are performed in other places with other populations. We shall not know how much children can be helped by interventions of this sort until objective studies evaluate the process more fully. With inappropriate management, it is likely that they worsen.

A variety of technical problems, such as improving methods of assessment and intervention, must be overcome. We must disagree strongly with the critic who offered the opinion that the individual differences model in mental health "has been relatively exhausted" (Carek, 1992). The opportunities for fruitful advancement probably have been only minimally realized to date.

In the meanwhile, let us celebrate the useful lives of Stella and Alex for suggesting new directions in our thinking and for their friendship.

REFERENCES

American Psychiatric Association. (1990). Report of the APA Task Force on Prevention Research. *American Journal of Psychiatry, 147*, 1701–1704.

Carek, D. J. (1992). [Book review of Carey & McDevitt (1989)]. *Journal of Child and Adolescent Psychiatry, 31*, 375–376.

Carey, W. B. (1982). Clinical use of temperament data in paediatrics. In R. Porter & G. M. Collins (Eds.), *Temperamental differences in infants and young children*. London: Pitman.

Carey, W. B. (1992). Temperament issues in the school-aged child. In M. D. Levine & E. Christophersen (Eds.), *Pediatric Clinics of North America, 39*, 569–584.

Carey, W. B., & McDevitt, S. C. (Eds.). (1989). *Clinical and educational applications of temperament research*. Amsterdam/Lisse, The Netherlands: Swets & Zeitlinger.

Chess, S., & Thomas, A. (1984). *Origins and evolution of behavior disorders*. New York: Brunner/Mazel.

Chess, S., & Thomas, A. (1986). *Temperament in clinical practice*. New York: Guilford Press.

Chess, S., & Thomas, A. (1992). Dynamics of individual behavioral development. In M. D. Levine, W. B. Carey, & A. C. Crocker (Eds.), *Developmental-behavioral pediatrics* (2nd ed.). Philadelphia: W. B. Saunders.

Rutter, M. L. (1987). Temperament, personality and personality disorder. *British Journal of Psychiatry, 150*, 443–458.

Thomas, A. (1981). Current trends in developmental theory. *American Journal of Orthopsychiatry, 51*, 580–609.

Thomas, A., & Chess, S. (1977). *Temperament and development*. New York: Brunner/Mazel.

APPENDIX*

TEMPERAMENT CHARACTERISTICS

Activity: The amount of physical motion during sleep, eating, play, dressing, bathing, etc.

Rhythmicity: The regularity of physiologic functions such as hunger, sleep, and elimination.

Approach/Withdrawal: The nature of initial responses to new stimuli—people, situations, places, foods, toys, procedures.

Adaptability: The ease or difficulty with which reactions to stimuli can be modified in a desired way.

Intensity: The energy level of responses regardless of quality or direction.

Mood: Amount of pleasant and friendly or unpleasant and unfriendly behavior in various situations.

Persistence/Attention Span: The length of time particular activities are pursued by the child with or without obstacles.

Distractibility: The effectiveness of extraneous enviromental stimuli in interfering with ongoing behaviors.

Sensory threshold: The amount of stimulation, such as sounds or light, necessary to evoke discernable responses in the child.

---

*Derived from: A. Thomas & S. Chess (1977), *Temperament and Development*. New York: Brunner/Mazel.

NEW YORK LONGITUDINAL STUDY BIBLIOGRAPHY

BOOKS

Thomas, A., Birch, H. G., Chess, S. Hertzig, M. E., & Korn, S. (1963). *Behavioral individuality in early childhood.* New York: New York University Press.

Chess, S., Thomas, A., & Birch, H. G. (1965). *Your child is a person.* New York: Viking Press.

Thomas, A., Chess, S., & Birch, H. G. (1968). *Temperament and behavior disorders in children.* New York: New York University Press.

Thomas, A., & Chess, S. (1977). *Temperament and development.* New York: Brunner/Mazel.

Thomas, A., & Chess, S. (1980). *Dynamics of psychological development.* New York: Brunner/Mazel.

Chess, S., & Thomas, A. (1984). *Origins and evolution of behavior disorders.* New York: Brunner/Mazel.

Chess, S., & Thomas, A. (1986). *Temperament in clinical practice.* New York: Guilford Press.

Chess, S., & Thomas, A. (1987). *Know your child.* New York: Basic Books.

MONOGRAPHS

Thomas, A., & Chess, S. (1957). An approach to the study of sources of individual differences in child behavior. *Journal of Clinical and Experimental Psychopathology and Quarterly Review of Psychiatry and Neurology, 18,* 347–357.

Chess, A., & Thomas, A. (1959). The importance of nonmotivational behavior patterns in psychiatric diagnosis and treatment. *Psychiatric Quarterly, 33,* 326–334.

Thomas, A., Chess, S., & Birch, H. G. (1959). Characteristics of the individual child's behavioral responses to the environment. *American Journal of Ortho-psychiatry, 24*(4), 791–802.

Chess, S., Thomas, A., Birch, H. G., & Hertzig, M. E. (1960). Implications of a longitudinal study of child development for child psychiatry. *American Journal of Psychiatry, 117,* 434–441.

Thomas, A., Chess, S., Birch, H. G., & Hertzig, M. E. (1960). A longitudinal study of primary reaction patterns in children. *Comprehensive Psychiatry, 1*(8), 103–112.

Thomas, A., Birch, H. G., Chess, S., & Robbins, L. (1961). Individuality in responses of children to similar environmental situations. *American Journal of Psychiatry, 117*, 798–803.

Thomas, A., Birch, H. G., Chess, S., & Hertzig, M. E. (1961). The developmental dynamics of primary reaction characteristics in children. *Proceedings of the Third World Congress of Psychiatry, 1*, 722–726. Montreal: University of Toronto Press.

Birch, H. G., Thomas, A., Chess, S., & Hertzig, M. E. (1962). Individuality in the development of children. *Developmental Medicine and Child Neurology, 4*, 370–379.

Chess, S., Hertzig, M. E., Birch, H. G., & Thomas, A. (1962). Methodology of a study of adaptive functions to the preschool child. *Journal of the American Academy of Child Psychiatry, 2*, 236–245.

Chess, S., Thomas, A., Rutter, M., & Birch, H. G. (1963). Interaction of temperament and environment in the production of behavioral disturbances in children. *American Journal of Psychiatry, 120*, 142–147.

Rutter, M., Korn, S., & Birch, H. G. (1963). Genetic and environmental factors in the development of primary reaction patterns. *British Journal of Clinical and Social Psychology, 2*, 161.

Robbins, L. (1963). The accuracy of parental recall of aspects of child development and child-rearing practices. *Journal of Abnormal and Social Psychology, 66*, 261–270.

Rutter, M., Birch, H. G., Thomas, A., & Chess, S. (1964). Temperamental characteristics in infancy and the later development of behavioral disorders. *British Journal of Psychiatry, 110*, 651–661.

Birch, H. G., Thomas, A., & Chess, S. (1964). Behavioral development in brain-damaged children. *Archives of General Psychiatry, 11*, 596–603.

Thomas, A. (1965). Emotional expressiveness of nursery school children as it relates to formal learning. In *Going to school*, Massachusetts Chapter of the American Academy of Pediatrics, Committee on Mental Health.

Chess, S. (1966). Individuality in children: Its importance to the pediatrician. *Journal of Pediatrics, 69*, 676–684.

Chess, S., Thomas, A., & Birch, H. G. (1966). Distortions in developmental reporting made by parents of behaviorally disturbed children. *Journal of the Academy of Child Psychiatry, 5*, 226–234.

Chess, S. (1967). The role of temperament in the child's development. *Acta Paedopsychiatrica, 34*, 91–103.

Chess, S., Thomas, A., & Birch, H. G. (1967). Behavior problems revisited: Findings of an anterospective study. *Journal of the American Academy of Child Psychiatry, 6*, 321–331.

Gordon, E. M., & Thomas, A. (1967). Children's behavioral style and the teacher's appraisal of their intelligence. *Journal of School Psychology, 5*, 292–300.

Chess, S. (1967). Temperament in the normal infant. In J. Hellmuth (Ed.), *Exceptional infant: Normal infant*. Seattle: Special Child Publications.

Hertzig, M. E., Birch, H. G., Thomas, A., & Mendez, O. A. (1968). Class and ethnic differences in the responsiveness of preschool children to cognitive demands. *Monographs of the Society for Research in Child Development* (Serial No. 117).

Raph, J., Thomas, A., Chess, S., & Korn, S. J. (1968). The influence of nursery school on social interactions. *American Journal of Orthopsychiatry, 38*, 144–152.

Chess, S. (1968). Temperament and learning ability of school children. *American Journal of Public Health, 58*, 2231–2239.

Thomas, A. (1968). Variations in temperament as a factor generating psychological deprivation. R. Jersir & S. Richardson (Eds.), In *Perspectives on human deprivation: Biological, psychological and sociological.* Washington, D.C.: National Institute of Child Health and Human Development.

Thomas, A. (1968). Significance of temperamental individuality for school functioning. In J. Hellmuth (Ed.), *Learning disorders.* Seattle: Special Child Publications.

Chess, S. (1969). Individuality and baby care. *Developmental Medicine and Child Neurology, 11*, 749–754.

Marcus, J., Thomas, A., & Chess, S. (1969). Behavioral individuality in kibbutz children. *The Israel Annals of Psychiatry and Related Disciplines, 7*, 43–54.

Chess, S. (1969). Genesis of behavior disorders. In J.G. Howells (Ed.), *Modern perspectives in international child psychiatry.* Edinburgh: Oliver & Boyd.

Chess, S. (1970). The influence of temperament on education of mentally retarded children. *Journal of Special Education, 4*, 13–27.

Thomas, A., & Chess, S. (1970). Behavioral individuality in childhood. In L. R. Aronson, E. Tobach, D. S. Lehman, & J. S. Rosenblatt (Eds.), *Development and evolution of behavior.* San Francisco: W. H. Freeman.

Thomas, A., Chess, S., & Birch, H. G. (1970). Origins of personality. *Scientific American, 223*(2), 102–109.

Thomas, A. (1970). Purpose vs. consequence in the analysis of behavior. *American Journal of Psychotherapy, 24*, 49.

Thomas, A., Hertzig, M. E., Dryman, I., & Fernandez, P. (1971, October). Examiner effect in I.Q. testing of Puerto Rican working-class children. *American Journal of Orthopsychiatry, 41*(4).

Thomas, A. (1971). Impact of renewed interest in earliest individual differences. In H. E. Rie (Ed.), *Behavior disorders in children: Changing concepts and practices.* New York: Aldin-Alherson.

Chess, S., & Thomas, A. (1972). Differences in outcome with early intervention with behavior disorders. In M. Roff, L. Robbins, & M. Pollack (Eds.), *Life history research in psychopathology* (Vol. 2, pp. 35–46). Minneapolis: University of Minnesota Press.

Thomas, A., & Chess, S. (1972). Development in middle childhood. *Seminars in Psychiatry, 4*, 331–341.

Chess, S., & Thomas, A. (1973). Temperament in the normal infant. In J. Westman (Ed.), *Individual differences in children* (pp. 83–104). New York: John Wiley.

Thomas, A., Chess, S., Sillen, J., & Mendez, O. A. (1974). Cross-cultural studies of behavior in children with special vulnerabilities to stress. In *Life history research in psychopathology* (Vol. 3, pp. 53–67). Minneapolis: University of Minnesota Press.

Thomas, A., & Chess, S. (1975). A longitudinal study of three brain damaged children. *Archives of General Psychiatry, 32*, 457–465.

Thomas, A. (1976). Behavioral individuality in childhood. In A. R. Kaplan (Ed.), *Human behavior genetics* (pp. 151–163). Springfield, IL: Charles C. Thomas.

Chess, S., Thomas, A., & Cameron, M. (1976). Temperament: Its significance for early schooling. *New York University Educational Quarterly, 73*, 24–29.

Chess, S., & Fernandez, P. (1976). Temperament and the rubella child. In S. Jastrzembaka (Ed.), *On the effects of blindness and other impairments on early childhood development* [Proceedings of conference], pp.186–200. American Foundation for the Blind.

Thomas, A., & Chess, S. (1976). Evolution of behavior disorders into adolescence. *American Journal of Psychiatry, 133*, 539–542.

Thomas, A., Chess, S., & Cameron, M. (1976). Sexual attitudes and behavior patterns in a middle-class adolescent population. *American Journal of Orthopsychiatry, 46*, 689–701.

Chess, S. (1976, November). Mood in infancy. *Proceedings from Conference on Affective States in Infants and Young Children.* Bethesda, MD: National Institute of Mental Health.

Chess, S., & Thomas, A. (1977). Temperamental traits and parent guidance. In L. E. Arnold (Ed.), *Helping parents help their children* (pp. 135–144). New York: Brunner/Mazel.

Chess, S., & Thomas, A. (1977). Temperament and the parent-child interaction. *Pediatric Annals,* September.

Chess, S., & Thomas, A. (1977). Temperamental individuality from childhood into adolescence. *Journal of the American Academy of Child Psychiatry, 16*, 218–226.

Chess, S. (1977). Temperament and the handicapped child. *Proceedings of the Second International Conference on Developmental Screening.* Santa Fe, NM.

Thomas, A., & Chess, S. (1978). Emergence of individuality. In Wolman (Ed.), *International encyclopedia of neurology, psychiatry, psychoanalysis and psychology.* New York: Aesculapius.

Chess, S. (1979). Developmental theory revisited: Findings of a longitudinal study [Academic lecture]. *Canadian Journal of Psychiatry, 24*, 101–112.

Kim, S., Ferrara, A., & Chess, S. (1980). Temperament and asthmatic children. A preliminary study. *Journal of Pediatrics, 97*, 483–486.

Thomas, A., & Chess, S. (1981). The role of temperament in the contributions of individuals to their development. In R. M. Lerner & N. A. Busch-Rossnage (Eds.), *Individuals as producers of their development.* New York: Academic Press.

Thomas, A. (1981). Current trends in developmental theory. *American Journal of Orthopsychiatry, 51*, 580–609.

Thomas, A., Chess, S., & Korn, S. J. (1982). The reality of difficult temperament. *Merrill-Palmer Quarterly, 28*(1), 1–20.

Thomas, A., & Chess. S. (1982). Temperament and follow-up to adulthood. In R. Porter & G. Collins (Eds.), *Temperamental differences in infants and young children.* London: Pitman.

Thomas, A., Korn, S. J., Mittelman, M., Cohen, J., & Chess, S. (1982). A temperament questionnaire for early adult life. *Educational and Psychological Measurement, 42*, 593–600.

Chess, S., Thomas, A., Korn, S. J., Mittelman, M., & Cohen, J. (1983). Early parental attitudes, divorce and separation, and early adult outcome. Findings of a longitudinal study. *Journal of the American Academy of Child Psychiatry, 22*(1), 47–51.

Chess, S., Thomas, A., & Hassibi, M. (1983). Depression in childhood and adolescence:

A prospective study of six cases. *Journal of Nervous and Mental Disease, 171*(7), 411–420.

Chess, S., & Thomas, A. (1983). Dynamics of individual behavioral development. In M. D. Levine, W. B. Carey, A. C. Crocker, & R. T. Gross (Eds.), *Developmental-behavioral pediatrics* (pp. 158–174). Philadelphia: W. B. Saunders. (Second edition 1992)

Thomas, A., & Chess, S. (1984). Genesis and evolution of behavioral disorders: From infancy to early adult life. *American Journal of Psychiatry, 141*, 1–9.

Chess, S., & Thomas, A. (1985). Temperamental differences: A critical concept in child health care. *Pediatric Nursing, 11*(3), 167–171.

Chess, S. (1986). Early childhood development and its implications for analytic theory. *American Journal of Psychoanalysis, 46*(2), 123–148.

Chess, S., & Thomas, A. (1987, October). *Continuities and discontinuities in temperament.* Paper presented at the meeting of Life History Research Society, St. Louis, MO.

Thomas, A., & Chess, S. (1986). The New York Longitudinal Study: From infancy to early adult life. In R. Plomin & J. Dunn (Eds.), *The study of temperament: Change, continuities and challenges.* Hillside, NJ: Lawrence Erlbaum.

Lerner, J. V., Hertzog, C., Hooker, K. A., Hassibi, M., & Thomas, A. (1988). A longitudinal study of negative emotional states and adjustments from early childhood through adolescence. *Child Development, 59*, 356–366.

Chess, S., & Thomas, A. (1989). The practical application of temperament to psychiatry. In W. B. Carey & S. C. McDevitt (Eds.), *Clinical and educational applications of temperament research.* Amsterdam/Lisse, The Netherlands: Swets & Zeitlinger.

Chess, S., & Thomas, A. (1989). Temperament and its functional significance. In S. I. Greenspan & G. H. Pollack (Eds.), *The course of life: Vol. II. Early childhood* (pp. 163–227). Madison, CT: International Universities Press.

Chess, S., & Thomas, A. (1990). Continuities and discontinuities in temperament. In L. Robbins & M. Rutter (Eds.), *Straight and deviant pathways from childhood to adulthood* (pp. 205–226). Cambridge: Cambridge University Press.

Chess, S., & Thomas, A. (1990). The New York Longitudinal Study (NYLS): The young adult period. *Canadian Journal of Psychiatry, 35*, 557–561.

Chess, S. (1990). Pathogenesis of adjustment disorders: Vulnerabilities due to temperamental factors. In J. D. Noshpitz & R. D. Coddington (Eds.), *Stressors and adjustment disorders* (pp. 457–476). New York: John Wiley.

Chess, S. (1990). Studies in temperament: A paradigm in psychosocial research. *Yale Journal of Biology and Medicine, 63*, 313–324.

Chess, S., & Thomas, A. (1991). Temperament and the concept of goodness of fit. In J. Strelau & A. Angleitner (Eds.), *Explorations in temperament* (pp. 15–28). New York: Plenum Press.

NAME INDEX

SUBJECT INDEX

For Product Safety Concerns and Information please contact our EU
representative GPSR@taylorandfrancis.com
Taylor & Francis Verlag GmbH, Kaufingerstraße 24, 80331 München, Germany